SAUNDERS

Fundamentals of Medical Assisting

STUDENT MASTERY MANUAL

Sue Hunt, MN, RN, CMA
Professor and Coordinator
Medical Assisting Program
Middlesex Community College
Lowell, Massachusetts

Jon H. Zonderman, BA, MSJ
Contributing Writer
Orange, Connecticut

SAUNDERS
An Imprint of Elsevier

SAUNDERS

An Imprint of Elsevier

The Curtis Center
Independence Square West
Philadelphia, Pennsylvania 19106

All photos throughout this text, unless specified as borrowed from other sources, are from the Harcourt Health Sciences Medical Assisting Photo Collection.

FUNDAMENTALS OF MEDICAL ASSISTING
STUDENT MASTERY MANUAL

ISBN 0-7216-9226-5

Printed in the United States of America

Last digit is the print number: 9 8 7 6 5 4 3

Contents

Chapter 1

Introduction

The student mastery manual is an important tool as you learn the theoretical material and master the entry-level competencies to become a medical assistant. Each chapter has been organized into five sections.

1. **CHAPTER FOCUS:** This section is a brief review of the key points of the chapter.

2. **TERMINOLOGY REVIEW:** This section contains exercises to review the vocabulary words and abbreviations at the beginning of each chapter. You may be asked to match the vocabulary word with its definition (Vocabulary Matching), add the vocabulary word being defined in a sentence (Definitions), or expand an abbreviation (Abbreviations). It is essential that you learn to understand, spell, and use the terminology in common use in your chosen profession. When you are reading the textbook, make a list of the vocabulary words (highlighted in boldface type). Define them, either from what you have read, the definitions in the text, or from the definitions in the Glossary at the back of the book. Then test your mastery by completing the exercises in this section.

3. **CONTENT REVIEW:** These are questions to determine whether you understand and remember the information presented in the chapter. Some students outline each chapter as they read it in order to reinforce their understanding and retention of chapter material. You should read the chapter carefully first, outline it if that is helpful to you, and answer the content review questions at the end of the chapter. Then you should try to complete the questions in your workbook without looking at the text, check your answers against the textbook, and correct any errors. Most people have a preferred learning style, which is either visual, auditory, or sensory-motor (by doing). People with a visual learning style usually learn best by seeing something, either in writing, in a picture, or in real life. When they try to remember something that they have learned recently, they bring a mental picture to mind. If a person with a visual learning style had to learn the names of ten students, he or she would learn best if given a list of the names. These people learn well by reading a textbook and examining the pictures.

People with an auditory learning style learn best by hearing new information. If someone tells them something, they remember it better than if they had read it. If a person with a visual learning style had to learn the names of ten students, he or she would do best if each student said his or her name. These individuals can benefit by reading out loud, by tape recording lectures, and by studying in groups with verbal review.

People with a sensory-motor learning style learn best by doing and sometimes have difficulty learning rules or abstract information. These individuals should pantomime practice as they read and always try to link rules or definitions in their mind with specific things to do. Sometimes writing things down while reading helps this type of learner remember the information.

Describe how you learn best and identify your preferred learning style.

____

____

____

____

____

____

4. CRITICAL THINKING: Questions in this section ask you to use information from the chapter and, sometimes, additional information from your experience or research to reflect and probe deeper into real life or social implications. Working as a professional medical assistant requires making decisions about what to do and when to do it, predicting the consequences of actions, evaluating how effective activities have been, and planning for the future. This means that it is essential to develop your ability to think critically. Students often become frustrated by this type of question because the answer is not immediately obvious, or there may be no single correct answer. The effort you make to improve your skill in this area will improve not only your performance as a medical assistant but also your ability to learn and to express your knowledge. Take the opportunity to challenge yourself by completing these questions to the best of your ability.

Answer the following as a critical thinking activity:

Give reasons to agree or disagree with the following statement: Thinking about things is one of my strong points. (Remember, the thinking part is identifying and arranging reasons to convince the reader that your position is correct.)

____

____

____

____

____

____

5. PRACTICAL APPLICATIONS: This section contains questions and activities to help you review practical knowledge and apply what you have learned to real-life situations. Discussing your answers with your classmates can encourage you to consider alternative approaches. Many of the activities in this section will help you to learn and/or practice all or part of the procedures presented in the textbook. In addition, this section will tell you when you should complete additional practice activities on the *Virtual Medical Office Challenge CD-ROM* from the back inside cover of your textbook.

UNIT 1

The Medical Office

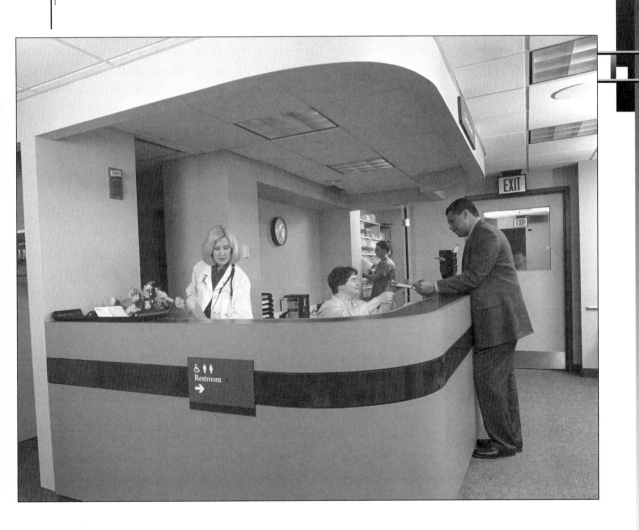

Chapter 3

What Kinds of Care Do Patients Look for and Why?

CHAPTER FOCUS

In this chapter you learned some basic psychological theory and how it can influence the expectations patients have when they seek health care. You also learned about the structure of health care in Western societies for specific medical specialties. Western medical tradition is contrasted with other medical traditions and correlated to cultural influences on patients' behavior and expectations.

TERMINOLOGY REVIEW

Vocabulary Matching: Match each term with its definition.

___ 1. empathy
___ 2. palliative
___ 3. acting out
___ 4. self-actualization
___ 5. anxiety
___ 6. denial
___ 7. projection
___ 8. ego defense mechanisms
___ 9. physiologic needs
___ 10. hierarchy

A. To translate feelings into inappropriate activity
B. A feeling of dread
C. Failure to acknowledge the reality of a situation
D. Unconscious mental processes and behavioral strategies that offer psychological protection
E. The ability to identify the feelings of need a person has; to understand those needs in an emotional way
F. An arrangement in order of importance or with a series of levels
G. Seeking to relieve or alleviate symptoms without curing the underlying condition
H. Basic biological needs for survival
I. To believe that another person is feeling or experiencing feelings that are really one's own
J. Fulfillment of a person's potential

CONTENT REVIEW QUESTIONS

1. Identify the needs on each level of Maslow's hierarchy of needs.
   a. Level 1 (lowest level): ____________________
   b. Level 2: ____________________
   c. Level 3: ____________________
   d. Level 4: ____________________
   e. Level 5: ____________________

2. When can a person devote energy to fulfilling higher level needs from Maslow's hierarchy?

   ____

   ____

   ____

3. Why is it important for medical assistants to identify the unmet needs of patients?

   ____

   ____

   ____

4. How do people use ego defense mechanisms?

   ____

   ____

   ____

5. What are three things that patients often expect when they seek health care?
   a. ____________________
   b. ____________________
   c. ____________________

6. Identify three medical specialties that provide primary care (are the patient's primary care provider)?
   a. ____________________
   b. ____________________
   c. ____________________

7. How long does the residency period of a physician's training last?

   ____

   ____

   ____

8. What are two different ways for physicians to form a group practice?

   ____

   ____

   ____

9. What are disadvantages for the physician in solo practice?

____

____

____

10. What are advantages for the patient when a practice contains physicians from several specialties?

____

____

____

11. Briefly describe the following types of medical care, which are often used to supplement scientific medical practice:

a. osteopathy ____

____

b. chiropractic ____

____

c. podiatry ____

____

d. psychotherapy ____

____

e. acupuncture/acupressure ____

____

f. nutrition therapy ____

____

g. biofeedback ____

____

h. hypnosis ____

____

i. relaxation techniques ____

____

j. therapeutic touch ____

____

k. massage ____

____

l. postural therapies ____

____

m. herbal medicine ____

____

n. prayer and meditation ______________________________

____

12. Identify three systems of alternative medicine (i.e., often used instead of Western scientific medicine).

a. ______________________________

b. ______________________________

c. ______________________________

13. What are differences between Western medicine and traditional medical systems such as Chinese medicine, Ayurvedic medicine, or Native American medicine?

____

____

____

____

14. When patients come from different cultural backgrounds, how can the medical assistant demonstrate respect for their beliefs about disease and medical practice?

____

____

____

____

CRITICAL THINKING QUESTIONS

1. How does belief and expectation influence a person's response to health care? Do research to find out about the "placebo effect."

____

____

____

____

____

____

2. Discuss times you have been disappointed with a doctor visit or a visit to another type of health practitioner. Identify your own priorities (what things were most important to you), then try to identify the priorities of the health practitioner (what things were most important to him or her). If your priorities did not agree, how was the care affected? Was your health affected?

____

____

____

3. What are advantages and disadvantages for patients of the fact that there are so many medical specialties in our medical system? Try to think of at least five advantages and five disadvantages. Discuss with your classmates whether the advantages outweigh the disadvantages.

4. Discuss the reasons why you are sure that there are living beings too small to see that can live in food or water and can cause disease if they enter the body. Consider why you believe that your belief in this phenomenon (which cannot be seen with the naked eye) is more valid than a belief in bad spirits that can cause disease.

PRACTICAL APPLICATIONS

1. Identify specific health practices of various cultural groups based either on research or interviews. Some possible interview questions that can form a basis for discussion are as follows:
   a. Are there any special things you were taught to do or foods to eat during pregnancy and after delivery?
   b. What things do you do when you are sick besides going to the doctor?
   c. Do you believe that illness can be caused by bad spirits or evil people? If so, what do you do about that kind of problem?
   d. Do people in your family (culture) use herbs or special plants to prevent or cure illness? Where do you buy them? How do you know what to use?
   e. Do you think your doctor understands people from your culture? How do you decide what doctor to choose?
2. Discuss with your classmates any complementary or alternative types of medical treatment that they have tried. How effective do they think they were? How did they determine the skill level of the practitioner?

3. Notice the educational qualifications of the doctors and other health practitioners that you go to. Ask your physician how difficult it is to become board certified. Obtain information about medical schools and residency programs in your area from the web sites of local hospitals and medical schools.

4. Locate medical specialists in your area. Discuss how would you choose a surgeon if you needed an appendectomy, a knee replacement, or removal of a brain tumor. How could you evaluate the qualifications of a specialist?

____

____

____

____

____

____

____

____

SELF-EVALUATION

UNIT 2

Basic Concepts: Professionalism & Law, Communication, and Safety

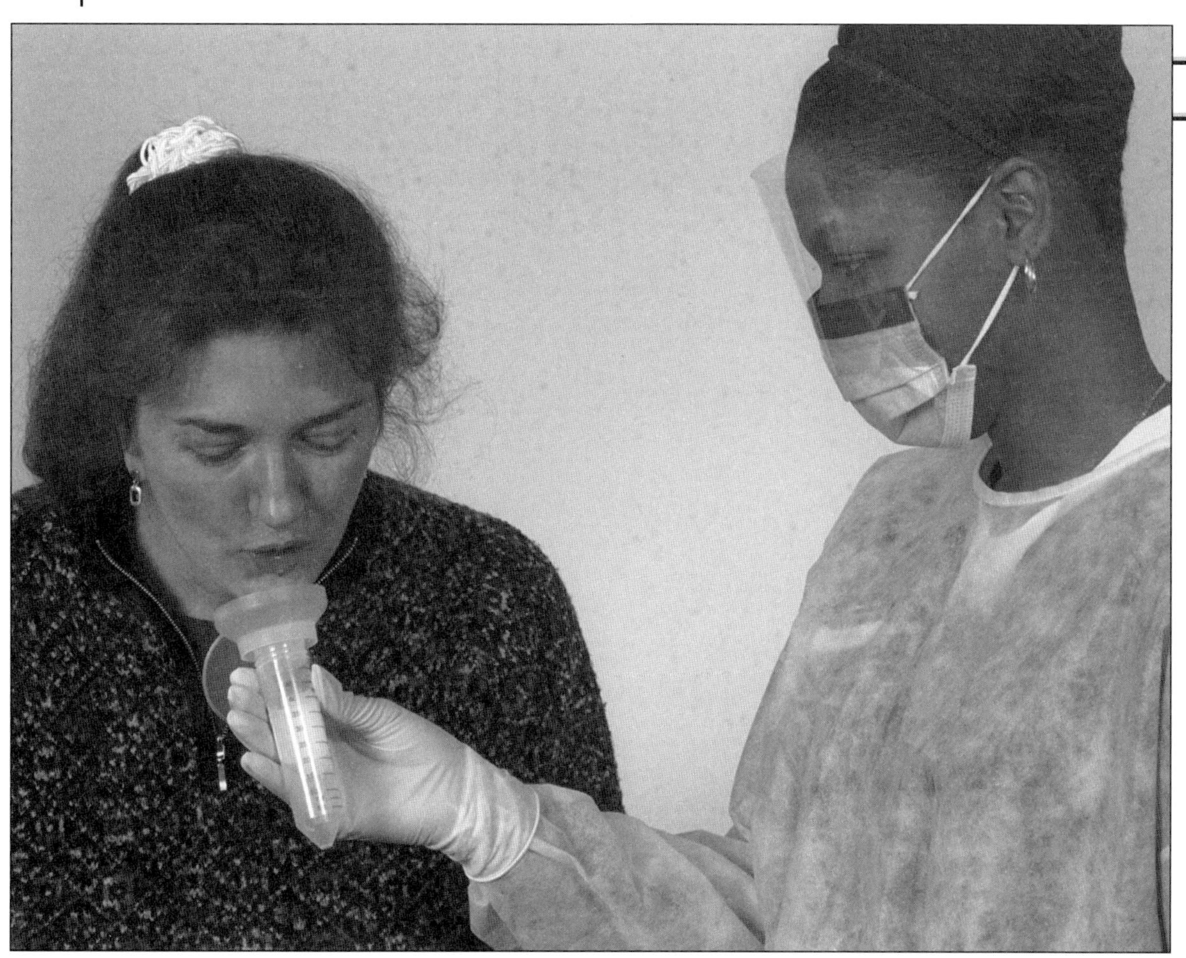

Chapter 4

Professionalism and the Law: How Do You Behave in the Workplace?

CHAPTER FOCUS

In this chapter you learned about what it means to be a professional medical assistant, and how a professional behaves in the workplace. The behavior of the medical assistant is influenced by laws that regulate medical offices and by patient rights such as confidentiality and the right to give informed consent.

TERMINOLOGY REVIEW

Vocabulary Matching: Match each term with its definition.

___ 1. professionalism
___ 2. informed consent
___ 3. liability
___ 4. sexual harassment
___ 5. slander
___ 6. Good Samaritan Act
___ 7. statute
___ 8. certification
___ 9. criminal law

A. A person who speaks up for another person or group of people
B. A law passed by a legislative body
C. A process by which a professional organization verifies a certain level of education and training
D. The set of laws that deals with disputes between two people or groups of people; between people and organizations; and between organizations
E. A mutual agreement to do or refrain from doing something that is legal in exchange for consideration or payment
F. The set of laws that protect society in a large sense, such as laws against robbery, rape, or driving under the influence of alcohol
G. Legal responsibility
H. Laws that protect health professionals from being sued for giving emergency care
I. Deliberately making someone uncomfortable

___ 10. invasion of privacy	J. Consent to perform a procedure or test granted by a patient after he or she has received information about the procedure or a test's risks
___ 11. civil law	K. Release of information about a person, or release of photographs, without that person's permission
___ 12. advocate	L. Written release of false information about a person
___ 13. licensure	M. The process by which a governmental body grants permission for a person to practice a profession after examination of the person's qualifications
___ 14. medical practice act	N. A group of laws that regulate the practice of medicine in each state
___ 15. libel	O. Behavior based on a body of knowledge and ethical standards
___ 16. reciprocal licensure	P. The ability to be granted a license in one state because you hold a license in another state
___ 17. contract	Q. "Let the master answer"; that is, the employer is legally responsible for the negligent actions of his or her employees
___ 18. doctrine of *respondeat superior*	R. When a person of the opposite sex or the same sex makes intentional and clearly understood statements or takes clearly understood actions that cause another person to feel that his or her job is at risk if the other person's sexual advances are not accepted
___ 19. intimidation	S. Verbal release of false information about a person
___ 20. objectivity	T. Not allowing one's personal point of view to influence decisions

Definitions: Insert the correct word to complete the sentence.

1. When a doctor terminates the doctor/patient relationship, but the patient is still under the belief that the relationship exists, if the patient suffers injury because of lack of care, he or she may sue the doctor for ______________________.
2. A contract that is not formally agreed to but is obvious from the circumstances is called an ______________________.
3. Legal responsibility is called ______________________.
4. Professional negligence is often called ______________________.
5. The failure to act—or refrain from acting—as a reasonable person would act in a similar circumstance, is called ______________________.
6. A ______________________ contract is one that is agreed to in words but not written down.
7. A ______________________ contract is a contract on a piece of paper that has been signed by the parties to the contract.

CONTENT REVIEW QUESTIONS

Directions: Answer the questions in the space provided.

1. The four most important character traits of a professional medical assistant are:

   ______________________ ______________________

   ______________________ ______________________

2. Personality traits of a successful medical assistant include ______________________ and ______________________.

3. Identify three reasons why neatness and good grooming are important for the medical assistant.

   a. ______________________

   b. ______________________

   c. ______________________

4. Identify how the medical assistant can demonstrate initiative.

   ____

   ____

5. How do health professionals identify the ethical standards that should guide their behavior? What is an example for medical assistants?

   ____

   ____

   ____

6. Identify five areas of ethical behavior that are important for medical assistants in your own words.

   a. ______________________

   b. ______________________

   c. ______________________

   d. ______________________

   e. ______________________

7. Briefly describe the following three types of law:

   a. Criminal law ______________________

   b. Civil law ______________________

   c. Contract law ______________________

8. If a state requires a health professional to be licensed, what are common requirements?

   ____

   ____

9. What are the four basic requirements for a physician to be licensed in most states?

   a. ______________________

   b. ______________________

   c. ______________________

   d. ______________________

10. What are grounds for suspending or revoking a license to practice medicine?

a. ______________________________

b. ______________________________

c. ______________________________

11. What is the difference between licensure and certification?

____

____

12. What two organizations certify medical assistants and what credential does the medical assistant receive?

a. ______________________________

b. ______________________________

13. Describe what a mandated report is and give five examples of mandated reports for physicians.

____

____

____

____

____

____

14. What is required in order to release information about a patient (except for mandated reports)?

____

____

____

15. Define the term *intentional tort* and give three examples.

____

____

____

____

____

16. Identify how the doctor–patient relationship meets the definition of a contract.

____

____

____

17. Give examples of each of the following types of contracts:

a. implied ______________________________

b. verbal ______________________________

c. written ______________________________

18. When can a physician terminate care to a patient?

____

____

____

19. How should the physician notify the patient that he or she is terminating care? Why?

____

____

____

20. Why is informed consent usually verified by having the patient sign a consent form?

____

____

____

21. What is the medical assistant's role in obtaining a signature on a consent form?

____

____

22. Why is negligence called an unintentional tort?

____

____

23. The name for negligence by a professional is:

____

____

24. What does the term "standard of care" mean?

____

____

25. What four elements must be proved in order to prove liability for malpractice?

a. ______________________________

b. ______________________________

c. ______________________________

d. ______________________________

26. What are two reasons for physicians to purchase professional liability insurance?

a. ______________________________

b. ______________________________

27. How do measures to prevent mistakes and/or reduce the impact of mistakes fit into the overall process of risk management?

CRITICAL THINKING QUESTIONS

1. When patients are scheduled for surgery or invasive procedures, they are often frightened when they learn about possible problems that could occur, especially serious complications. Discuss this aspect of informed consent. Do you think that it could prevent a person from having a test or procedure that would be beneficial? How can information be presented to minimize this effect?

2. One of the overhead costs that has great impact on the medical office is the cost of professional liability insurance. Costs have risen because of increasing numbers of malpractice lawsuits and the fear of insurance companies that courts will award large settlements. Discuss the impact of this trend on patients.

3. Describe the role of the medical assistant related to the doctor–patient relationship.

PRACTICAL APPLICATIONS

1. Discuss with your classmates what you as a "reasonably prudent person" would be expected to do in the following situations:

a. Your elderly neighbor slips and falls on a patch of ice in your driveway. She appears unable to get up and complains of pain in her left hip.

b. You are in the washroom at work and you notice that the handle on the hot water tap is not working properly so that very hot water is constantly dripping into the sink. You see another person head for that sink to wash her hands.

c. You spill some coffee on a tile floor at your school.

2. In the situations above, if you fail to act as a "reasonable prudent person," what can happen?

3. If you are working as a medical assistant, describe how you may be held to a standard higher than that expected of a reasonable prudent person.

4. Decide whether the following situations would most likely be examples of invasion of privacy, slander, libel, negligence, breach of contract, or none of the above. Discuss what the legal consequences may be.

   a. In a casual conversation, an acquaintance says: "That dentist is totally incompetent. He can't even put in a filling that won't fall out."

   b. A person stops making car payments because he lost his job and can no longer afford them.

c. While backing up in his car, a person hits her neighbor's mailbox and knocks it over.

____

____

____

d. An employee of a medical office informs a journalist that a well-known person in the community has received a positive test for HIV.

____

____

____

5. Identify what laws in your state regulate health care professions and especially the medical assisting profession.

____

____

____

____

____

SELF-EVALUATION

Chapter 5

Communication: How Do You Speak in the Workplace?

CHAPTER FOCUS

In this chapter you learned the fundamentals of communication, then how to apply these fundamentals in the health care setting when interviewing patients and establishing caring relationships with patients. You also learned how to adapt your normal communication style when barriers to communication exist.

TERMINOLOGY REVIEW

Vocabulary Matching: Match each term with its definition.

___ 1. non-verbal	A. A person who pays attention with his or her entire mind to what is being said
___ 2. body language	B. Control over one's own circumstances; ability to make decisions for one's self
___ 3. closed questions	C. Elements that interfere with effective communication
___ 4. perception	D. The way a person's body signals feelings and emotions
___ 5. reflecting	E. Questions that can be answered with one word or a few words
___ 6. active listener	F. Expression without words, using body language, facial expressions, and other means
___ 7. autonomy	G. Questions that encourage the person being asked to open up and talk
___ 8. barriers to communication	H. Expressed in words
___ 9. open-ended questions	I. Using your own words to restate the verbal or written words of someone else
___ 10. summarizing	J. The way a person experiences a situation or believes things are

___ 11. verbal — K. Turning a question or statement around to give the speaker the opportunity to continue

___ 12. paraphrasing — L. Restating the main points of a statement in a shorter form

CONTENT REVIEW QUESTIONS

Directions: Answer the questions in the space provided.

1. Give four examples of different types of verbal communication:

   ____________________ ____________________

   ____________________ ____________________.

2. Give four examples of non-verbal communication:

   a. ____________________

   b. ____________________

   c. ____________________

   d. ____________________

3. Emotions that can interfere with communication include:

   ____________________ ____________________

   ____________________ ____________________.

4. What are four ways to be a good receiver of communication?

   a. ____________________

   b. ____________________

   c. ____________________

   d. ____________________

5. Describe active listening.

   ____

   ____

   ____

6. How can the medical assistant use eye contact and body posture to facilitate communication?

   ____

   ____

   ____

7. When is it appropriate to use closed questions during an interview?

   ____

   ____

   ____

When are open-ended questions more useful?

____

____

____

8. What are six communication techniques you can use to draw patients out and encourage them to tell you more?

   a. _______________
   b. _______________
   c. _______________
   d. _______________
   e. _______________
   f. _______________

9. What are three common underlying feelings of ill patients?

   a. _______________
   b. _______________
   c. _______________

10. How can the medical assistant use empathy to help patients deal with feelings and emotions resulting from their medical conditions?

____

____

____

11. How can a medical assistant communicate caring to a patient?

____

____

____

12. Identify four types of situations where barriers to effective communication can arise.

   a. _______________
   b. _______________
   c. _______________
   d. _______________

CRITICAL THINKING

1. In any interaction, a significant part of communication is non-verbal and includes individual interpretation of non-verbal cues. Examine each of the following photographs and summarize your assumptions about each person in the photograph: Who is each person? What is he or she feeling? What might be happening between the two people in the photograph? What is the location pictured in the photograph? Distinguish between assumptions that you are sure of and those you would need more information to confirm.

a. 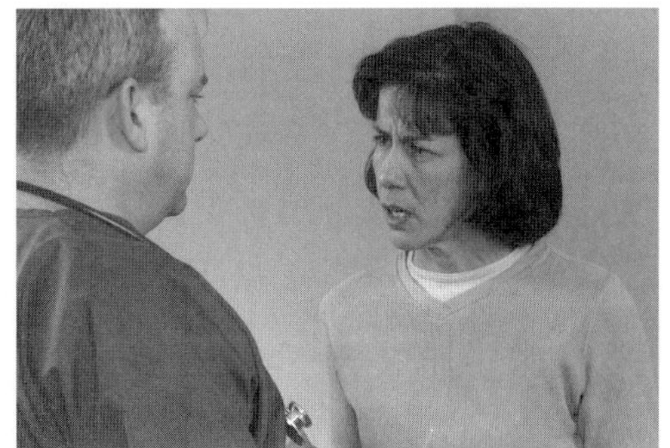

b. 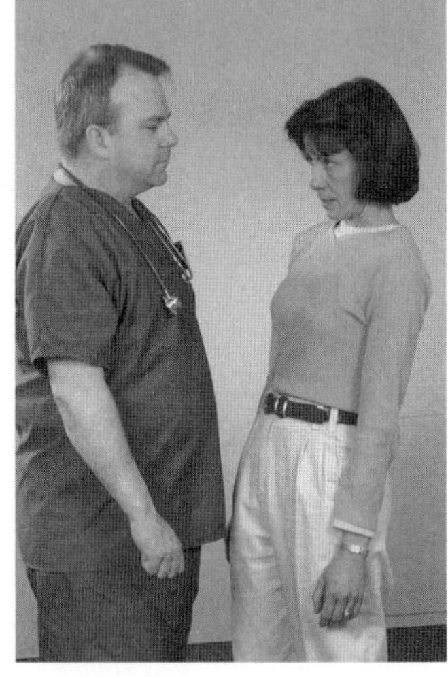

c. 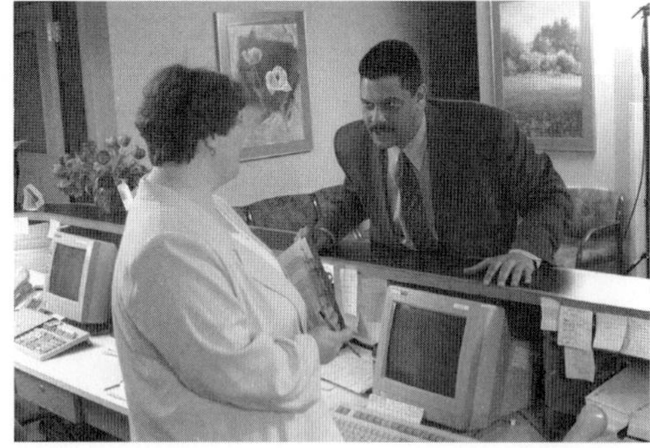

d.

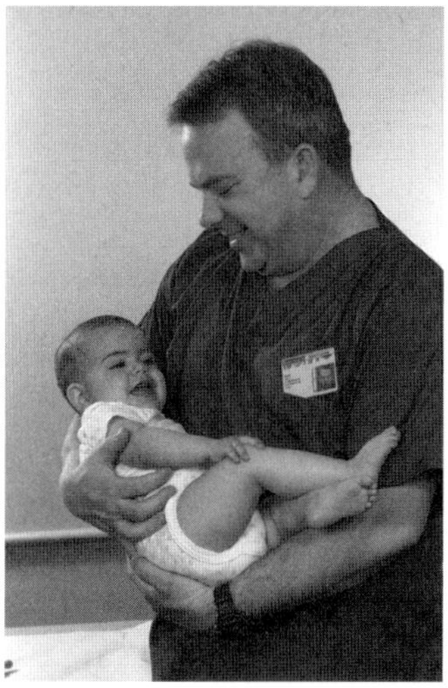

2. Describe how assumptions may facilitate communication. How can they interfere with effective communication? Give examples.

PRACTICAL APPLICATIONS

1. After you take the vital signs of Valerie Hoffman, a 34-year-old teacher, Valerie says, "I don't know if I'm sick or not. I mean, I hope that Dr. Hughes finds something wrong with me to explain why I feel so bad. I don't have any energy, you know. I get up in the morning, when I can finally get myself up, and in about ten minutes I'm ready to go back to bed for a nap. Everything just seems like it takes so much effort." Give an example of a response you could make that demonstrates each of the following communication techniques:

   a. Paraphrasing

   b. Translating into feelings

   c. Reflecting

   d. Summarizing

   e. Repeating or restating

2. Discuss how you feel about role-playing with a partner. Include previous experience, feelings about being in a "pretend situation," etc. Have one person talk for several sentences while the partner listens actively. When you are the listener, try to encourage the other person to keep talking. You may ask questions, but do not give your own opinion. When the first person has expressed him or herself completely, the second person should talk for several sentences while the partner encourages complete expression. Discuss how it feels to talk and listen for longer periods than usual in casual conversation.

3. Reflect on the discussion above. Describe the difference between a normal conversation where each participant usually responds with his or her own feelings and ideas, and the conversation you had with your partner where your partner waited until you had completely finished expressing your thoughts and opinions. How would you apply what you have experienced to being a medical assistant?

____

____

____

____

____

____

____

____

SELF-EVALUATION

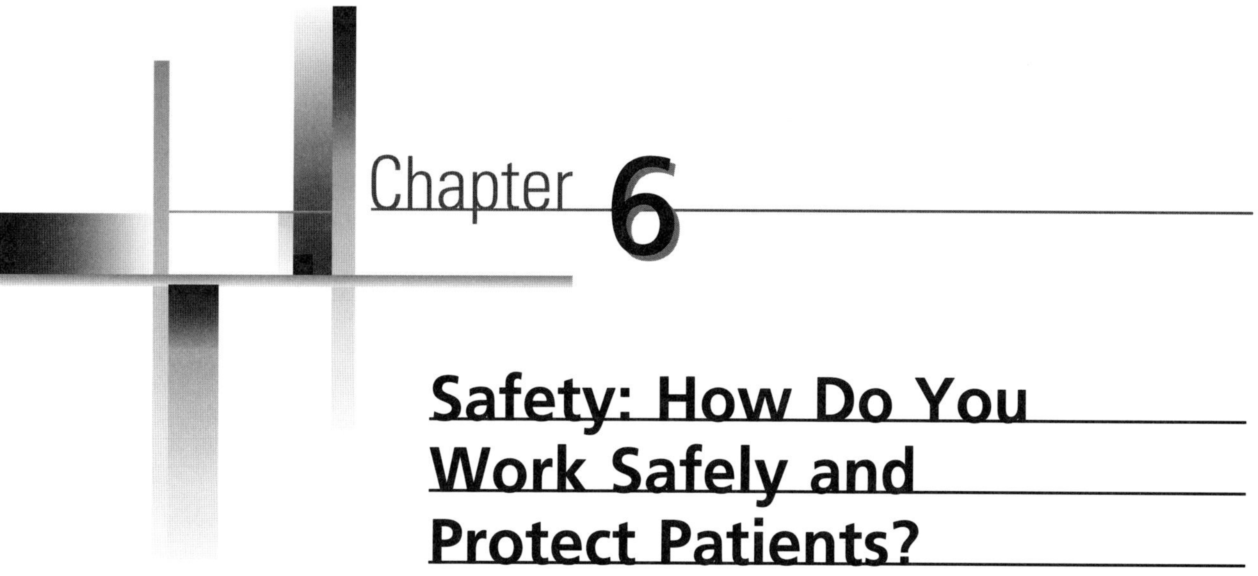

Chapter 6

Safety: How Do You Work Safely and Protect Patients?

CHAPTER FOCUS

In this chapter you learned about measures to protect the safety of both patients and employees in the medical office. In addition to general safety measures, this includes use of good body mechanics and ergonomics as well as measures to prevent exposure to dangerous chemicals or microorganisms. Measures to prevent the spread of infection (standard precautions) are used in all health care facilities for the protection of patients and staff.

TERMINOLOGY REVIEW

Vocabulary Matching: Match each term with its definition.

___	1. contact precautions	A.	Precautions used for patients with a known diagnosis of illness transported by airborne droplet nuclei
___	2. biohazard	B.	Materials that may be able to transmit infection
___	3. body mechanics	C.	The way the body moves when performing particular tasks
___	4. HIV	D.	Precautions used for serious skin and wound infections caused by a variety of microorganisms
___	5. personal protective equipment (PPE)	E.	Precautions used for patients known to have or suspected of having illnesses transported by airborne droplet nuclei
___	6. standard precautions	F.	The study of maximizing work efficiency by adapting the work environment for optimum physical and mental function
___	7. HBV	G.	The virus that causes hepatitis B
___	8. droplet precautions	H.	The virus that causes acquired immunodeficiency syndrome (AIDS)

___ 9. isolation precautions

___ 10. airborne precautions

___ 11. ergonomics

___ 12. sharps

I. Precautions used when there is a high risk of exposure to a specific disease

J. Equipment used to protect a health care worker from exposure to pathogens

K. Items such as needles, glass slides, and scalpel blades

L. Safety precautions used whenever a health care worker comes in contact with body fluid or non-intact skin

CONTENT REVIEW QUESTIONS

1. Identify general principles for storage of boxes and use of filing cabinets in the medical office.

____

____

____

2. What measures should be taken to ensure the safety of electrical equipment?

____

____

____

3. What measures should be taken for fire safety?

____

____

____

4. What emergency telephone numbers should be posted at every telephone?

____

____

____

5. What is the reason for setting up work areas so that people can work with good ergonomics?

____

____

____

6. Describe good body posture.

____

____

____

7. Describe the position for working at a computer or desk that helps minimize strain on the body.

____

8. What does the term "good body mechanics" mean? Give examples.

9. How does stress affect body physiology?

10. What may happen if a person is subject to chronic stress?

11. Identify six measures the medical assistant can use to cope with stress on the job.
    a.
    b.
    c.
    d.
    e.
    f.

12. What are five physical and mental exercises that can be used to reduce stress?
    a.
    b.
    c.
    d.
    e.

13. What standard of the Occupational Safety and Health Administration (OSHA) helps protect employees of medical offices from contracting diseases? How?

14. How can a medical office employee find out if he or she is at risk from potentially hazardous chemicals?

15. When should a medical assistant use standard precautions to prevent contact with material that might spread disease?

____

____

____

16. What are seven specific guidelines for using personal protective equipment (PPEs)?

 a. _______________
 b. _______________
 c. _______________
 d. _______________
 e. _______________
 f. _______________
 g. _______________

17. What is the proper method for disposal of biohazardous waste?

____

____

____

18. Describe each of the following category specific isolation precautions:

 a. Airborne precautions _______________
 b. Droplet precautions _______________
 c. Contact precautions _______________

CRITICAL THINKING QUESTIONS

1. Do research and find information to answer one of the following questions. After obtaining information, discuss how this information may affect your own behavior.

 a. What is the likelihood that a person who keys information into a computer for a significant part of the day will suffer a repetitive strain injury such as carpal tunnel syndrome?

____

____

____

____

____

____

b. What is the likelihood that a health professional will contract hepatitis B, hepatitis C, or HIV from a needlestick injury?

____

____

____

____

____

____

c. What is the likelihood that a health professional will suffer a back or neck injury from job-related causes?

____

____

____

____

____

____

2. What factors make working in a medical office stressful? What measures can employers and employees take to reduce the stress?

____

____

____

____

____

____

3. The federal government has given OSHA the mandate to actively regulate the work environment of every American to be sure that it is safe. It can make unannounced inspections and require large fines from employers who fail to meet its standards. Is this appropriate in a democracy? Discuss this topic and identify at least three reasons to support OSHA's power and at least three reasons why it can be seen as interfering with the rights of businesses and/or citizens.

____

____

____

____

____

____

PRACTICAL APPLICATIONS

1. Identify the PPE (personal protective equipment) that a medical assistant should wear for the following procedures and discuss how to dispose of any supplies used:

   a. Cleaning a counter on which small amount of blood has spilled. ______________________

   ____

   b. Cleaning open wounds for a patient who has several cuts on the arm. ______________________

   ____

   c. Transferring urine from a urine specimen container to a test tube. ______________________

   ____

   d. Preparing a patient with possible active tuberculosis for examination. ______________________

   ____

   e. Drawing blood from a patient. ____

   ____

   f. Cleaning up after a physician has performed a minor surgical procedure to stitch a wound.

   ____

   ____

2. Discuss the body position of the person in each of the following two pictures in relation to head position, posture, hand and arm position, and leg position (if shown). Is the person using good body mechanics? What suggestions would you make?

a. ______________________________

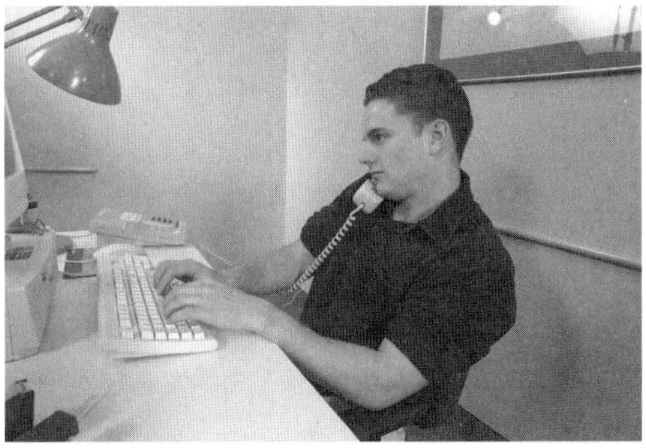

b. ______________________________

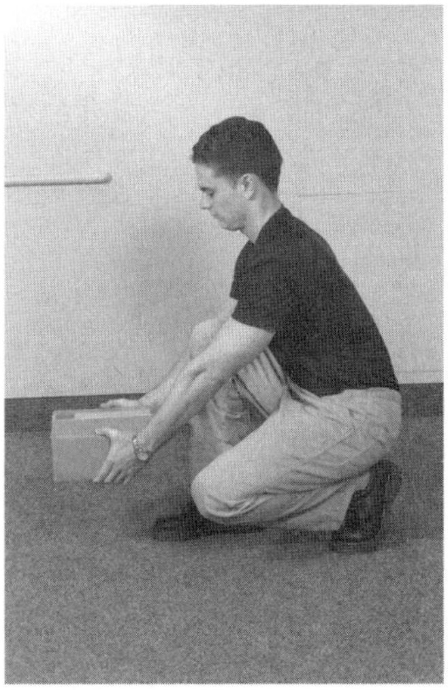

3. Obtain a material safety data sheet for a chemical used in your medical assisting lab (or look at Figure 6-5) and identify safety precautions that should be taken if this chemical is used.

4. Practice conscious muscle relaxation for the neck, shoulders and upper back, arms, facial muscles, and leg muscles of the front and back of the upper and lower leg. It may be helpful to tense and then relax various muscle groups. Notice which muscles are tense even when they are not in use.

SELF-EVALUATION

UNIT 3

Preparing for the Patient

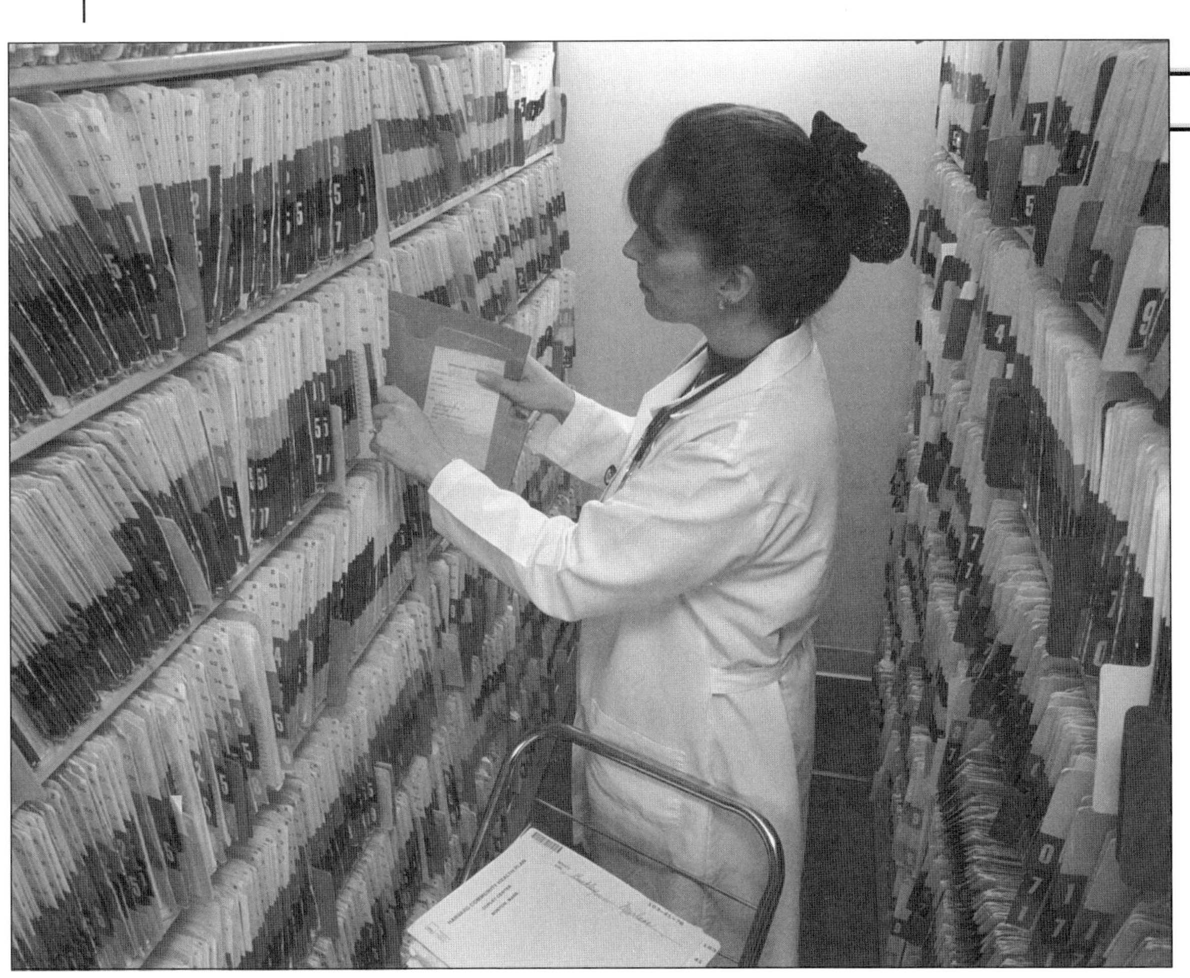

PRACTICAL APPLICATIONS

1. Take messages for the following conversations on the forms given on the next page. Identify any information that the medical assistant should have gotten to take a complete message. Use the current date and time:
   a. *Joanne:* This is Joanne at Blackburn Primary Care Associates. How can I help you?
      Mary: This is Mary Kingston. I am running out of my pills, and the pharmacist told me that I don't have any more refills.
      Joanne: What is the name of the medication?
      Mary: I am taking Lipitor, and like I said, I only have a few pills left.
      Joanne: How many milligrams? And how often do you take it?
      Mary: They are 10-milligram tablets and I take one every morning.
      Joanne: What pharmacy do you use?
      Mary: West River Pharmacy in Blackburn. . . .
   b. *Caller:* Can I speak to Dr. Hughes please?
      Joanne: This is Joanne, Dr. Hughes' medical assistant. The doctor is not available right now. Can I take a message for her?
      Caller: I was wondering if she had gotten the results of the test I had on Monday.
      Joanne: What type of test was it?
      Caller: It was an x-ray, I think they called it an upper GI.
      Joanne: Did you have the test at Memorial Hospital?
      Caller: Yes, I did.
      Joanne: I will leave a message for Dr. Hughes. Can you give me a number where you can be reached this afternoon?
      Caller: I'll be at work. That's 777-7543.
   c. *Caller:* Could I speak to someone about an order you placed for urinalysis dipsticks?
      Joanne: The office manager, Diane Stuart, would normally handle that, but she is at lunch. Can I take a message?
      Caller: Yes, would you ask her to call Sandy at Williams Medical Supply about this order? It is purchase order #7099.
      Joanne: What is your telephone number?
      Caller: She can reach me at 777-2282, extension 4402.
      Joanne: I'll give her the message as soon as she returns . . .

2. Compose a message for an answering machine for the office of Blackburn Primary Care Associates that could be used when office personnel are at lunch.

   ____

   ____

   ____

   ____

   ____

   ____

3. Working with a partner and using the telephone, practice the following scenarios. If possible, use a tape recorder to record the conversations for later analysis. Each person should practice being the caller and being the medical assistant. You can assume that the medical practice is Blackburn Primary Care Associates. The office is located at 1990 Turquoise Drive, Blackburn, WI. The telephone number is 459-8857. After the calls have been recorded, listen to the tapes

MESSAGE FROM

For Dr. | Name of Caller | Ref. to pt. | Patient | Pt. Age | Pt. Temp. | Message Date / / | Message Time AM PM | Urgent ❑ Yes ❑ No

Message: | Allergies

Respond to Phone # | Best Time to Call AM PM | Pharmacy Name / # | Patient's Chart Attached ❑ Yes ❑ No | Patient's chart # | Initials

DOCTOR - STAFF RESPONSE

Doctor's / Staff Orders / Follow-up Action

Call Back ❑ Yes ❑ No | Chart. Mes. ❑ Yes ❑ No | Follow-up Date / / | Follow-up Completed-Date/Time / / AM PM | Response By:

Product # 78-9156-Pkg, #78-9157-Pads, Bibbero Systems, Inc., Petaluma, CA. To order, call toll free 800-BIBBERO (800 242-2376) OR FAX 800-242-9330.

MESSAGE FROM

For Dr. | Name of Caller | Ref. to pt. | Patient | Pt. Age | Pt. Temp. | Message Date / / | Message Time AM PM | Urgent ❑ Yes ❑ No

Message: | Allergies

Respond to Phone # | Best Time to Call AM PM | Pharmacy Name / # | Patient's Chart Attached ❑ Yes ❑ No | Patient's chart # | Initials

DOCTOR - STAFF RESPONSE

Doctor's / Staff Orders / Follow-up Action

Call Back ❑ Yes ❑ No | Chart. Mes. ❑ Yes ❑ No | Follow-up Date / / | Follow-up Completed-Date/Time / / AM PM | Response By:

Product # 78-9156-Pkg, #78-9157-Pads, Bibbero Systems, Inc., Petaluma, CA. To order, call toll free 800-BIBBERO (800 242-2376) OR FAX 800-242-9330.

MESSAGE FROM

For Dr. | Name of Caller | Ref. to pt. | Patient | Pt. Age | Pt. Temp. | Message Date / / | Message Time AM PM | Urgent ❑ Yes ❑ No

Message: | Allergies

Respond to Phone # | Best Time to Call AM PM | Pharmacy Name / # | Patient's Chart Attached ❑ Yes ❑ No | Patient's chart # | Initials

DOCTOR - STAFF RESPONSE

Doctor's / Staff Orders / Follow-up Action

Call Back ❑ Yes ❑ No | Chart. Mes. ❑ Yes ❑ No | Follow-up Date / / | Follow-up Completed-Date/Time / / AM PM | Response By:

Product # 78-9156-Pkg, #78-9157-Pads, Bibbero Systems, Inc., Petaluma, CA. To order, call toll free 800-BIBBERO (800 242-2376) OR FAX 800-242-9330.

Courtesy of Bibbero Systems.

to be sure that the medical assistant has maintained a pleasant tone of voice and obtained complete information.

a. The caller is a patient of Dr. Lopez named Jorge Santos. He has a cut on his finger that is not healing and he would like an appointment. Dr. Lopez has an opening at 3:00 this afternoon. This is a difficult time for Mr. Santos. There are no other open appointments today although there is an appointment tomorrow morning.

b. The caller is a patient named Winifred Post who has a question about her bill. The medical assistant should inform Ms. Post that the insurance has not paid the bill at this time, although the insurance form has been sent. The medical assistant should instruct Ms. Post to contact the insurance company directly.

c. The caller is the wife of a patient named James Mansfield. The wife wants to obtain the test results from an MRI that her husband had two weeks ago.

d. The medical assistant is calling a patient, Diane Rice, to remind her of an appointment at 2:00 PM tomorrow. The telephone is answered by the patient's eight-year-old daughter. The medical assistant gives her the message.

e. Melissa Sanderson calls because her teen-age daughter, a patient of Dr. Lawler, has fallen and twisted her leg and ankle in the hall. The daughter, whose name is Kelsey, cannot get up and is complaining of severe pain in her right ankle. There is no doctor in the office when the call is received.

f. One of the physicians asks the medical assistant to call an ambulance for a patient in the office who is complaining of severe chest pain. Prepare a list of all the information the medical assistant should have ready to give to the emergency operator and simulate the call.

g. The medical assistant is placing a call for Dr. Lawler to the office of Dr. Gulbrandson. When she first places the call, the medical assistant at that office asks her to hold. After about 30 seconds, she tells her that Dr. Gulbrandson will take the call momentarily.

4. Use the CD-ROM and complete the activities for answering the telephone in Cases 1 and 4.

PROCEDURE PERFORMANCE CHECKLISTS

Procedure 7-1: Answering Incoming Calls

Performance Objective

Task: Demonstrate proper telephone technique

Conditions: Given a telephone, message pad, pen or pencil, clock or watch

Standards: Complete the procedure within 5 minutes and achieve a satisfactory score on the procedure performance checklist

*Scoring Key: (**S**)atisfactory, (**U**)nsatisfactory, (**NA**) Not Applicable*
◆ *Denotes a critical element for a satisfactory score on the procedure*

Procedure Steps	1st trial	2nd trial	3rd trial
1. Answer the telephone within the first three rings.			
2. Identify the practice in the proper manner.			
3. Give your name.			
4. Speak distinctly and at a moderate rate.			
5. Ask for the caller's name.			
6. If you can handle the call, do so promptly.			
7. If you need to transfer the call, place the caller on hold, noting the caller's name and telephone number.			
8. Transfer the call correctly according to the telephone system you are using.			
9. If another call comes in while you are still talking, ask to put the first call on hold, and wait for the caller to agree.			
10. After pressing the hold button, pick up the ringing line and explain you are on another line.			
11. Give the second caller the option to hold or call again.			
12. Don't leave a caller on hold for more than 30 seconds.			
13. Return to the first call and provide the information or service.			
14. End the call in a professional manner.			
15. Return to the second call and provide the information or service.			
16. End the call in a professional manner.			
17. Complete the procedure within 5 minutes. ◆			

Evaluator Comments:

Score Calculation:

For each procedural step marked U (Unsatisfactory) deduct 6 points
For each procedural step (◆) marked U (Unsatisfactory) deduct 20 points

Score calculation	100 points			
	– points missed	1st	2nd	3rd
	Total score			

Satisfactory score: 85 or above

Procedure 7-2: Taking a Telephone Message

Performance Objective

Task: Demonstrate proper technique for taking a telephone message

Conditions: Telephone, message pad, pen or pencil, clock or watch

Standards: Complete the procedure within 5 minutes, and achieve a satisfactory score on the procedure performance checklist

Scoring Key: **(S)***atisfactory,* **(U)***nsatisfactory,* **(NA)** *Not Applicable*
◆ *Denotes a critical element for a satisfactory score on the procedure*

Procedure Steps	1st trial	2nd trial	3rd trial
1. Answer the telephone within the first three rings.			
2. Identify the practice in the proper manner.			
3. Give your name.			
4. Speak pleasantly, distinctly, and at a moderate rate.			
5. Ask for the caller's name.			
6. If the person the caller wants to speak to is not available, offer to take a message.			
7. Give the caller a reason why the person cannot take the call.			
8. On the message form, fill in the caller's name, business affiliation, if any, date and time, and telephone number including area code.			
9. Indicate the action desired by the caller and write out a message if necessary.			
10. Verify the information with the caller.			
11. Initial the message form in case there are any questions.			
12. End the call in a professional manner.			
13. Complete the procedure within 5 minutes. ◆			

Evaluator Comments:

Score Calculation:

For each procedural step marked U (Unsatisfactory) deduct 6 points
For each procedural step (◆) marked U (Unsatisfactory) deduct 20 points

Score calculation	100 points			
	− points missed	1st	2nd	3rd
	Total score			

Satisfactory score: 85 or above

Procedure 7-3: Taking Requests for Medication or Prescription Refills

Performance Objective

Task: Demonstrate proper technique for taking a message requesting medication or a refill

Conditions: Telephone, message pad, pen or pencil, clock or watch

Standards: Complete the procedure within 5 minutes, and achieve a satisfactory score on the procedure performance checklist

Scoring Key: (**S**)*atisfactory,* (**U**)*nsatisfactory,* (**NA**) *Not Applicable*
◆ *Denotes a critical element for a satisfactory score on the procedure*

Procedure Steps	1st trial	2nd trial	3rd trial
1. Answer the telephone within the first three rings.			
2. Identify the practice in the proper manner.			
3. Give your name.			
4. Speak distinctly and at a moderate rate.			
5. Identify the caller and telephone number.			
6. Identify if the caller is a patient or a pharmacy.			
7. Write a message including the date and time, patient's name and address, medication and dose requested, and the name and telephone number of the pharmacy to be called.			
8. Inform the caller when the physician is likely to handle the message.			
9. End the call in a professional manner.			
10. Complete the procedure within 5 minutes. ◆			

Evaluator Comments:

Score Calculation:

For each procedural step marked U (Unsatisfactory) deduct 6 points
For each procedural step (◆) marked U (Unsatisfactory) deduct 20 points

Score calculation 100 points

− points missed

Total score

1st	2nd	3rd

Satisfactory score: 85 or above

Notes

Procedure 7-4: Procedure for Emergency Calls

Performance Objective

Task: Answer, assess, and respond appropriately to an emergency telephone call

Conditions: Telephone, message pad, pen or pencil, procedure manual, list of emergency telephone numbers

Standards: Complete the action within 10 minutes, and achieve a satisfactory score on the procedure performance checklist

*Scoring Key: (**S**)atisfactory, (**U**)nsatisfactory, (**NA**) Not Applicable*
◆ *Denotes a critical element for a satisfactory score on the procedure*

Procedure Steps	1st trial	2nd trial	3rd trial
1. Answer the telephone within the first three rings.			
2. Identify the practice in the proper manner.			
3. Give your name.			
4. Speak distinctly and at a moderate rate.			
5. Ask for the caller's name.			
6. If the caller states that a problem is an emergency or urgent, assess the situation immediately.			
7. Remain calm.			
8. Write on the message pad the caller's name, phone number, who has the problem (name, age, and relationship to the caller), symptoms and current condition, brief history of symptoms or accident, and whether any treatment has been given.			
9. Read back the details to confirm.			
10. Decide if the call is an emergency.			
11. If the call is an emergency, transfer the call immediately to a doctor or other licensed medical professional in the office. ◆			
12. If the call is an emergency and there is no licensed person in the office, tell the caller to call an ambulance immediately. ◆			
13. If the emergency is a poisoning, give the caller the number of the local Poison Control Center.			
14. Repeat the instructions and any follow-up that you have agreed to take.			
15. End the call in a professional manner.			
16. Chart your actions in the medical record, including the date, time, information about the patient, your actions, and your planned follow-up.			
17. Complete the procedure within 10 minutes. ◆			

Charting

DATE	

Evaluator Comments:

Score Calculation:

For each procedural step marked U (Unsatisfactory) deduct 6 points
For each procedural step (◆) marked U (Unsatisfactory) deduct 20 points

Score calculation 100 points

− ___ points missed

Total score

1st	2nd	3rd

Satisfactory score: 85 or above

Procedure 7-5: Activating the Emergency Medical Services (EMS) System

Performance Objective

Task: Activate the EMS system by telephone

Conditions: Telephone, completed message form or notes, list of emergency telephone numbers, pen or pencil

Standards: Complete the action within 10 minutes, and achieve a satisfactory score on the procedure performance checklist

Scoring Key: (**S**)*atisfactory*, (**U**)*nsatisfactory*, (**NA**) *Not Applicable*
◆ *Denotes a critical element for a satisfactory score on the procedure*

Procedure Steps	1st trial	2nd trial	3rd trial
1. Determine that you need to activate the EMS system, either by instructions from a licensed professional or by your own assessment.			
2. Dial the correct number.			
3. Inform the person who answers the telephone that you would like to report an emergency.			
4. Remain calm.			
5. Identify the nature of the emergency.			
6. Provide your name and telephone number (including area code).			
7. Give the address and telephone number you are calling from.			
8. Identify who has the problem (name, age, and relationship to caller).			
9. Identify the location of the person with the problem.			
10. Describe the medical emergency including a brief history of symptoms or illness, treatment that has been given, and any medication the patient has taken recently.			
11. State that you will have someone wait at the street entrance for the ambulance and direct the emergency personnel to the patient.			
12. End the call in a professional manner.			
13. Complete the procedure within 10 minutes. ◆			

Evaluator Comments:

Score Calculation:

For each procedural step marked U (Unsatisfactory) deduct 6 points
For each procedural step (◆) marked U (Unsatisfactory) deduct 20 points

Score calculation	100 points			
	− points missed	1st	2nd	3rd
	Total score			

Satisfactory score: 85 or above

Procedure 7-6: Placing Outgoing Telephone Calls

Performance Objective

Task: Use correct technique for placing an outgoing phone call

Conditions: Telephone, scratch pad, pen or pencil, and any information necessary to place the call (i.e., phone book, order information, insurance information, patient record, etc.)

Standards: Complete the action within 10 minutes, and achieve a satisfactory score on the procedure performance checklist

Scoring Key: (**S**)*atisfactory,* (**U**)*nsatisfactory,* (**NA**) *Not Applicable*
◆ *Denotes a critical element for a satisfactory score on the procedure*

Procedure Steps	1st trial	2nd trial	3rd trial
1. Organize material including telephone number and any information needed to conduct the call.			
2. Write the telephone number on a piece of scratch paper, including area code and country code if necessary.			
3. Choose a time and location free from distractions.			
4. Choose a location where the call will not be overheard by patients.			
5. Listen for a dial tone and dial the number.			
6. When the call is answered, ask for your party.			
7. Identify yourself and your practice name.			
8. Clearly state the reason for your call.			
9. Conduct business efficiently and politely.			
10. Confirm information by repeating it.			
11. End the call in a professional manner.			
12. Complete the procedure within 10 minutes. ◆			

Evaluator Comments:

Score Calculation:

For each procedural step marked U (Unsatisfactory) deduct 6 points
For each procedural step (◆) marked U (Unsatisfactory) deduct 20 points

Score calculation	100 points			
	– points missed	1st	2nd	3rd
	Total score			

Satisfactory score: 85 or above

SELF-EVALUATION

Chapter 8

Computers in the Medical Office

CHAPTER FOCUS

In this chapter you reviewed the parts of a computer and how a computer works, and learned how computers are used in a medical office. In addition you learned how to care for computer equipment and maintain a computer system. As computers are used for more tasks in the medical office, it becomes increasingly important for the medical assistant to improve computer skills and knowledge.

TERMINOLOGY REVIEW

Vocabulary Matching: Match each term with its definition.

___ 1. gigabyte	A. The programs that allow you to perform specific tasks, such as database management, desktop publishing, and insurance processing
___ 2. database	B. To create a copy of the data and information that resides on the computer's hard drive
___ 3. mouse	C. To turn on the computer
___ 4. operating system	D. The "guts" of the computer, where all of the microcircuitry sits that allows a computer to do what it does
___ 5. boot	E. The flashing dot that appears where the next character will be written in
___ 6. log on/log in	F. Set of records or information
___ 7. application software	G. The slot where a floppy disk or CD-ROM fits into the case of the computer. Also the device for reading floppy disks or CD-ROM disks
___ 8. motherboard	H. An set of information comprising one document, image, spreadsheet, etc.
___ 9. megabyte	I. A collection of computer files, stored together

____ 10. icon
____ 11. file
____ 12. hardware
____ 13. central processing unit
____ 14. cursor
____ 15. folder
____ 16. back up
____ 17. disk drive
____ 18. monitor
____ 19. keyboard
____ 20. network

J. 1,000 megabytes of memory
K. The physical components of the computer
L. Small graphic on the computer screen that links to a file, folder, or piece of application software
M. The device with which information is typed into the computer, laid out the same way a typewriter is
N. To enter into a computer system or specific program
O. 2^{20} bytes of computer memory
P. The screen on which computer information is displayed
Q. Printed circuit board inside the CPU on which all of the computer's microcircuitry sits
R. A device that allows a computer user to manipulate the cursor without using the up, down, left, or right cursor arrows
S. A group of computers tied together
T. The code that contains the computer's basic operating instructions and tells a computer how to interact with application software

Definitions: Insert the correct word to complete the sentence.

1. A ____________________ is an individual code consisting of letters and/or numbers that allows access to particular information stored on a computer.
2. A ____________________ allows you to make paper copies of the information stored on the computer.
3. ____________________ is the kind of memory that can store information while your computer is on, but which is wiped clear as soon as your computer is turned off.
4. ____________________ controls the computer and does not allow you to discard information and write over it with new information.
5. Data is arranged into a matrix using ____________________ software.
6. A partially completed document that is created to provide formatting, placement of document sections, and sometimes general language is called a ____________________.
7. The computer version of typing, used to compose documents, is called ____________________.

Abbreviations: Expand each abbreviation to its complete form.

1. CPU ______________________________
2. CD-ROM ______________________________
3. DOS ______________________________

4. GB ______________________________
5. LAN ______________________________
6. MB ______________________________
7. RAM ______________________________
8. ROM ______________________________
9. WAN ______________________________
10. HIPAA ______________________________

CONTENT REVIEW QUESTIONS

1. Describe the following elements of a computer system briefly:
   a. Input devices ______________________________
   ____
   b. Central processing unit ______________________________
   ____
   c. Output devices ______________________________
   ____
   d. Storage devices ______________________________
   ____
2. How is computer memory measured? Differentiate between ROM (read-only memory) and RAM (random-access memory).
   ____
   ____
   ____
   ____
3. Describe the following types of information storage for the computer:
   a. Floppy disk ______________________________
   b. CD-ROM ______________________________
   c. Hard drive ______________________________
   d. Magnetic tape drives ______________________________
   e. Zip disk ______________________________
4. Identify the type of output device that would be most useful for each of the following tasks:
   a. To produce a copy of a term paper to hand in to a teacher. ______________________________
   b. To edit and proofread a report while you are working on it. ______________________________
   c. To transfer a file to the computer of a friend who lives five miles from your house.
   ____

5. What are advantages of linking computers into a network?

____

____

____

____

6. Describe the most common computer operating system in current use.

____

____

____

____

7. The type of software that is used to produce and edit documents is ____________ ____________ software. The type that is used to arrange data in a matrix, often for computation, is ____________ software, and the type used to keep sets of related records is ____________ software.

8. Describe briefly how medical billing programs and appointment scheduling programs work.

____

____

____

____

____

____

9. Identify common uses for the computer in the medical office.

a. ____

b. ____

c. ____

d. ____

e. ____

f. ____

10. Identify four areas that are important to keep a computer running properly.

a. ____

b. ____

c. ____

d. ____

11. Identify and describe the three areas of computer maintenance that should be performed regularly.

a. ____

____

b. ______________________________

____

c. ______________________________

____

12. How is patient information kept confidential on an office computer?

____

____

____

CRITICAL THINKING QUESTIONS

1. What methods can be used to limit access to patient data and prevent unauthorized individuals from changing information in a computer system? Are commonly used data protection methods adequate to protect patient information? Give reasons to support your answer.

____

____

____

____

____

____

2. How important are the computer skills of a medical assistant in the job market? How can they affect the medical assistant's ability to specialize within the medical office?

____

____

____

____

____

____

3. Assess your own computer skills and identify strengths and weaknesses. Include a description of your skills in the following areas: a. basic familiarity with the computer, disks, mouse, etc.; b. use of specific software packages; c. use of the Internet to communicate and to find information; d. ability to perform maintenance functions including backing up data, fixing computer errors, and running maintenance programs; and e. familiarity with computer networks and network functions. Identify your two top priorities for improving your computer skills.

____

____

____

PRACTICAL APPLICATIONS

1. Review the following skills at the computer. Practice until you can perform all of the following tasks independently:

   a. Turn on the computer and peripherals (such as a monitor, printer and/or speakers).

   b. Use the mouse to open icons on the Windows desktop. Use the mouse to maximize screen size of a window, close a program, and close a window without closing the program. The left mouse button is usually used to click on an item to highlight it or to double-click on it to open it. The right mouse button has different functions depending on the software you are using. Many computers have a tutorial to help you use the mouse if you are unfamiliar with it. Your instructor can help you if necessary.

   c. Use the Help function to locate information, for example information on how to use the right button on the mouse. Click on the start menu at the bottom of the computer screen. Move the mouse until the arrow on the screen highlights the Help line. Double-click on Help. Type "mouse buttons" to locate the specific topic.

   d. Use the floppy disk drive (A drive). Insert a disk. Review how to open a file or program on a floppy disk, how to format a disk, and how to copy a disk.

      Insert a 3.5″ disk with the label facing up and the metal plate going into the drive first. After insertion, double-click the My Computer icon, then the 3.5″ floppy (A:) icon to view the contents of the disk. To open a program or file, double-click on its icon.

      To format or copy a floppy disk, right click on the 3.5″ floppy (A:) icon. Highlight the appropriate command and follow directions on the screen. If you are copying a disk, be sure that the disk you want to copy from is in the disk drive when you begin to make the copy. This helps you avoid accidentally erasing or replacing files.

   e. Use a word processing program such as Microsoft Word. Click on the Start menu located at the bottom of the computer screen. Highlight Programs with your mouse. A new menu of programs opens. Move the mouse up or down the list until you find the word processing program on your computer. Double-click on the name of the word processing program.

      When the program opens, set up a letter with 2-inch margins on all sides using the New York font, size 12 points. Write a letter to your instructor informing her that you are practicing computer skills using the *Student Mastery Manual.* Use italics for the name of the book. Save the letter to a file on the hard drive. Save a copy on a floppy disk. Print the letter.

      If you have difficulty using the word processing program, you may use the help feature in the program. Highlight Help on the menu bar and click to view the menu options. Click on your selection.

   f. Exit all open applications and turn off the computer. Click Exit on the File menu or click the box containing an X in the upper right-hand corner to exit an application. To turn off the computer correctly, click on the Start menu and highlight Shut Down. When the Shut Down Window opens, click on OK.

SELF-EVALUATION

Chapter 9

Scheduling Appointments

CHAPTER FOCUS

In this chapter you learned how to set up an appointment matrix and schedule appointments for new and established patients. The appointment schedule may be maintained in an appointment book or using a computer program, but no matter what system is used, appointments must be scheduled correctly in order for the medical office to function efficiently.

TERMINOLOGY REVIEW

Vocabulary Matching: Match each term with its definition.

___ 1. matrix

___ 2. blocked

___ 3. suture

___ 4. clustering

___ 5. no-show

___ 6. wave

___ 7. triage

___ 8. fixed scheduling

___ 9. double booking

___ 10. modified wave

A. Grouping patients with similar problems or conditions on certain days or at certain times of the day

B. Booking two people into a single time slot

C. Crossed out of the appointment schedule

D. Dividing each hour into equal periods of 10 or 15 minutes, and assigning each patient to a time slot

E. A form or arrangement for information, such as appointments

F. A scheduling method that uses both fixed appointments and more than one patient scheduled for the same appointment time

G. A person who does not appear for his or her appointment

H. The process of sorting patients according to their need for care

I. Scheduling three or four patients every half-hour, who are seen in the order in which they arrive

J. Using stitches to hold the edges of a wound together

CONTENT REVIEW QUESTIONS

1. Identify six guidelines to follow when making appointments.

   a. ______________________________

   b. ______________________________

   c. ______________________________

   d. ______________________________

   e. ______________________________

   f. ______________________________

2. Identify two ways of recording scheduled appointments.

   a. ______________________________

   b. ______________________________

3. Why must the daily appointment sheet record any changes in the schedule and/or patients who miss appointments in ink? How long must it be kept by the office?

   ____

   ____

   ____

4. What factors must be considered when setting up the appointment matrix?

   ____

   ____

   ____

5. How are new patients treated differently from established patients when setting up appointments?

   ____

   ____

   ____

6. Identify four categories of medical problems that are usually referred to an emergency room.

   a. ______________________________

   b. ______________________________

   c. ______________________________

   d. ______________________________

7. Identify eight types of medical problems for which patients would usually be given an immediate appointment.

   a. ______________________________

   b. ______________________________

   c. ______________________________

   d. ______________________________

   e. ______________________________

   f. ______________________________

g. ________________

h. ________________

8. What should a medical assistant do if an appointment needs to be changed?

____

____

____

9. Identify three common methods to help patients remember appointments.

a. ________________

b. ________________

c. ________________

10. How should the medical assistant handle a patient who comes to the office without an appointment?

____

____

____

CRITICAL THINKING QUESTIONS

1. Write a paragraph stating your position on the following statement: *Most doctors today are well advised to follow an appointment schedule so that patients normally do not have to wait longer than 15 minutes.* Remember to introduce data and/or logical arguments for and against this statement and find a way to refute those of the position that you consider weaker.

____

____

____

____

____

____

____

____

____

2. How does the appointment schedule get slowed down during the course of office visits? Identify as many ways that this happens as you can. Discuss ways to help keep appointments on schedule.

____

____

____

____

____

3. Discuss the resources that are available in the medical office to help an inexperienced medical assistant distinguish between serious medical problems that require care in the emergency room, urgent problems that will be treated in the medical office as soon as possible, problems that require care the same day, and medical problems that can wait for the next open appointment.

PRACTICAL APPLICATIONS

1. Using one of the blank forms at the end of this chapter, set up the appointment matrix for Blackburn Primary Care Associates for Monday October 12, 20XX. Dr. Lawler and Dr. Hughes are scheduled for hospital rounds early in the morning and will begin appointments at 9:00 AM. They will take their lunch break from 12:00 noon until 1:10 PM. Dr. Lawler has a regular Monday meeting from 4:00 to 5:00 PM at the hospital. Dr. Lopez is scheduled at the satellite office in the morning. His first scheduled appointment will be at 1:10 PM after the lunch break. The appointment times from 3:20 through 3:40 PM are blocked out for Dr. Hughes and Dr. Lopez as catch-up time. After you have completed this exercise, you can check your work by looking at Figure 9-3 in your textbook.
2. Using one of the blank forms at the end of this chapter set up an appointment matrix with the following alterations. Dr. Lawler will be at a conference for the entire afternoon. Dr. Hughes has a meeting scheduled at the hospital from 9:00 to 10:00 AM. Dr. Lopez will do hospital rounds from 8:00 to 9:00 AM and be in the main office for appointments from 9:00 through 11:50 AM and will take the usual lunch break. Otherwise the appointment schedule is the same as described in Question 1.
3. Using one of the blank forms at the end of this chapter, set up an appointment matrix with the following alterations from the schedule described in Question 1. Dr. Lopez will be on vacation for the entire day. Dr. Lawler's afternoon meeting has been canceled. Dr. Hughes needs to leave the office at 4:00 PM and does not want any appointments scheduled after 3:20 PM.
4. Make appointments for the following patients on the page from the appointment book for October 13 at the end of the chapter. Assume that established patients will be given 20-minute appointments and new patients will be given 30-minute appointments (except for Dr. Lawler whose new patients

are seen for 40 minutes). Use the abbreviation PE for examinations and the abbreviation re √ for patients who are returning for follow-up. Include the patient's day telephone number. All telephone numbers are in the same area code as the office.

a. June St. Cyr, an established patient, calls for an appointment with Dr. Hughes. She is working and wants to come as late as possible. Her home telephone number is 648-3333 and her work telephone number is 722-1212.

b. William Reardon makes an appointment for follow-up. He is retired and his telephone number is 648-9292. He is to see Dr. Lopez as early in the day as possible.

c. Diana Starr telephones for an appointment for an examination. She is a new patient who has recently moved to the area. Her home telephone has not yet been connected, but her work telephone number is 731-1998. She asks to see Dr. Hughes and requests a late afternoon appointment. She cannot arrive before 5:00 PM.

d. Douglas Wright telephones for an appointment because he has been having dizziness and feeling weak. He has never had an appointment with Dr. Lawler before, but a friend told him that Dr. Lawler is very experienced. He would prefer to come before lunch or as early in the day as possible. His home telephone number is 731-8282 and his work telephone number is 932-1415.

e. Angela Newton needs an appointment for follow-up with Dr. Lopez. She is in high school and cannot arrive before 3:00. Her home telephone number is 452-2001.

5. Add or delete the following patients to the computer generated schedule at the end of the chapter for Dr. Lawler for 10/13/XX. Include information about the visit. Note that this schedule blocks out 20-minute visits so a new patient is scheduled for 40 minutes and an established patient for 20 minutes.

   a. Douglas Wright telephones for an appointment because he has been having dizziness and feeling weak. He has never had an appointment with Dr. Lawler before, but a friend told him that Dr. Lawler is very experienced. He would prefer to come before lunch or as early in the day as possible. His home telephone number is 731-8282 and his work telephone number is 932-1415.

   b. Corrine Davis has been running a fever of 102°F since yesterday and has been off work. She would like to come as early as possible. Her home telephone number is 648-9010. Her work telephone number is 452-8100, ext. 2000. She is a patient of Dr. Lawler's.

   c. Peter Williams hurt his finger after slamming it in his car door this morning. He has gone to work, but it is hurting more now and he would like to come as soon as possible. His work telephone number is 932-6554. His home telephone number is 452-9980. He is a patient of Dr. Lawler.

6. Fill in the appointment cards at the end of the chapter for the two patients from Question 3 who have rechecks.

   a. William Reardon

   b. Angela Newton

7. Use the CD-ROM and schedule Mr. Shapiro for a new patient appointment (Case Study 1).

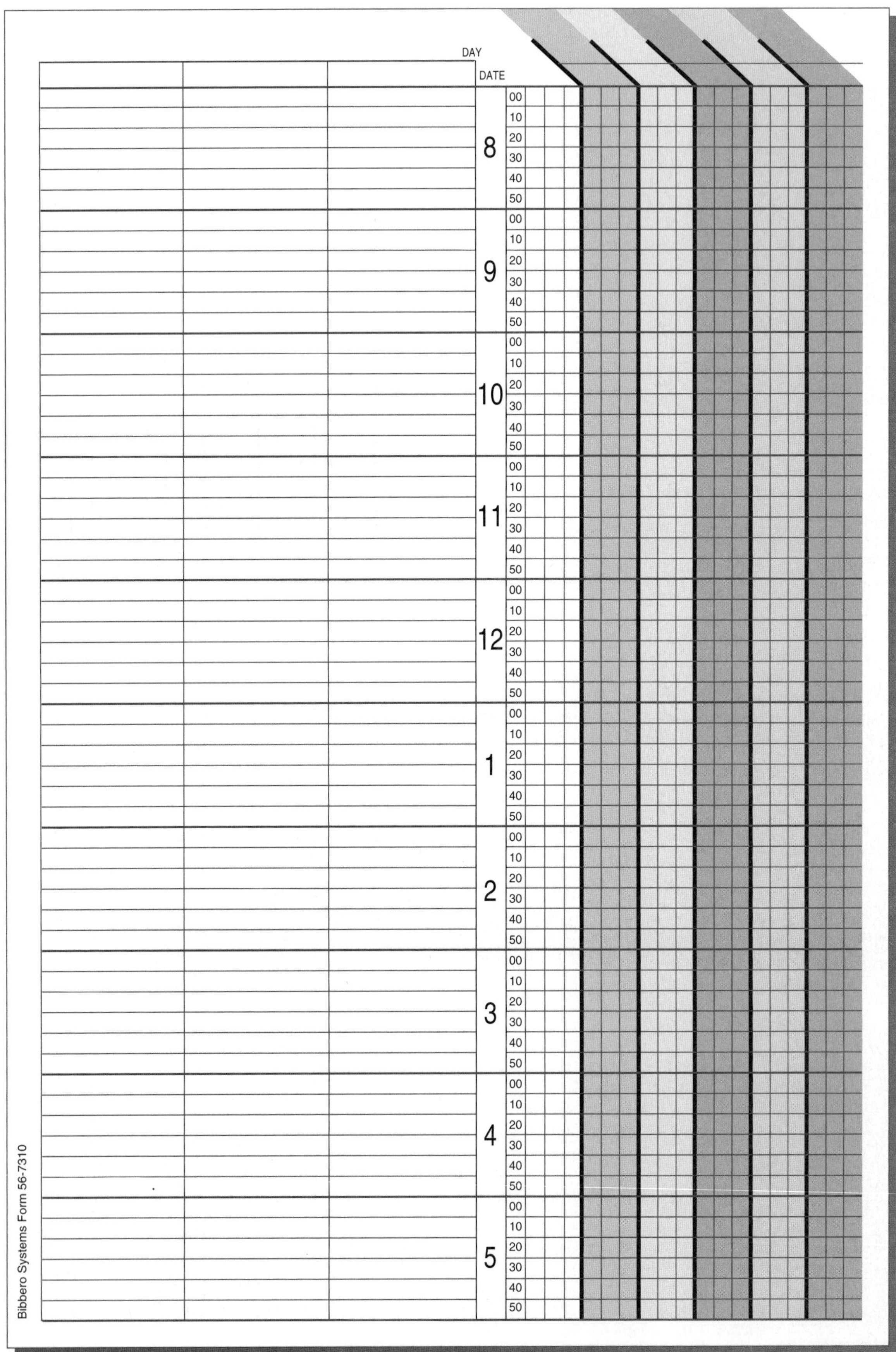

DAY

DATE

Hour	Minutes
8	00, 10, 20, 30, 40, 50
9	00, 10, 20, 30, 40, 50
10	00, 10, 20, 30, 40, 50
11	00, 10, 20, 30, 40, 50
12	00, 10, 20, 30, 40, 50
1	00, 10, 20, 30, 40, 50
2	00, 10, 20, 30, 40, 50
3	00, 10, 20, 30, 40, 50
4	00, 10, 20, 30, 40, 50
5	00, 10, 20, 30, 40, 50

Bibbero Systems Form 56-7310

Courtesy Bibbero Systems.

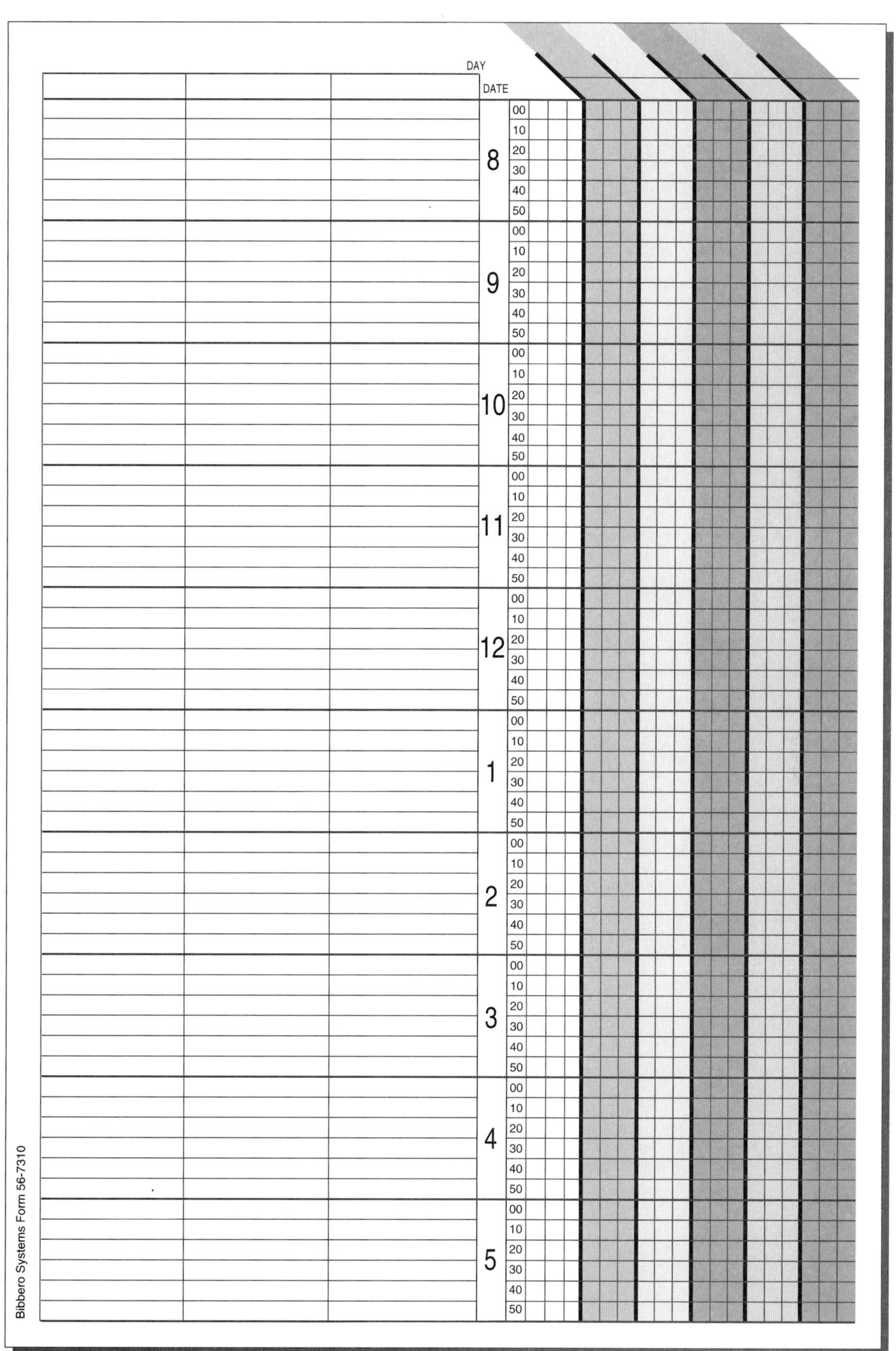

DAY

DATE

8: 00, 10, 20, 30, 40, 50

9: 00, 10, 20, 30, 40, 50

10: 00, 10, 20, 30, 40, 50

11: 00, 10, 20, 30, 40, 50

12: 00, 10, 20, 30, 40, 50

1: 00, 10, 20, 30, 40, 50

2: 00, 10, 20, 30, 40, 50

3: 00, 10, 20, 30, 40, 50

4: 00, 10, 20, 30, 40, 50

5: 00, 10, 20, 30, 40, 50

Bibbero Systems Form 56-7310

Courtesy Bibbero Systems.

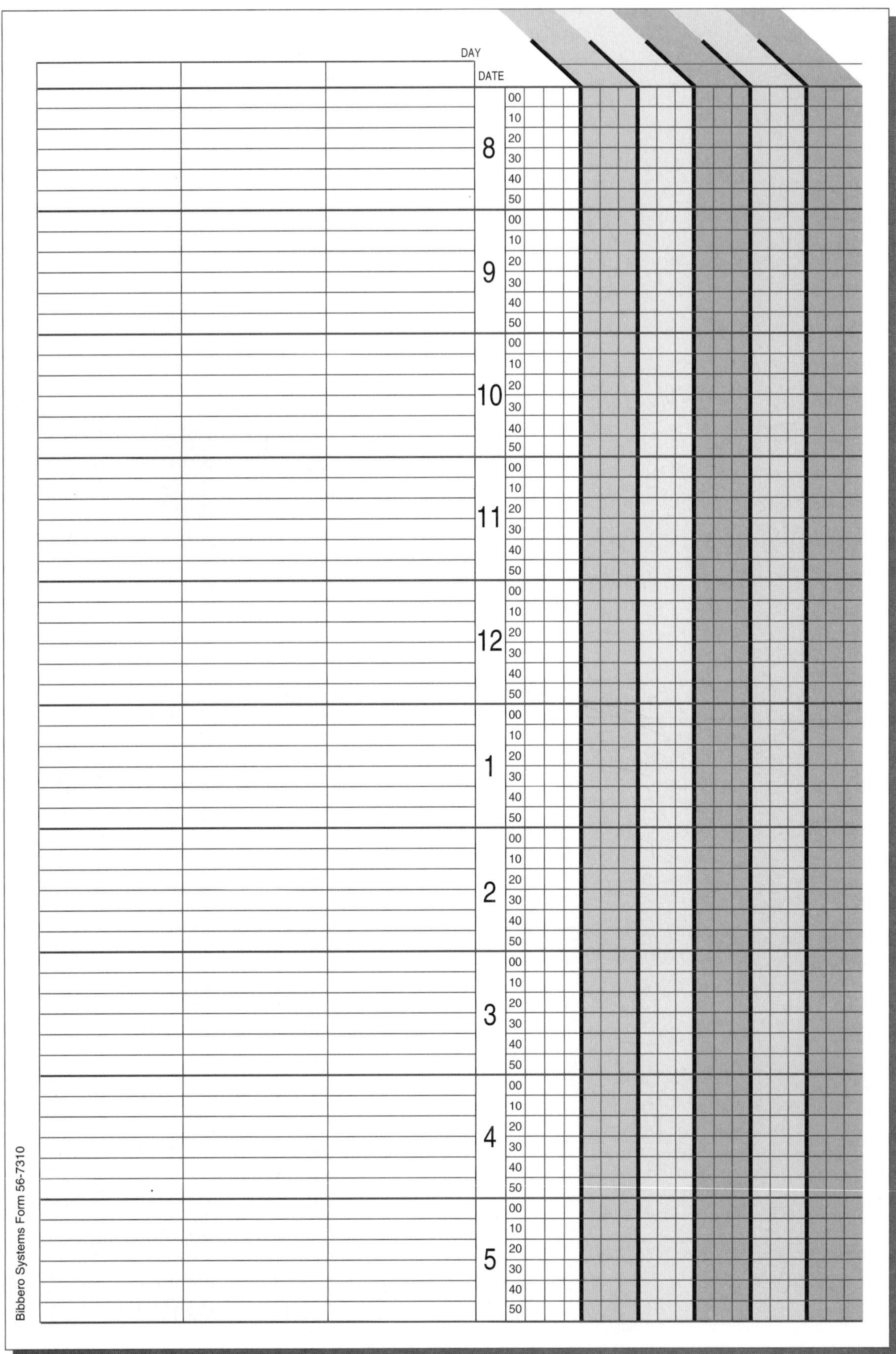

DAY

DATE

Hour	Minutes
8	00
	10
	20
	30
	40
	50
9	00
	10
	20
	30
	40
	50
10	00
	10
	20
	30
	40
	50
11	00
	10
	20
	30
	40
	50
12	00
	10
	20
	30
	40
	50
1	00
	10
	20
	30
	40
	50
2	00
	10
	20
	30
	40
	50
3	00
	10
	20
	30
	40
	50
4	00
	10
	20
	30
	40
	50
5	00
	10
	20
	30
	40
	50

Bibbero Systems Form 56-7310

Courtesy Bibbero Systems.

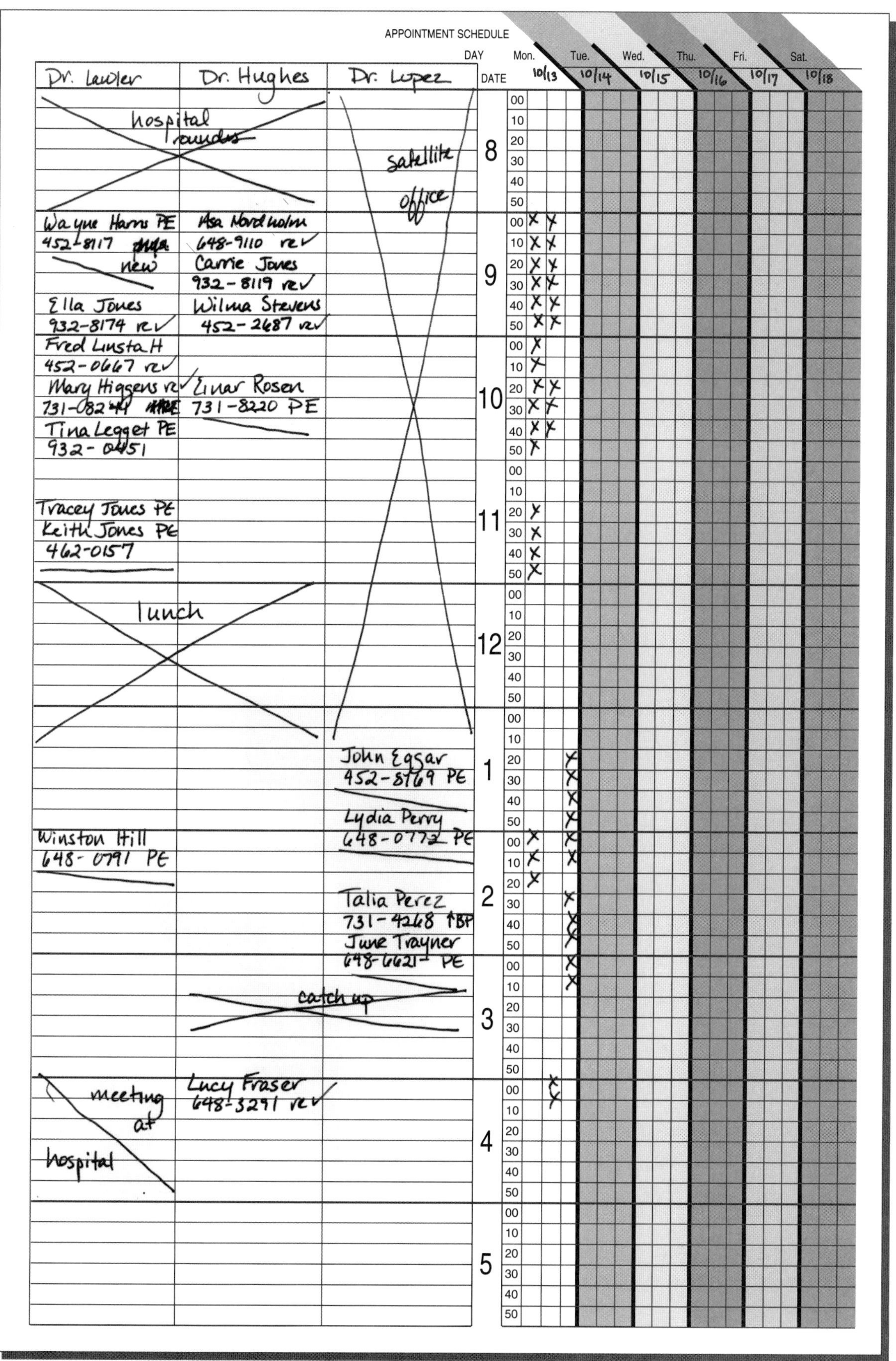

APPOINTMENT SCHEDULE

DAY	Mon.	Tue.	Wed.	Thu.	Fri.	Sat.
DATE	10/13	10/14	10/15	10/16	10/17	10/18

Time	Dr. Lawler	Dr. Hughes	Dr. Lopez
8:00–8:50	hospital rounds	hospital rounds	satellite office
9:00	Wayne Harris PE 452-8117 new	Asa Nordholm 648-9110 rev✓	satellite office
9:20		Carrie Jones 932-8119 rev✓	satellite office
9:40	Ella Jones 932-8174 rev✓	Wilma Stevens 452-2687 rev✓	satellite office
10:00	Fred Linstatt 452-0667 rev✓		satellite office
10:20	Mary Higgens rev✓ 731-8244	Einar Rosen 731-8220 PE	satellite office
10:40	Tina Legget PE 932-0451		satellite office
11:20	Tracey Jones PE		satellite office
11:30	Keith Jones PE 462-0157		satellite office
12:00–12:50	lunch	lunch	satellite office
1:20			John Egsar 452-8169 PE
1:50			Lydia Perry 648-0772 PE
2:00	Winston Hill 648-0791 PE		
2:30			Talia Perez 731-4268 TBP
2:50			June Trayner 648-6621 PE
3:10–3:30		catch up	catch up
4:00	meeting at hospital	Lucy Fraser 648-3291 rev✓	
5:00–5:50			

Schedule for 10/13/XX For Dr. Howard Lawler

Time	Patient	Phone	Comments
8:00a	HOSPITAL ROUNDS		
8:20a	↓		
8:40a	↓		
9:00a	Wayne Harris	452-8117	New Patient; Complete Physical
9:20a	****************		
9:40a	~~Ella Jones~~	~~932-8174~~	~~recheck~~ cancel 8am 10/13
10:00a	Fred Linstatt	452-0667	recheck
10:20a	Mary Higgens	731-8241	recheck; URI 2 weeks ago
10:40a	Tina Leggett	931-0451	PE
11:00a			
11:20a	Tracey Jones	462-0157	2yr PE; father Robert
11:40a	Keth Jones		3 yr PE
12:00p	LUNCH		
12:20p	↓		
12:40p	↓		
1:00p	↓		
1:20p			
1:40p			
2:00p	Winston Hill	648-0791	PE
2:20p			
2:40p			
3:00p			
3:20p			
3:40p			
4:00p	Meeting at hospital		
4:20p	↓		
4:40p	↓		
5:00p			
5:20p			
5:40p			

Blackburn Primary Care Associates, PC

1990 Turquiose Drive • Blackburn, WI 54937 • 608-459-8857

has an appointment on provider

date time

Please telephone one day in advance if you will be unable to keep the appointment

Blackburn Primary Care Associates, PC

1990 Turquiose Drive • Blackburn, WI 54937 • 608-459-8857

has an appointment on provider

date time

Please telephone one day in advance if you will be unable to keep the appointment

PROCEDURE PERFORMANCE CHECKLISTS

Procedure 9-1: Setting Up the Appointment Matrix

Performance Objective

Task: Set up an appointment matrix using the office's guidelines

Conditions: Appointment book or computer program, pen, doctors' schedules, office calendar

Standards: Complete the action within 5 minutes, and achieve a satisfactory score on the procedure performance checklist

Scoring Key: (**S**)*atisfactory,* (**U**)*nsatisfactory,* (**NA**) *Not Applicable*
◆ *Denotes a critical element for a satisfactory score on the procedure*

Procedure Steps	1st trial	2nd trial	3rd trial
1. Mark an X through times when the office is not open to see patients.			
2. For each doctor, mark an X through times when he or she is not available to see patients.			
3. For each doctor, mark times when he or she does particular types of procedures or exams (if applicable).			
4. According to office policy, block out time for each doctor for urgent visits, phone calls, or catch-up.			
5. Complete the procedure within 5 minutes. ◆			

Evaluator Comments:

Score Calculation:

For each procedural step marked U (Unsatisfactory) deduct 6 points
For each procedural step (◆) marked U (Unsatisfactory) deduct 20 points

Score calculation	100 points			
	− points missed	1st	2nd	3rd
	Total score			

Satisfactory score: 85 or above

Notes

Procedure 9-2: Making an Appointment

Performance Objective

Task: Arrange a patient appointment

Conditions: Appointment book or computer program, pencil

Standards: Complete the action within 5 minutes, and achieve a satisfactory score on the procedure performance checklist

Scoring Key: (**S**)*atisfactory,* (**U**)*nsatisfactory,* (**NA**) *Not Applicable*
◆ *Denotes a critical element for a satisfactory score on the procedure*

Procedure Steps	1st trial	2nd trial	3rd trial
1. Obtain information from the patient: which doctor the patient would like to see, the purpose of the appointment, and any scheduling preference.			
2. Offer the patient a date and time for an appointment. Keep locating appointment times until you and the patient agree on a date and time.			
3. Obtain the information necessary to fill in the appointment book: name, reason for the visit, daytime phone number, and date of birth (especially for common names).			
4. Enter all the information in pencil and block out the correct amount of time for the required visit.			
5. If the patient is a new patient, also collect insurance company, group number, and ID number, and a referral number if applicable.			
6. Offer travel and parking directions.			
7. Confirm the information by repeating it to the caller.			
8. Complete the procedure within 5 minutes. ◆			

Evaluator Comments:

Score Calculation:

For each procedural step marked U (Unsatisfactory) deduct 6 points
For each procedural step (◆) marked U (Unsatisfactory) deduct 20 points

Score calculation 100 points
− ___ points missed

	1st	2nd	3rd
Total score			

Satisfactory score: 85 or above

SELF-EVALUATION

CRITICAL THINKING QUESTIONS

1. Discuss what a medical assistant might be directly responsible for in relation to the routine maintenance of a medical office.

2. Identify at least five potential safety hazards in a medical office and the responsibilities of a medical assistant in preventing injuries from these potential hazards.

3. Discuss what can happen when a medical office does not have adequate storage space for office and medical supplies. How can this affect the medical assistants who work in the office? How can it affect the smooth function of the office as a whole?

4. Obtain samples of five different brands of adhesive bandages that are 3/4″ × 3″. Compare the bandages for price, ease of opening, size, ease of application and ability to adhere. Which bandage would you recommend for use in a medical office.

5. How can the process of applying for accreditation help an organization to improve procedures and service?

____

____

____

____

____

____

PRACTICAL APPLICATIONS

1. As a class activity, create an inventory control system for the supplies used for the administrative or clinical portion of your medical assisting program. Identify all supplies used, the amount necessary for a 6-month period, and reorder points for each item. Identify a possible supplier for each item. Create an inventory card for each item to take inventory.

2. Obtain catalogs for medical supplies or identify a medical supply company on the Internet. You can use a resource from the Web sites listed for the section **If You Were the Medical Assistant** in Chapter 11 of your textbook. Prepare an order for the following supplies using the purchase order form at the end of the chapter and complete the procedure performance checklist for Procedure 11-3. Enter the name and address of the vendor, and use Net 30 days for the terms of payment. Be sure to add tax and/or shipping costs as directed by the vendor. Purchase the least expensive product that meets the description below.

Latex gloves - small	6 boxes
non-Latex gloves - medium - powder free	6 boxes
alcohol swabs - small	10 boxes of 100
universal spill kit	2
nonsterile gauze squares 2″ × 2″	2000

3. Obtain product information from the Internet or a catalog for three tympanic thermometers including a description of the product, cost, cost and packaging of probe covers, and type and cost of batteries and/or charger. Discuss with your classmates which model you would recommend for a medical office that expects to use the thermometer at least ten times daily.

PURCHASE ORDER

No. 1554

Bill to:

Blackburn Primary Care Associates. PC
1990 Turquoise Drive
Blackburn, WI 54937

Ship to:

Blackburn Primary Care Associates, PC
1990 Turquoise Drive
Blackburn, WI 54937

Vendor: ______________________

____

____

Terms: ______________________

ORDER #	DESCRIPTION	QTY.	COLOR	SIZE	UNIT PRICE	TOTAL PRICE
					SUBTOTAL	
					TAX	
					SHIPPING	
					TOTAL	

PURCHASE ORDER

No. 1554

Bill to:

Blackburn Primary Care Associates. PC
1990 Turquoise Drive
Blackburn, WI 54937

Ship to:

Blackburn Primary Care Associates, PC
1990 Turquoise Drive
Blackburn, WI 54937

Vendor: ______________________

____

____

Terms: ______________________

ORDER #	DESCRIPTION	QTY.	COLOR	SIZE	UNIT PRICE	TOTAL PRICE
					SUBTOTAL	
					TAX	
					SHIPPING	
					TOTAL	

PROCEDURE PERFORMANCE CHECKLISTS

Procedure 11-1: Taking a Supply Inventory

Performance Objective

Task: Take a supply inventory using an inventory card system, inventory notebook, or computer printout

Conditions: Inventory cards or notebook, supplies to inventory, pen

Standards: Complete the action within 10 minutes, and achieve a satisfactory score on the procedure performance checklist

Scoring Key: (**S**)*atisfactory,* (**U**)*nsatisfactory,* (**NA**) *Not Applicable*
◆ *Denotes a critical element for a satisfactory score on the procedure*

Procedure Steps	**1st trial**	**2nd trial**	**3rd trial**
1. Obtain list of items in inventory—either an inventory notebook, box of inventory cards, or computer printout.			
2. Considering the supplies on hand in both examining rooms and storage, check expiration dates and dispose of supplies that have expired.			
3. Count the number of one item and enter the number in the appropriate place on the card, in notebook, or on printout.			
4. Check the number of supplies on hand against the number listed as the reorder point. If there are fewer on hand than the reorder point, flag the item to be ordered.			
5. Check that the information on the inventory record is correct and complete with regard to size, color, order number, and manufacturer.			
6. Repeat steps 2 through 5 for each item to be inventoried.			
7. Tidy storage space as needed to make it easy to find items.			
8. Place inventory record in the appropriate place for follow-up, including ordering and updating computer information.			
9. Complete the procedure within 10 minutes. ◆			

Evaluator Comments:

Score Calculation:

For each procedural step marked U (Unsatisfactory) deduct 6 points
For each procedural step (◆) marked U (Unsatisfactory) deduct 20 points

Score calculation 100 points

		1st	2nd	3rd
−	points missed			
	Total score			

Satisfactory score: 85 or above

Procedure 11-2: Stocking the Supply Closet

Performance Objective

Task: Stock the supply cabinet and dispose of expired supplies

Conditions: Inventory card, notebook, or printout, new supplies, invoice or packing list, pen or pencil

Standards: Complete the action within 10 minutes, and achieve a satisfactory score on the procedure performance checklist

Scoring Key: (**S**)*atisfactory,* (**U**)*nsatisfactory,* (**NA**) *Not Applicable*
◆ *Denotes a critical element for a satisfactory score on the procedure*

Procedure Steps	1st trial	2nd trial	3rd trial
1. Bring box of supplies to the area where they are going to be stored (i.e., supply room, copy room, staff area).			
2. Unpack supplies and check each item received against packing slip.			
3. Shelve supplies by type in the location they are usually stored. Place older supplies in front of newer supplies.			
4. Check expiration dates of supplies on the shelf (if any) and discard expired supplies.			
5. For each type of supply, note in the inventory record the amount of supplies added to inventory. Deduct any expired supplies discarded.			
6. Continue until all supplies have been placed in storage.			
7. Note on the packing slip any supplies that were not included with the order.			
8. File invoice/packing slips in the proper file for payment.			
9. Complete the procedure within 10 minutes. ◆			

Evaluator Comments:

Score Calculation:

For each procedural step marked U (Unsatisfactory) deduct 6 points
For each procedural step (◆) marked U (Unsatisfactory) deduct 20 points

Score calculation	100 points			
	– points missed	1st	2nd	3rd
	Total score			

Satisfactory score: 85 or above

Procedure 11-3: Preparing a Purchase Order

Performance Objective

Task: Prepare a purchase order for supplies

Conditions: Inventory record, purchase order form, pen, list of items "flagged" as in need of reorder, catalog or on-line supply web site, copier, and communication (phone, fax, or computer) if needed

Standards: Complete the action within 15 minutes, and achieve a satisfactory score on the procedure performance checklist

Scoring Key: (**S**)*atisfactory,* (**U**)*nsatisfactory,* (**NA**) *Not Applicable*
◆ *Denotes a critical element for a satisfactory score on the procedure*

Procedure Steps	1st trial	2nd trial	3rd trial
1. Collect a list of regularly purchased items and supplies that have been flagged for reorder.			
2. Look up items in a catalog or at an on-line supply web site to identify catalog number, description, size, color, and unit price.			
3. Enter each item either on a form provided by the vendor or an office-generated and vendor-approved form including the catalog number, description, quantity, color, size, and unit price.			
4. For each item, multiply the quantity times the unit price to obtain the total price.			
5. Add the total price of all items to obtain a subtotal.			
6. Calculate the correct tax for your state and enter on the correct line.			
7. Calculate the shipping according to the supplier's directions and enter on the correct line.			
8. Calculate the total for the entire order.			
9. Make a copy of the order for your records.			
10. Leave the order and copy for the office manager to place the order.			
11. If your inventory system has flags to indicate when an item is on order, so indicate for all items ordered.			
12. Complete the procedure within 15 minutes. ◆			

Evaluator Comments:

Score Calculation:

For each procedural step marked U (Unsatisfactory) deduct 6 points
For each procedural step (◆) marked U (Unsatisfactory) deduct 20 points

Score calculation 100 points

− ___ points missed

Total score

1st	2nd	3rd

Satisfactory score: 85 or above

SELF-EVALUATION

Chapter 12

Opening the Office and Checking Patients In

CHAPTER FOCUS

In this chapter you learned how to open the office, pick up messages from an answering machine or answering service, prepare for the day's activities and check patients in. If the check in process is handled smoothly and professionally, it benefits both the medical practice and the patient. It reassures the patient that office staff are caring and competent. In addition, when proper information and signatures have been obtained, the billing process proceeds smoothly.

TERMINOLOGY REVIEW

Vocabulary Matching: Match each term with its definition.

___ 1. encounter form

___ 2. co-payment

___ 3. point-of-service (POS) device

___ 4. assignment of benefits

___ 5. call-in times

A. When the office accepts payment directly from the insurance company

B. A fixed amount of money that the patient is required to pay each time he or she receives a medical treatment

C. The form on which information about the visit, including the diagnosis, and the charge for visit, is recorded

D. A small machine in the doctor's office connected via telephone to the insurance company's database, which can verify insurance benefits while the patient is in the office

E. Times when the physician takes telephone calls

CONTENT REVIEW QUESTIONS

1. Identify five tasks that are performed when the medical office is first opened in the morning.

   a. ______________________________

   b. ______________________________

   c. ______________________________

   d. ______________________________

   e. ______________________________

2. Identify two ways that patients might leave messages when the office is closed.

   a. ______________________________

   b. ______________________________

3. To prepare for patient visits, office staff must find the ______________________ for each patient and prepare a ______________________.

4. What are four tasks that may be necessary to prepare examination or treatment rooms?

   a. ______________________________

   b. ______________________________

   c. ______________________________

   d. ______________________________

5. To maintain confidentiality of a patient who is checking in, the medical assistant can

   ____

   ____

6. Identify at least six areas of information about the practice that new patients should be oriented to.

   a. ______________________________

   b. ______________________________

   c. ______________________________

   d. ______________________________

   e. ______________________________

   f. ______________________________

7. Why is it helpful if the practice has a patient information booklet?

   ____

   ____

   ____

   ____

8. Identify four different types of information and/or signatures that are usually collected from new patients.

   a. ______________________________

   b. ______________________________

c. ______________________________

d. ______________________________

9. How does the medical assistant verify insurance eligibility and information?

____

____

____

____

10. How does the medical assistant inform office staff that a patient is waiting to be seen?

____

____

CRITICAL THINKING QUESTIONS

1. Identify general guidelines that a medical office could use to deal with situations where the physicians are running late with appointments and/or out of the office for emergencies.

____

____

____

____

____

____

2. Discuss advantages and disadvantages of using an answering service, voice mail, or answering machine to take messages.

____

____

____

____

____

____

3. Do you think it is worth the effort to take five or ten minutes with a new patient to orient the patient to how the practice works? Do you think this happens in reality? Describe how you would respond if you went to a first appointment and office staff provided such information during your visit.

____

____

____

____

4. Should physicians maintain Web sites on the Internet? What would be advantages and disadvantages? Would patients use them? What information could be provided? Finding examples may help you answer this question.

PRACTICAL APPLICATIONS

1. Role-play the following situations:
   a. Explaining to a patient that the service he or she is requesting may not be covered by insurance, and requesting the patient to sign a form agreeing to pay for the service if insurance does not.
   b. Explaining to a patient that the doctor is running 30 minutes late. If you are role-playing the patient, pretend to have another important appointment.
   c. Requesting a new patient to fill out a patient information sheet. Provide all supplies needed to complete your request.
   d. Calling an answering service for messages and explaining that the office is now open.
   e. Calling an insurance company for authorization for a specific service, such as a proctosigmoidoscopy or a referral to a chiropractor.
2. Fill out a new patient information sheet (located at the end of this section) and clarify any questions that you do not understand.
3. Describe the entire process for checking in an established patient and a new patient.

REGISTRATION
(PLEASE PRINT)

Home Phone: ____________________ Today's Date: ______________

PATIENT INFORMATION

Name ______________________________ (Last Name) (First Name) (Initial) Soc. Sec.# ______________

Address ______________________________

City ______________ State ______________ Zip ______________

Single ___ Married ___ Widowed ___ Separated ___ Divorced ___ Sex M___ F___ Age ___ Birthdate ______________

Patient Employed by ______________ Occupation ______________

Business Address ______________ Business Phone ______________

By whom were you referred? ______________

In case of emergency who should be notified? ______________ (Last Name) (Relationship to Patient) Phone ______________

PRIMARY INSURANCE

Person Responsible for Account ______________________________ (Last Name) (First Name) (Initial)

Relation to Patient ______________ Birthdate ______________ Soc. Sec.# ______________

Address (if different from patient's) ______________ Phone ______________

City ______________ State ______________ Zip ______________

Person Responsible Employed by ______________ Occupation ______________

Business Address ______________ Business Phone ______________

Insurance Company ______________

Contract # ______________ Group # ______________ Subscriber # ______________

Name of other dependents covered under this plan ______________

ADDITIONAL INSURANCE

Is patient covered by additional insurance? ___ Yes ___ No

Subscriber Name ______________ Relationship to Patient ______________ Birthdate ______________

Address (if different from patient's) ______________ Phone ______________

City ______________ State ______________ Zip ______________

Subscriber Employed by ______________ Business Phone ______________

Insurance Company ______________

Contract # ______________ Group # ______________ Subscriber # ______________

Name of other dependents covered under this plan ______________

ASSIGNMENT AND RELEASE

I, the undersigned, certify that I (or my dependent) have insurance coverage with ______________ (Name of Insurance Company(ies))

and assign directly to Dr. ______________ insurance benefits, if any, otherwise payable to me for services rendered. I understand that I am financially responsible for all charges whether or not paid by insurance. I hereby authorize the doctor to release all information necessary to secure the payment of benefits. I authorize the use of this signature on all insurance submissions.

______________ ______________ ______________
Responsible Party Signature Relationship Date

ORDER# 58-8426 • © 1996 BIBBERO SYSTEMS, INC. • PETALUMA, CALIFORNIA • TO REORDER CALL TOLL FREE: (800) 242-9330

REGISTRATION
(PLEASE PRINT)

Home Phone: ________________ Today's Date: ____________

PATIENT INFORMATION

Name ____________________ Soc. Sec.# ____________
Last Name First Name Initial

Address ____________________

City ____________ State ____________ Zip ____________

Single ___ Married ___ Widowed ___ Separated ___ Divorced ___ Sex M___ F___ Age___ Birthdate ____________

Patient Employed by ____________ Occupation ____________

Business Address ____________ Business Phone ____________

By whom were you referred? ____________

In case of emergency who should be notified? ____________ Phone ____________
Last Name Relationship to Patient

PRIMARY INSURANCE

Person Responsible for Account ____________
Last Name First Name Initial

Relation to Patient ____________ Birthdate ____________ Soc. Sec.# ____________

Address (if different from patient's) ____________ Phone ____________

City ____________ State ____________ Zip ____________

Person Responsible Employed by ____________ Occupation ____________

Business Address ____________ Business Phone ____________

Insurance Company ____________

Contract # ____________ Group # ____________ Subscriber # ____________

Name of other dependents covered under this plan ____________

ADDITIONAL INSURANCE

Is patient covered by additional insurance? ____Yes ____ No

Subscriber Name ____________ Relationship to Patient ____________ Birthdate ____________

Address (if different from patient's) ____________ Phone ____________

City ____________ State ____________ Zip ____________

Subscriber Employed by ____________ Business Phone ____________

Insurance Company ____________

Contract # ____________ Group # ____________ Subscriber # ____________

Name of other dependents covered under this plan ____________

ASSIGNMENT AND RELEASE

I, the undersigned, certify that I (or my dependent) have insurance coverage with ____________
Name of Insurance Company(ies)

and assign directly to Dr. ____________ insurance benefits, if any, otherwise payable to me for services rendered. I understand that I am financially responsible for all charges whether or not paid by insurance. I hereby authorize the doctor to release all information necessary to secure the payment of benefits. I authorize the use of this signature on all insurance submissions.

____________ ____________ ____________
Responsible Party Signature Relationship Date

ORDER# 58-8426 • © 1996 BIBBERO SYSTEMS, INC. • PETALUMA, CALIFORNIA • TO REORDER CALL TOLL FREE: (800) 242-9330

PROCEDURE PERFORMANCE CHECKLISTS

Procedure 12-1: Taking Messages from an Answering Machine

Performance Objective

Task: Retrieve, record, and assess the importance of messages from an answering machine

Conditions: Answering machine, telephone message pad, pen, clock, or watch

Standards: Complete the action within 5 minutes, and achieve a satisfactory score on the procedure performance checklist

Scoring Key: (**S**)*atisfactory,* (**U**)*nsatisfactory,* (**NA**) *Not Applicable*
◆ *Denotes a critical element for a satisfactory score on the procedure*

Procedure Steps	**1st trial**	**2nd trial**	**3rd trial**
1. Whenever the office has been closed, check answering machine as soon as the office reopens to see if there are new messages.			
2. Listen to the messages in order, writing down on a message pad the pertinent information from each message.			
3. Place initials on all messages in case there are any questions.			
4. After taking all messages, cancel messages and reset the answering machine to the day message (if one is used).			
5. Arrange messages in order of importance.			
6. After dealing with urgent messages, pull medical records for calls from patients and place messages (with records if appropriate) for doctors and/or other staff to review them.			
7. Complete the procedure within 5 minutes. ◆			

Evaluator Comments:

Score Calculation:

For each procedural step marked U (Unsatisfactory) deduct 6 points
For each procedural step (◆) marked U (Unsatisfactory) deduct 20 points

Score calculation 100 points
− ___ points missed

	1st	2nd	3rd
Total score			

Satisfactory score: 85 or above

Notes

Procedure 12-2: Taking Messages from an Answering Service

Performance Objective

Task: Retrieve, record, and assess importance of calls from the answering service

Conditions: Telephone message pad, pen, clock or watch

Standards: Complete the action within 5 minutes, and achieve a satisfactory score on the procedure performance checklist

Scoring Key: (**S**)*atisfactory,* (**U**)*nsatisfactory,* (**NA**) *Not Applicable*
◆ *Denotes a critical element for a satisfactory score on the procedure*

Procedure Steps

Procedure Steps	1st trial	2nd trial	3rd trial
1. Call the answering service and identify yourself and the practice.			
2. State that you are in the office and would like any messages for the practice.			
3. Write down pertinent information for each message on message slips.			
4. Confirm information by repeating it to the person at the answering service.			
5. Place your initials on the slips in case there are any questions.			
6. Terminate the call in a professional manner.			
7. Arrange messages in order of importance.			
8. After dealing with urgent messages, pull medical records for calls from patients and place messages (with records if appropriate) for doctors and/or other staff to review them.			
9. Complete the procedure within 5 minutes. ◆			

Evaluator Comments:

Score Calculation:

For each procedural step marked U (Unsatisfactory) deduct 6 points
For each procedural step (◆) marked U (Unsatisfactory) deduct 20 points

Score calculation 100 points
− points missed

	1st	2nd	3rd
Total score			

Satisfactory score: 85 or above

Notes

Procedure 12-3: Checking Patients In

Performance Objective

Task: Check patients in for office visits

Conditions: Charge slip, medical record, pen, appointment schedule and, for new patients, patient information form, authorization to release information to insurance company, assignment of benefits form, patient information booklet, photocopy machine

Standards: Complete the action within 10 minutes, and achieve a satisfactory score on the procedure performance checklist

Scoring Key: (**S**)*atisfactory,* (**U**)*nsatisfactory,* (**NA**) *Not Applicable*
◆ *Denotes a critical element for a satisfactory score on the procedure*

Procedure Steps	1st trial	2nd trial	3rd trial
1. Greet each person who enters the office. If helping someone else, ask the new arrival to have a seat and say that you will see him or her in a moment.			
2. Establish if the new arrival is a patient.			
3. Find the patient's name on the appointment schedule and determine if it is a new or established patient.			
4. If it is a new patient, ask the patient to fill out forms used by your office for new patients. Give the person the office's information packet.			
5. When the patient returns the completed forms, review them for completeness and accuracy.			
6. Ask for the patient's insurance card and make a photocopy of both sides.			
7. Confirm patient eligibility for insurance coverage if necessary.			
8. If the patient is a referral, request a referral form and confirm that it is correctly filled out.			
9. If the visit will not be covered by insurance, discuss the patient's financial responsibility.			
10. If the patient is an established patient, ask if there are any changes in basic information, such as address or phone, or any change in insurance coverage.			
11. Collect the co-payment if there is one, and enter the amount collected on the charge slip.			
12. Use a pen or highlighter to check off the person's name on the patient master appointment list.			

Procedure Steps	1st trial	2nd trial	3rd trial
13. Insert any new forms into the medical record and place it with the charge slip.			
14. Ask the patient to have a seat and inform the patient approximately how long the wait will be.			
15. Place the chart and charge slip in the designated place to indicate to the doctor and or clinical assistant that the patient is in the waiting room ready to be seen.			
16. Complete the procedure within 10 minutes. ◆			

Evaluator Comments:

Score Calculation:

For each procedural step marked U (Unsatisfactory) deduct 6 points
For each procedural step (◆) marked U (Unsatisfactory) deduct 20 points

Score calculation 100 points

− points missed

Total score

1st	2nd	3rd

Satisfactory score: 85 or above

SELF-EVALUATION

UNIT 4

The Patient Visit

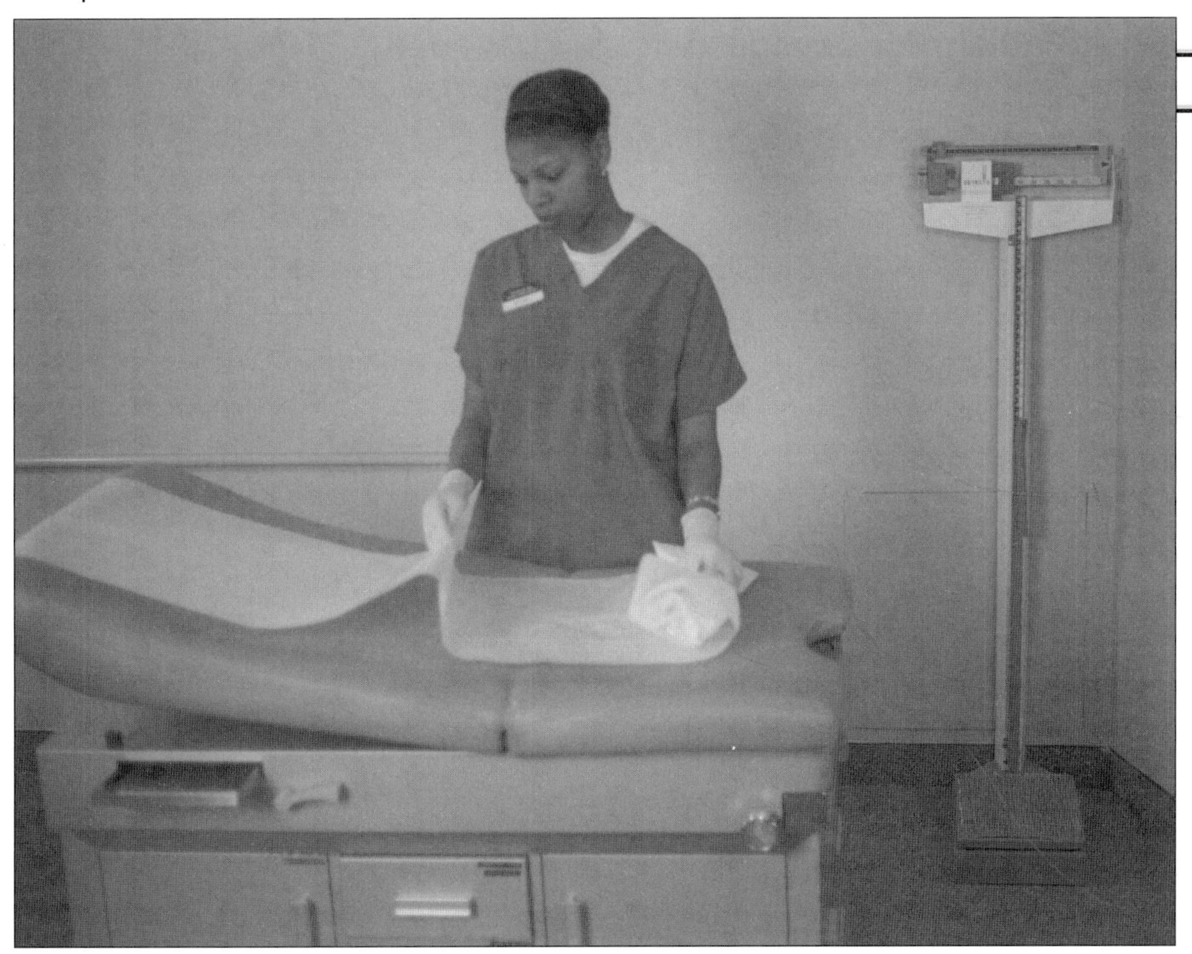

Chapter 13

Medical Asepsis and Infection Control

CHAPTER FOCUS

In this chapter you learned about microorganisms that cause disease, the infection cycle, how the body resists infection, and measures taken in the medical office to prevent the transmission of infectious disease. You learned when to use medical asepsis by sanitizing and/or disinfecting instruments, equipment, or surfaces, and when to use surgical asepsis including sterile technique and sterilization. Infection control measures are practiced by all health professionals in the medical office, including the medical assistant.

TERMINOLOGY REVIEW

Vocabulary Matching: Match each term with its definition.

___ 1. vector

___ 2. natural immunity

___ 3. medical asepsis

___ 4. resistance

___ 5. humoral immune response

___ 6. artificial immunity

___ 7. surgical asepsis

___ 8. virulent

A. A specific protein that attaches itself to an antigen

B. A protein recognized by the immune system cells as foreign

C. Temporary immunity acquired from antibodies of another person, such as the immunity of a nursing infant

D. Immunity that occurs when a person produces his or her own antibodies

E. A type of lymphocyte produced in bone marrow and found in the spleen and lymph nodes

F. A response to antigens that is effective against viruses, fungi, cancerous cells, and foreign tissue grafts

G. Cells that destroy foreign antigens, sometimes called "killer" cells

H. Treating with chemicals or heat to kill pathogens

___ 9. disinfection	I. An inanimate object that can transmit disease
___ 10. sanitizing	J. Measures taken to destroy all microorganisms, pathogenic or nonpathogenic, on an object in order to keep sterile objects from coming into contact with unsterile objects
___ 11. sterilization	K. Cleaning any body part or surface that has been exposed to pathogens and reducing transfer of microorganisms
___ 12. B cells	L. Immunity developed as a response to contracting a disease
___ 13. active immunity	M. Immunity that is achieved by immunization without the person having the disease
___ 14. antigen	N. The ability to defend against infection
___ 15. T cells	O. Washing with soap and water
___ 16. cytotoxic	P. Killing all microorganisms including bacteria, viruses, and spores
___ 17. fomite	Q. An immune response that produces antibodies specific to target antigens
___ 18. cell-mediated immune response	R. A type of lymphocyte produced in the thymus gland, or that has passed through the thymus gland in order to mature
___ 19. antibody	S. An insect or animal that transmits a disease
___ 20. passive immunity	T. Able to cause an infection

Definitions: Insert the correct word to complete the sentence.

1. A microorganism that needs oxygen to live is called an ______________________ organism.
2. ______________________ diseases are caused by pathogenic microorganisms such as bacteria, viruses, parasites, and fungi.
3. A ______________________ is the smallest infectious agent containing either DNA or RNA, but not both.
4. ______________________ are about ten times as large as bacteria, and can be single- or multi-celled. One common type is found in bread, but others can cause disease.
5. Cocci, bacilli, and spirochetes are three types of ______________________.
6. A microorganism that can cause disease is called a ______________________.
7. ________________ ______________________ are those microorganisms that normally live on the skin, in the gastrointestinal tract, and in the respiratory tract.
8. A microorganism that can live in the absence of oxygen is called an ______________________ organism.
9. Single-celled parasites such as *Trichomonas* are called ______________________.
10. A ______________________ is a dormant form of a bacteria that has formed a thick capsule around itself and is highly resistant to heat or chemicals.

CONTENT REVIEW QUESTIONS

1. List seven reasons why it is important to prevent the spread of infection, especially in outpatient settings.

   a. ______________________________

   b. ______________________________

   c. ______________________________

   d. ______________________________

   e. ______________________________

   f. ______________________________

   g. ______________________________

2. Arrange the following types of microorganisms in size from largest to smallest. Give a specific example of each and place a star beside all that can be grown in culture in the laboratory: bacteria, specialized bacteria, viruses, fungi.

Type of microorganism (largest to smallest)	Example
a. ______________	______________
b. ______________	______________
c. ______________	______________
d. ______________	______________

3. How do each of the following help the body fight off harmful microorganisms?

   a. normal flora ______________________________

   b. intact skin ______________________________

   c. mucous membranes ______________________________

   d. secretions ______________________________

4. List six physiologic responses that help prevent infection.

   a. ______________________________

   b. ______________________________

   c. ______________________________

   d. ______________________________

   e. ______________________________

   f. ______________________________

5. Identify the four classic symptoms of inflammation.

   a. ______________________________

   b. ______________________________

   c. ______________________________

   d. ______________________________

6. What four types of cells recognize pathogens in the cell-mediated immune response?

   a. ______________________________

   b. ______________________________

   c. ______________________________

   d. ______________________________

7. What is the role of antibodies in the immune response?

   ____

   ____

   ____

   ____

8. How does the immune system prevent people from getting certain diseases a second time?

   ____

   ____

   ____

   ____

9. Give an example of each of the following types of immunity.

   a. genetic immunity ______________________________

   b. natural active immunity ______________________________

   c. natural passive immunity ______________________________

   d. artificial passive immunity ______________________________

   e. artificial active immunity ______________________________

10. What part(s) of the infection cycle do each of the following items of personal protective equipment interrupt?

    a. mask ______________________________

    b. gloves ______________________________

    c. safety glasses or goggles ______________________________

    d. gown ______________________________

11. List five factors that can influence how susceptible a person is to infection.

    a. ______________________________

    b. ______________________________

c. ______________________________

d. ______________________________

e. ______________________________

12. What is the difference between medical asepsis and surgical asepsis?

____

____

____

____

13. What are the important elements of effective handwashing?

____

____

14. What are five other ways to maintain medical asepsis?

a. ______________________________

b. ______________________________

c. ______________________________

d. ______________________________

e. ______________________________

15. Why are instruments usually soaked in disinfectant solution until they can be cleaned?

____

____

16. Describe the standard used to categorize chemicals as

a. low-level disinfectants ______________________________

b. intermediate-level disinfectants ______________________________

c. high-level disinfectants ______________________________

17. Can instruments be sterilized by boiling? Why or why not?

____

____

18. What must happen in order for moist heat to provide effective sterilization?

____

____

19. Why are instruments usually wrapped in cloth, paper, or plastic before being sterilized?

____

____

20. List two methods that are used to indicate that effective sterilization has occurred.

   a. ______________________________

   b. ______________________________

21. After the autoclave reaches a temperature of 250°F at 15 pounds of pressure, how long should each of the following be sterilized?

   a. unwrapped items ______________________________

   b. wrapped instrument packages ______________________________

   c. large double-wrapped surgical packs ______________________________

22. Why should items be placed in the autoclave with space between items? Why should bowls or containers be placed on their side or upside down?

____

____

23. Can items be removed from the autoclave if the wrapping is wet? Why or why not?

____

____

CRITICAL THINKING QUESTIONS

1. Why is it important for medical assistants to understand different types of microorganisms that can cause disease? Give at least three examples.

____

____

____

____

____

____

2. When should medical instruments be cleaned (sanitized)? Is simple cleaning usually sufficient? Why or why not? Describe what measures should be taken for stethoscopes, glass thermometers, metal vaginal speculums, and instruments used for surgery.

____

____

____

____

____

____

3. Identify several reasons why doctors' offices and clinics tend to use disposable instruments and disposable surgical packs while hospitals still sterilize the instruments and packs used for surgery.

4. Develop a plan for a medical office with an autoclave to test routinely whether the autoclave is sterilizing effectively.

5. Research the cost of paper wrap for instruments, cloth wraps, and various type of plastic peel packs. What would you recommend for a medical office that plans to sterilize ten small packages (for single instruments) and two large packages (for bowls or packs) per day? Why?

6. Discuss the actual use of handwashing in the medical office. Do you believe that health personnel always follow the procedure you have been taught? Do you believe that they wash their hands as often as recommended? What areas do you think may be neglected? Give reasons to justify your answer.

PRACTICAL APPLICATIONS

1. Which items of personal protective equipment should the medical assistant use to do each of the following tasks:

   a. Sanitizing equipment used to remove sutures from a surgical incision.

   b. Using a 1 : 10 bleach solution to clean a counter where urine has been spilled.

   c. Loading wrapped packages into the autoclave.

   d. Placing a closed container of urine into a plastic biohazard lab bag.

   e. Measuring a patient's height.

   f. Removing wrapped packages from the autoclave and placing them in examination and treatment rooms.

2. Give the reason why it is important to carry out each of the following parts of the medical aseptic handwash.

   a. Remove jewelry, watch, etc.

   b. Use foot pedals or paper towel to turn faucets on and off.

   c. Use warm water rather than hot or cold water.

   d. Clean under fingernails and around cuticle area.

e. Rub hands briskly, interlacing fingers for 1 to 2 minutes.

____

____

f. Rinse hands thoroughly with fingers pointing down.

____

____

3. Describe how soiled gloves should be removed and discarded.

____

____

____

____

4. Place a C before each item in the following list for which it is enough to sanitize it. Place a D if the item should be disinfected. Place an S before each item that should be sterilized.

_____ a. Surgical scissors

_____ b. Vaginal speculum

_____ c. Coffeepot in the break room

_____ d. Counter that has had blood spilled on it

_____ e. Glass thermometer

_____ f. Bowl to hold solution during surgery

_____ g. Plastic toy in waiting room

_____ h. Lab coat that has not come in contact with body fluids

Procedure 13-1: Medical Aseptic Handwashing

Performance Objective

Task: Perform a medical aseptic handwash

Conditions: Sink, liquid soap, paper towels, nail stick or brush, and wastebasket

Standards: Complete the procedure in 5 minutes, and achieve a satisfactory score on the procedure performance checklist

Scoring Key: **(S)***atisfactory,* **(U)***nsatisfactory,* **(NA)** *Not Applicable*
◆ *Denotes a critical element for a satisfactory score on the procedure*

Procedure Steps	1st trial	2nd trial	3rd trial
1. Remove rings, watch, bracelets.			
2. Stand near sink but do not touch.			
3. Turn on water to a comfortable temperature.			
4. If hand-controlled, use paper towel.			
5. Wet hands.			
6. Pump 1 tablespoon liquid soap.			
7. Work soap to lather.			
8. Rub hands and wrists briskly.			
9. Clean hands, fingers, and wrists.			
10. Use a circular motion.			
11. Interlace fingers at least ten times.			
12. Use a clean orangewood stick or stiff brush to clean under nails.			
13. Rinse hands, wrists, and fingers thoroughly, keeping fingers below wrists.			
14. Repeat soaping and scrubbing if first wash of the day.			
15. Dry hands with paper towels, keeping fingers below wrists.			
16. Turn off faucets. If hand-controlled, use paper towel.			
17. Apply mild hand lotion as needed.			
18. Complete the procedure within 5 minutes. ◆			

Evaluator Comments:

Score Calculation:

For each procedural step marked U (Unsatisfactory) deduct 6 points
For each procedural step (◆) marked U (Unsatisfactory) deduct 20 points

Score calculation	100 points			
	– ___ points missed	1st	2nd	3rd
	Total score			

Satisfactory score: 85 or above

Procedure 13-2: Removing Soiled Gloves

Performance Objective

Task: Remove and dispose of soiled gloves

Conditions: Gloves, hazardous waste container

Standards: Complete the procedure within 2 minutes, and achieve a satisfactory score on the procedure performance checklist

*Scoring Key: (**S**)atisfactory, (**U**)nsatisfactory, (**NA**) Not Applicable*
◆ *Denotes a critical element for a satisfactory score on the procedure*

Procedure Steps	1st trial	2nd trial	3rd trial
1. Grasp outside of one soiled glove near the cuff with the other gloved hand. Do not touch skin above glove.			
2. Pull the soiled glove inside out as it is removed.			
3. Grasp removed glove in gloved hand.			
4. Contain removed glove inside fingers of other glove.			
5. Remove second glove, inside out over the other glove.			
6. Dispose of soiled gloves in biohazard waste container.			
7. Wash hands.			
8. Complete procedure within 2 minutes. ◆			

Evaluator Comments:

Score Calculation:

For each procedural step marked U (Unsatisfactory) deduct 6 points
For each procedural step (◆) marked U (Unsatisfactory) deduct 20 points

Score calculation 100 points
− points missed

	1st	2nd	3rd
Total score			

Satisfactory score: 85 or above

Notes

Procedure 13-3: Sanitizing Soiled Instruments

Performance Objective

Task: Wearing appropriate PPE, sanitize one or more soiled instruments before disinfection or sterilization

Conditions: Basin, gloves, PPE, detergent, scrub brush, paper towels

Standards: Complete the procedure within 10 minutes, and achieve a satisfactory score on the procedure performance checklist

*Scoring Key: (**S**)atisfactory, (**U**)nsatisfactory, (**NA**) Not Applicable*
◆ *Denotes a critical element for a satisfactory score on the procedure*

Procedure Steps	1st trial	2nd trial	3rd trial
1. Put on lab coat or apron.			
2. Put on eye and face protection.			
3. Put on heavy duty cleaning gloves (use disposable gloves if no cleaning gloves).			
4. Collect soiled instruments and rinse under cold water.			
5. Add detergent to basin.			
6. Fill with warm water.			
7. Scrub all instrument surfaces with scrub brush until visibly clean.			
8. Rinse each under running warm to hot water.			
9. Place each instrument on paper towels.			
10. Dry each instrument using paper towels.			
11. Check each instrument for proper working order.			
12. If using heavy duty cleaning gloves, wash outsides, rinse, remove, and store. **or**			
12. If using disposable gloves, follow procedure 13-2 for removing soiled gloves.			
13. Wash hands.			
14. Complete the procedure within 10 minutes. ◆			

Evaluator Comments:

Score Calculation:

For each procedural step marked U (Unsatisfactory) deduct 6 points
For each procedural step (◆) marked U (Unsatisfactory) deduct 20 points

Score calculation 100 points

− ____ points missed

Total score

1st	2nd	3rd

Satisfactory score: 85 or above

Procedure 13-4: Wrapping an Instrument for Sterilization

Performance Objective

Task: Using paper or cloth wrap and autoclave tape, wrap a previously sanitized instrument for autoclaving, and label

Conditions: Paper or cloth wrap, autoclave tape, instrument to wrap, pen with waterproof ink, sterilization indicator

Standards: Complete the procedure within 5 minutes, and achieve a satisfactory score on the procedure performance checklist

Scoring Key: (S)*atisfactory,* (U)*nsatisfactory,* (NA) Not Applicable
◆ Denotes a critical element for a satisfactory score on the procedure

Procedure Steps	1st trial	2nd trial	3rd trial
1. Wash hands.			
2. Select a piece of wrap of the appropriate size (cut paper wrap if necessary).			
3. Place wrap on a flat, dry surface with a corner facing you.			
4. Lay the object(s) about 1/3 of the way up the wrap, long ends toward corners.			
5. Keep instruments in open position when wrapping.			
6. If using paper wrap, protect instrument tips with gauze squares.			
7. Fold corner facing you toward the instrument(s).			
8. Fold the corner back toward yourself.			
9. Fold each side toward the center at the ends of the object(s) being wrapped.			
10. Fold 1 to 2 inches back toward the side to make small flaps on each side.			
11. Wrap the instrument(s) toward the final corner.			
12. If preparing a surgical pack, repeat to create a second layer of wrap the can be opened to provide a sterile inner pack.			
13. Secure final corner with autoclave tape.			
14. Extend tape at least 1 inch beyond each corner.			
15. Write contents of pack, data, and your initials on the tape.			
16. Complete the procedure within 5 minutes. ◆			

Evaluator Comments:

Score Calculation:

For each procedural step marked U (Unsatisfactory) deduct 6 points
For each procedural step (◆) marked U (Unsatisfactory) deduct 20 points

Score calculation 100 points

− ___ points missed

	1st	2nd	3rd
Total score			

Satisfactory score: 85 or above

Procedure 13-5: Operating the Autoclave

Performance Objective

Task: Load and operate autoclave

Conditions: Autoclave, distilled water, items to sterilize (manufacturer's manual for reference), tape containing sterilization indicator

Standards: Complete the procedure within 60 minutes, and achieve a satisfactory score on the procedure performance checklist

Scoring Key: (**S**)*atisfactory,* (**U**)*nsatisfactory,* (**NA**) Not Applicable
◆ Denotes a critical element for a satisfactory score on the procedure

Procedure Steps	1st trial	2nd trial	3rd trial
1. Fill reservoir to correct level with distilled water.			
2. Load autoclave so there is room for steam to circulate.			
3. Do not let packages or items touch each other.			
4. Containers should be placed on side or upside down.			
5. Using valve, allow water to flow into chamber to the level recommended by manufacturer.			
6. Close and tighten or lock the door.			
7. Turn on autoclave.			
8. Allow heat and pressure to rise to the level recommended by the manufacturer.			
9. Set timer for the approximate time to reach this level.			
10. When correct temperature and pressure are reached, adjust controls if necessary to maintain proper level.			
11. Set timer for correct sterilization time as recommended by the manufacturer. Use 30 minutes unless directed otherwise.			
12. When timer signals that sterilization is complete, vent autoclave.			
13. Allow pressure to drop completely.			
14. Open door carefully so steam can escape.			
15. Allow items to remain until fully dry. If autoclave has a drying cycle, set timer to turn off when cycle is complete.			
16. Remove items when all packages are completely dry.			

Procedure Steps	1st trial	2nd trial	3rd trial
17. Check each item's sterilization indicator to make sure sterilization is complete.			
18. Complete the procedure within 60 minutes. ◆			

Evaluator Comments:

Score Calculation:

For each procedural step marked U (Unsatisfactory) deduct 6 points
For each procedural step (◆) marked U (Unsatisfactory) deduct 20 points

Score calculation 100 points
− ____ points missed
Total score

1st	2nd	3rd

Satisfactory score: 85 or above

SELF-EVALUATION

3. Why is it important to try to obtain a complete list of the medications the patient is taking at every visit? Doesn't the physician know this already?

____

____

____

____

____

____

4. Discuss how factors that the medical assistant controls can influence how effectively he or she obtains the medical history and/or chief complaint. Identify as many factors as possible.

____

____

____

____

____

____

PRACTICAL APPLICATIONS

1. The following information has been obtained from the physician's notes. For each statement, indicate where on the patient's record you think this information is recorded. Choose your answers from the following headings:

CC - chief complaint
HPI - history of the present illness
PH - past history
FH - family history
SH - social or occupation history
ROS - review of systems

_____ a. The patient is a 24-year-old white male with left knee pain following a fall.

_____ b. The patient had her appendix removed in 1979.

_____ c. The patient's pain is midline, sharp, and improves temporarily after she eats. She has taken antacids without significant relief. She had an ulcer 3 years ago.

_____ d. "I have had severe headaches for the past 3 days."

_____ e. Related to the head and eyes, the patient says she does not have headaches or sinus pain and does not see flashes of light. She denies tearing or visual problems.

_____ f. Patient's parents are alive and well.

_____ g. Denies use of alcohol, tobacco, and drugs.

2. Label each of the following statements of a progress note as most likely *subjective, objective, assessment,* or *plan.*

   a. Return to office in 1 week for blood pressure check. ______________________

   b. Patient states "My headaches have stopped, but I still feel tired." ______________________

   c. BP 160/98, lungs clear, heart has regular rate and rhythm. ______________________

   d. Upper respiratory infection with pharyngitis, rule out strep throat. ______________________

   e. There is a 3-inch laceration on the lateral aspect of the right forearm. ______________________

   f. Will instruct patient to continue 1200-calorie diet until she has lost 10 more pounds.

   ____

   g. Patient states that she is now adjusting to the diet much better. ______________________

3. A patient tells you that her 3-year-old child has had an earache and fever for the past 2 days. List six questions you should ask the mother to learn more about this problem.

   a. ______________________

   b. ______________________

   c. ______________________

   d. ______________________

   e. ______________________

   f. ______________________

4. Jennifer Sortan says, "I have had pain in my arm (pointing to the left elbow) for about 3 weeks. It started when I hit my arm hard after I fell over on my bicycle when I was riding in the park. I had a few scrapes on my leg too, but those have healed. Anyway, my arm doesn't seem to be getting better at all, and I have trouble using it, especially if I have to lift it up above my head like to brush my hair. It really aches at night, and I take Extra-Strength Tylenol to sleep, but it doesn't really help that much. It hurts more if I have been trying to use it." When you look at the elbow, there are no marks or bruises, but it appears to be swollen and is bigger than the other elbow. Chart your observations concisely using medical terminology on the first sample progress note at the end of the chapter.

5. Julia Myers, an 82-year-old patient says, "My left foot is so swollen that I have trouble getting my shoe on." You observe that her foot is swollen and the ankle is about 2 inches bigger than the other ankle. She denies any trauma to the foot and says it does not hurt. She first noticed the problem about 3 days ago but thinks it may have started last week. You are able to feel a pulse in the dorsalis pedis artery, but it seems weaker than in the other foot. Chart your observations concisely using medical terminology on the second sample progress note at the end of the chapter.

6. Work with a classmate to obtain a patient history using the form at the end of the chapter. Remember that for the purposes of practice it is not necessary to disclose any personal medical information that you do not want to reveal. You may ask your classmate to fill out part of the form and ask questions while you fill in part of the form. Be sure to review any information filled out by a simulated patient.

PROCEDURE PERFORMANCE CHECKLISTS

Procedure 14-1: Assisting a Patient to Transfer to or From a Wheelchair

Performance Objective

Task: Assist a patient to transfer from a wheelchair to the examination table

Conditions: Wheelchair, patient, examination table

Standards: Complete the procedure in 5 minutes, and achieve a satisfactory score on the procedure performance checklist

Scoring Key: (**S**)*atisfactory,* (**U**)*nsatisfactory,* (**NA**) *Not Applicable*
◆ *Denotes a critical element for a satisfactory score on the procedure*

Procedure Steps	1st trial	2nd trial	3rd trial
1. Wash hands.			
2. Explain procedure to patient.			
3. Pull out exam table step. (If no step, place stool next to table.)			
4. Place wheelchair next to exam table with the patient's strong side positioned next to the table and step.			
5. Move both footrests out of way, or move footplate up.			
6. Lock wheelchair wheels. ◆			
7. Ask patient to place feet on floor.			
8. Ask patient to move forward in wheelchair.			
9. Hold patient while s/he is moving.			
10. Instruct patient to push up with arms.			
11. Assist patient to stand while holding patient securely. (Use gait belt if necessary.)			
12. Assist patient to place foot on exam table step or stool.			
13. Instruct patient to use his/her strong leg and push up on table with arm.			
14. While continuing support, assist patient to shift entire body weight up to the step.			
15. Continuing support, have patient pivot until back is to the table.			
16. Assist patient to sit on the table.			
17. Move wheelchair out of the way.			
18. Complete the procedure within 5 minutes. ◆			

Note: To move patient from table to chair, basically perform steps in reverse.

Evaluator Comments:

Score Calculation:

For each procedural step marked U (Unsatisfactory) deduct 6 points
For each procedural step (◆) marked U (Unsatisfactory) deduct 20 points

Score calculation 100 points

− points missed

Total score

1st	2nd	3rd

Satisfactory score: 85 or above

Procedure 14-2: Obtaining and Recording a Patient History

Performance Objective

Task: Obtain a complete and accurate medical history and/or information about current medical problem

Conditions: Health history questionnaire, pen, medical record or progress note sheet

Standards: Complete the procedure in 15 minutes, and achieve a satisfactory score on the procedure performance checklist

Scoring Key: (**S**)*atisfactory,* (**U**)*nsatisfactory,* (**NA**) Not Applicable
◆ Denotes a critical element for a satisfactory score on the procedure

Procedure Steps	1st trial	2nd trial	3rd trial
1. Ask the patient to accompany you to a private area.			
2. Seat patient and yourself comfortably.			
3. Explain the procedure and importance to the physician of having complete and accurate information.			
4. For new patient, go through medical history, either asking questions and filling in each answer or reviewing a questionnaire that the patient has filled out.			
5. Ask about the reason for the current visit and about current medications.			
6. Use open-ended questions if you want patient to talk freely.			
7. Use specific questions when you want "Yes" or "No" answers.			
8. Pronounce all terms on the questionnaire correctly, and give simple explanations if the patient has questions.			
9. Maintain eye contact, and show caring through active listening techniques.			
10. Document all answers or corrections in ink.			
11. When interview is complete, instruct patient about what to do next and give a realistic expectation of how long the patient must wait.			
12. Complete the procedure within 15 minutes. ◆			

Evaluator Comments:

Score Calculation:

For each procedural step marked U (Unsatisfactory) deduct 6 points
For each procedural step (◆) marked U (Unsatisfactory) deduct 20 points

Score calculation	100 points			
	− ____ points missed	1st	2nd	3rd
	Total score			

Satisfactory score: 85 or above

PROGRESS NOTES

Patient Name ______________________________

DATE	

PROGRESS NOTES

Patient Name ______________________________

DATE	

Identification Information

Today's Date ______________

Name______________________________ Date of Birth______________________________

Occupation ______________________________ Marital Status ______________________________

PART A – PRESENT HEALTH HISTORY

I. CURRENT MEDICAL PROBLEMS

Please list the medical problems for which you came to see the doctor. About when did they begin?

Problems	Date Began
______________________________	__________
______________________________	__________
______________________________	__________

What concerns you most about these problems?

____

____

If you are being treated for any other illness or medical problems by another physician, please describe the problems and write the name of the physician or medical facility treating you.

Illness or Medical Problem	Physician or Medical Facility	City
______________	______________	__________
______________	______________	__________

II. MEDICATIONS

Please list all medications you are now taking, including those you buy without a doctor's prescription (such as aspirin, cold tablets or vitamin supplements).

______________ ______________ ______________

______________ ______________ ______________

III. ALLERGIES AND SENSITIVITIES

List anything that you are allergic to such as certain foods, medications, dust, chemicals or soaps, household items, pollens, bee stings, etc., and indicate how each affects you.

Allergic To:	Effect	Allergic To:	Effect
__________	__________	__________	__________
__________	__________	__________	__________

IV. GENERAL HEALTH, ATTITUDE AND HABITS

How is your overall health now?	Health now:	Poor _____ Fair _____ Good _____ Excellent _____
How has it been most of your life?	Health has been:	Poor _____ Fair _____ Good _____ Excellent _____
In the past year:		
Has your appetite changed?	Appetite:	Decreased _____ Increased _____ Stayed same _____
Has your weight changed?	Weight:	Lost _____lbs. Gained _____lbs. No change _____
Are you thirsty much of the time?	Thirsty:	No _____ Yes _____
Has your overall 'pep' changed?	Pep:	Decreased _____ Increased _____ Stayed same _____
Do you usually have trouble sleeping?	Trouble sleeping:	No _____ Yes _____
How much do you exercise?	Exercise:	Little or none _____ Less than I need _____ All I need _____
Do you smoke?	Smokes:	No _____ Yes _____ If yes, how many years? _____
How many each day?		_____ Cigarettes _____ Cigars _____ Pipesfull
Have you ever smoked?	Smoked:	No _____ Yes _____ If yes, how many years? _____
How many each day?		_____ Cigarettes _____ Cigars _____ Pipesfull
Do you drink alcoholic beverages?	Alcohol:	No ____ Yes ____ I drink ____ Beers ____ Glasses of wine _____ Drinks of hard liquor - per day
Have you ever had a problem with alcohol?	Prior problem:	No _____ Yes _____
How much coffee or tea do you usually drink?	Coffee/Tea:	_____ cups of coffee or tea a day
Do you regularly wear seatbelts?	Seatbelts:	No _____ Yes _____

DO YOU:	Rarely/ Never	Occasionally	Frequently
Feel nervous?	_____	_____	_____
Feel depressed?	_____	_____	_____
Find it hard to make decisions?	_____	_____	_____
Lose your temper?	_____	_____	_____
Worry a lot?	_____	_____	_____
Tire easily?	_____	_____	_____
Have trouble relaxing?	_____	_____	_____
Have any sexual problems?	_____	_____	_____

DO YOU:	Rarely/ Never	Occasionally	Frequently
Ever feel like committing suicide?	_____	_____	_____
Feel bored with your life?	_____	_____	_____
Use marijuana?	_____	_____	_____
Use "hard drugs"?	_____	_____	_____

Do you want to talk to the doctor about a personal matter? No _____ Yes _____

STOCK NO. 19-742-4 8/95 Page 1

PART A – PRESENT HEALTH HISTORY (continued)

C O N F I D E N T I A L

IV. GENERAL HEALTH, ATTITUDE AND HABITS (continued)

Have you recently had any changes in your: If yes, please explain:

Marital status?	No______	Yes______	______
Job or work?	No______	Yes______	______
Residence?	No______	Yes______	______
Financial status?	No______	Yes______	______
Are you having any legal problems or trouble with the law?	No______	Yes______	______

PART B – PAST HISTORY

I. FAMILY HEALTH

Please give the following information about your immediate family:

Relationship	Age, if Living	Age At Death	State of Health Or Cause of Death
Father	______	______	______
Mother	______	______	______
Brothers and Sisters	______	______	______
	______	______	______
	______	______	______
Spouse	______	______	______
Children	______	______	______
	______	______	______
	______	______	______
	______	______	______

Have any **blood relatives** had any of the following illnesses? If so, indicate relationship (mother, brother, etc.)

Illness	Family Members
Asthma	______
Diabetes	______
Cancer	______
Blood Disease	______
Glaucoma	______
Epilepsy	______
Rheumatoid Arthritis	______
Tuberculosis	______
Gout	______
High Blood Pressure	______
Heart Disease	______
Mental Problems	______
Suicide	______
Stroke	______
Alcoholism	______
Rheumatic Fever	______

II. HOSPITALIZATIONS, SURGERIES, INJURIES

Please list all times you have been hospitalized, operated on, or seriously injured.

Year	Operation, Illness, Injury	Hospital and City
______	______	______
______	______	______
______	______	______

III. ILLNESS AND MEDICAL PROBLEMS

Please mark with an (X) any of the following illnesses and medical problems you have or have had and indicate the year when each started. If you are not certain when an illness started, write down an approximate year.

Illness	(x)	(Year)
Eye or eye lid infection	___	______
Glaucoma	___	______
Other eye problems	___	______
Ear trouble	___	______
Deafness or decreased hearing	___	______
Thyroid trouble	___	______
Strep throat	___	______
Bronchitis	___	______
Emphysema	___	______
Pneumonia	___	______
Allergies, asthma or hay fever	___	______
Tuberculosis	___	______
Other lung problems	___	______
High blood pressure	___	______
Heart attack	___	______
High cholesterol	___	______
Arteriosclerosis (Hardening of arteries)	___	______
Heart murmur	___	______
Other heart condition	___	______
Stomach/duodenal ulcer	___	______
Diverticulosis	___	______
Colitis	___	______
Other bowel problems	___	______
Hepatitis	___	______
Liver trouble	___	______
Gallbladder trouble	___	______

Illness	(x)	(Year)
Hernia	___	______
Hemorrhoids	___	______
Kidney or bladder disease	___	______
Prostate problem (male only)	___	______
Mental problems	___	______
Headaches	___	______
Head injury	___	______
Stroke	___	______
Convulsions, seizures	___	______
Arthritis	___	______
Gout	___	______
Cancer or tumor	___	______
Bleeding tendency	___	______
Diabetes	___	______
Measles/Rubeola	___	______
German measles/Rubella	___	______
Polio	___	______
Mumps	___	______
Scarlet fever	___	______
Chicken pox	___	______
Mononucleosis	___	______
Eczema	___	______
Psoriasis	___	______
Venereal disease	___	______
Genital herpes	___	______
HIV test	___	______
AIDS	___	______

STOCK NO. 19-742-4 8/95

PART C – BODY SYSTEMS REVIEW

MEN: Please answer questions 1 through 12, then skip to question 18.
WOMEN: Please start on question 6.

MEN ONLY

1. Have you had or do you have prostate trouble? . . . . No _____ . Yes _____
2. Do you have any sexual problems or a problem with impotency? . . . . No _____ . Yes _____
3. Have you ever had sores or lesions on your penis? . . . . No _____ . Yes _____
4. Have you ever had any discharge from your penis? . . . . No _____ . Yes _____
5. Do you ever have pain, lumps or swelling in your testicles? . . . . No _____ . Yes _____

Check here if you wish to discuss any special problems with the doctor . . . . ☐

MEN & WOMEN	Rarely/ Never	Occasionally	Frequently
6. Is it sometimes hard to start your urine flow?	_____	_____	_____
7. Is urination ever painful?	_____	_____	_____
8. Do you have to urinate more than 5 times a day?	_____	_____	_____
9. Do you get up at night to urinate?	_____	_____	_____
10. Has your urine ever been bloody or dark colored?	_____	_____	_____
11. Do you ever lose urine when you strain, laugh, cough or sneeze?	_____	_____	_____
12. Do you ever lose urine during sleep?	_____	_____	_____

WOMEN ONLY Do you:	Rarely/ Never	Occasionally	Frequently
13. a. Have any menstrual problems?	_____	_____	_____
b. Feel rather tense just before your period?	_____	_____	_____
c. Have heavy menstrual bleeding?	_____	_____	_____
d. Have painful menstrual periods?	_____	_____	_____
e. Have any bleeding between periods?	_____	_____	_____
f. Have any unusual vaginal discharge or itching?	_____	_____	_____
g. Ever have tender breasts?	_____	_____	_____
h. Have any discharge from your nipples?	_____	_____	_____
i. Have any hot flashes?	_____	_____	

14. How many times, if any, have you been pregnant? . . . . _____
15. How many children born alive? . . . . _____
16. Are you taking birth control pills? . . . . No_____ Yes _____
17. Do you examine your breasts monthly for lumps? . . . . No_____ Yes _____
17a. What was the date of your last menstrual period? . . . . Date _____

Check here if you wish to discuss any special problem with the doctor . . . . ☐

MEN & WOMEN 18. In the past year have you had any:	Rarely/ Never	Occasionally	Frequently
a. Severe shoulder pain?	_____	_____	_____
b. Severe back pain?	_____	_____	_____
c. Muscle or joint stiffness or pain due to sports, exercise or injury?	_____	_____	_____
d. Pain or swelling in any joints not due to sports, exercise or injury?	_____	_____	_____

19. Do you have dry skin or brittle fingernails? . . . . No_____ Yes _____
20. Do you bruise easily? . . . . No_____ Yes _____
21. Do you have any moles that have changed in color or in size? . . . . No_____ Yes _____
22. Do you have any other skin problems? . . . . No_____ Yes _____

23. In the last 3 months have you had:
    a. A fever that lasted more than one day? . . . . No_____ Yes _____
    b. Sores or cuts that were hard to heal? . . . . No_____ Yes _____
    c. Any cold sores (fever blisters)? . . . . No_____ Yes _____
    d. Any lumps in your neck, ampits or groin? . . . . No_____ Yes _____
    e. Do you ever have chills or sweat at night? . . . . No_____ Yes _____
24. Have you traveled out of the country in the last 2 years? . . . . No_____ Yes, Traveled in: _____
25. Write in the dates for the shots you have had: . . . . Measles _____ Smallpox _____ Mumps _____ Tetanus _____ Polio _____ Typhoid _____
26. Have you had a tuberculin (TB) skin test? . . . . No_____ Yes _____ Date _____
    If so, was it negative or positive? . . . . Neg ____ Pos _____
27. Have you had an HIV test for AIDS? . . . . No ____ Yes _____ Date _____
    If so, was it negative or positive? . . . . Neg ____ Pos _____

CONFIDENTIAL

29.	Do you wear contact lenses?	No_____	Yes_____	
30.	Has your vision changed in the last year?	No_____	Yes_____	
		Rarely/ Never	Occasionally	Frequently
31.	How often do you have:			
	a. Double vision?	_____	_____	_____
	b. Blurry vision?	_____	_____	_____
	c. Watery or itchy eyes?	_____	_____	_____
32.	Do you ever see colored rings around lights?	_____	_____	_____
33.	Do others tell you you have a hearing problem?	_____	_____	_____
34.	Do you have trouble keeping your balance?	_____	_____	_____
35.	Do you have any discharge from your ears?	_____	_____	_____
36.	Do you ever feel dizzy or have motion sickness?	_____	_____	_____
37.	Do you have any problems with your hearing?	No_____	Yes_____	Hearing Problems
38.	Do you ever have ringing in your ears?	No_____	Yes_____	Ringing in ears
		Rarely/ Never	Occasionally	Frequently
39.	How often do you have:			
	a. Head colds?	_____	_____	_____
	b. Chest colds?	_____	_____	_____
	c. Runny nose?	_____	_____	_____
	d. Stuffed up nose?	_____	_____	_____
	e. Sore/hoarse throat?	_____	_____	_____
	f. Bad coughing spells?	_____	_____	_____
	g. Sneezing spells?	_____	_____	_____
	h. Trouble breathing?	_____	_____	_____
	i. Nose bleeds?	_____	_____	_____
	j. Cough blood?	_____	_____	_____
40.	Have you ever worked or spent time:			
	a. On a farm?	No_____	Yes_____	
	b. In a mine?	No_____	Yes_____	
	c. In a laundry or mill?	No_____	Yes_____	
	d. In very dusty places?	No_____	Yes_____	
	e. With or near toxic chemicals?	No_____	Yes_____	
	f. With or near radioactive materials?	No_____	Yes_____	
	g. With or near asbestos?	No_____	Yes_____	
		Rarely/ Never	Occasionally	Frequently
41.	Do you get out of breath easily when you are active (like climbing stairs)?	_____	_____	_____
42.	Do you ever feel light-headed or dizzy?	_____	_____	_____
43.	Have you ever fainted or passed out?	_____	_____	_____
44.	Do you sometimes feel your heart is racing or beating too fast?	_____	_____	_____
45.	When you exercise do you ever get pains in your chest or shoulders?	_____	_____	_____
46.	Do you have any leg cramps or pain in your thighs or legs when walking?	_____	_____	_____
47.	Do you ever have to sit up at night to breathe easier?	_____	_____	_____
48.	Do you use two pillows at night to help you breathe easier?	_____	_____	_____
49.	Would you say you are a restless sleeper?	_____	_____	_____
50.	Are you bothered by leg cramps at night?	_____	_____	_____
51.	Do you sometimes have swollen ankles or feet?	_____	_____	_____
		Rarely/ Never	Occasionally	Frequently
52.	How often, if ever:			
	a. Are you nauseated (sick to your stomach)?	_____	_____	_____
	b. Do you have stomach pains?	_____	_____	_____
	c. Do you burp a lot after eating?	_____	_____	_____
	d. Do you have heartburn?	_____	_____	_____
	e. Do you have trouble swallowing your food?	_____	_____	_____
	f. Have you vomited blood?	_____	_____	_____
	g. Are you constipated?	_____	_____	_____
	h. Do you have diarrhea (watery stools)?	_____	_____	_____
	i. Are your bowel movements painful?	_____	_____	_____
	j. Are your bowel movements bloody?	_____	_____	_____
	k. Are your bowel movements dark or black?	_____	_____	_____
53.	Have you ever had a sigmoidoscopy?	No_____	Yes_____ Date_____	

Courtesy of Bibbero Systems.

SELF-EVALUATION

3. Are electronic sphygmomanometers widely used in the doctor's offices and/or hospitals in your area? Discuss the advantages and disadvantages of their use. Compare their cost to that of mercury or aneroid sphygmomanometers. If you were an office manager, would you encourage the practice to adopt them?

____

____

____

____

____

____

4. What are the long-term implications for a patient of treating high blood pressure aggressively versus an attitude that "As people get older, their blood pressure just gets higher"? Consider both positive and negative factors.

____

____

____

____

____

____

PRACTICAL APPLICATIONS

1. List four situations when you would not take a blood pressure on one of a patient's arms.

   a. ____

   b. ____

   c. ____

   d. ____

2. If you work in an office that does not take temperatures as a routine measurement on all patients, identify situations where you should take a temperature.

____

____

____

3. Fill in the correct temperatures in the thermometers below:
   a. 95.2°F

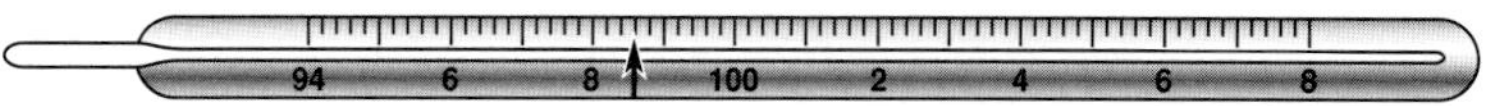

   b. 97.8°F

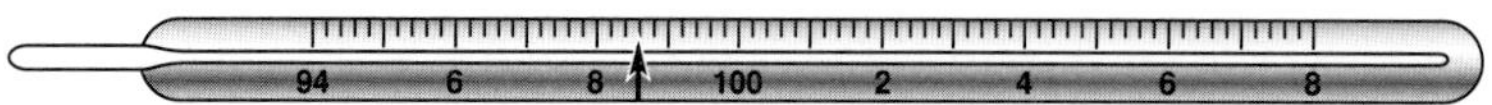

   c. 100.2°F

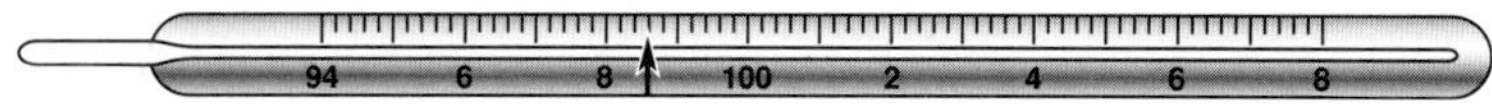

   d. 103.4°F

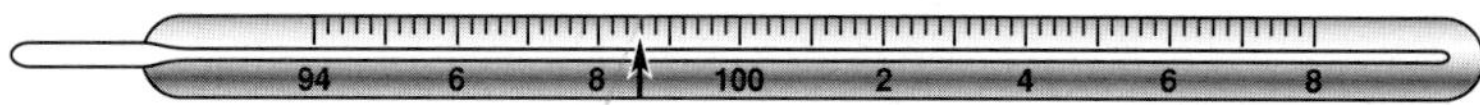

   f. 99.0°F

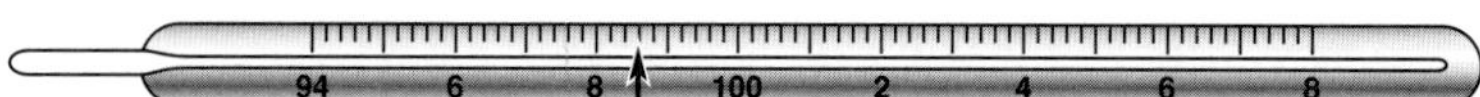

   g. 99.6°F

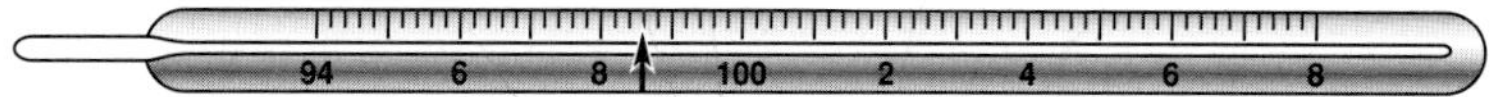

4. Mark the following blood pressures by drawing a vertical line at the mark corresponding to the blood pressure reading on the mercury sphygmomanometer below. Label each line with the blood pressure reading.
   a. 66
   b. 144
   c. 178
   d. 84
   e. 92
   f. 114

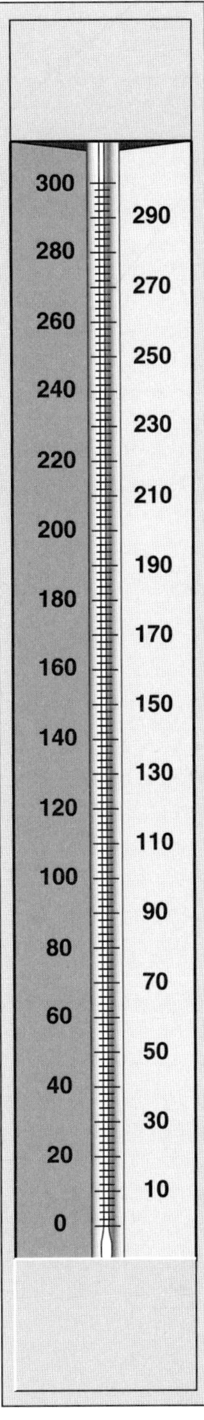

5. Mark the following blood pressures by drawing a slanted line through the mark corresponding to the blood pressure reading on the aneroid sphygmomanometer dial below. Label each line with the blood pressure reading.
   a. 58
   b. 94
   c. 116
   d. 122
   e. 168
   f. 192
   g. 230

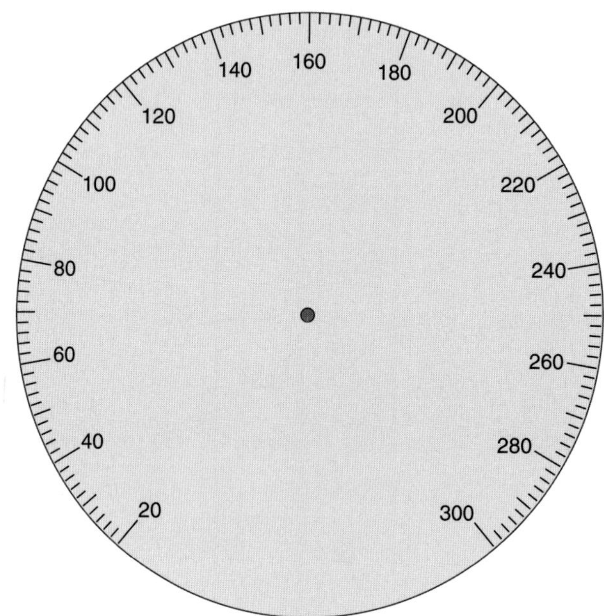

6. Read the height measured in the figure below. The height expressed in inches is ____________, or it can be expressed as ____________ feet, ____________ inches.

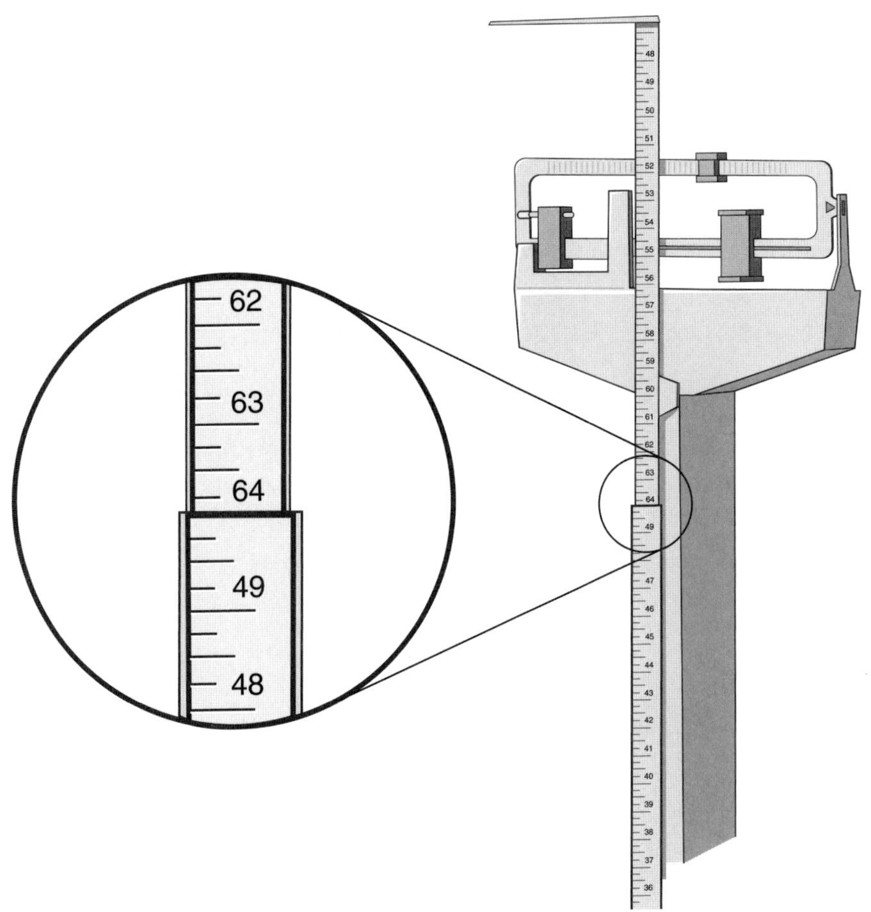

7. How high would you pump the blood pressure cuff for each of the following patients to measure blood pressure or how would you decide?

   a. Male patient whose former reading was 120/82. ____________________

   b. Female patient who has never been seen in your office. ____________________

   c. Child who is 10 years old. ____________________

   d. Elderly man whose former blood pressure was 150/94. ____________________

   e. Woman whose previous blood pressure was 230/114 but who has been placed on antihypertensive medication since her last visit. ____________________

8. Use CD-ROM to practice temperature, pulse, respirations, and blood pressure in the Clinical Skills section. Practice taking vital signs for Cases 1-4.

PROCEDURE PERFORMANCE CHECKLISTS

Procedure 15-1: Measuring Height

Performance Objective

Task: Measure height of an adult using measuring bar on a scale

Conditions: Balance scale with height bar, paper towel

Standards: Complete the procedure in 3 minutes, and achieve a satisfactory score on the procedure performance checklist

Scoring Key: (**S**)*atisfactory,* (**U**)*nsatisfactory,* (**NA**) *Not Applicable*
◆ *Denotes a critical element for a satisfactory score on the procedure*

Procedure Steps	1st trial	2nd trial	3rd trial
1. Wash hands.			
2. Identify patient.			
3. Explain procedure.			
4. Ask patient to remove shoes.			
5. Place a paper towel on the scale for the patient to step on.			
6. Raise height bar to a level well above patient's anticipated height.			
7. Ask patient to step on scale with back to measuring bar.			
8. Lower measuring bar to top of patient's head.			
9. Leaving measuring bar in place, ask patient to step down.			
10. Read height to the nearest 1/2 inch where top part of bar rises away from lower part.			
11. Lower measuring bar to closed position.			
12. Discard paper towel.			
13. Wash hands.			
14. Convert measurement to feet and inches, to nearest 1/2 inch.			
15. Record measurement in patient's medical record.			
16. The measurement recorded is identical to that obtained by the evaluator. ◆			
17. Complete the procedure within 3 minutes. ◆			

Charting

DATE	

Evaluator Comments:

Score Calculation:

For each procedural step marked U (Unsatisfactory) deduct 6 points
For each procedural step (◆) marked U (Unsatisfactory) deduct 20 points

Score calculation 100 points

− ____ points missed

Total score

1st	2nd	3rd

Satisfactory score: 85 or above

Procedure 15-2: Measuring Weight Using a Balance-Beam Scale

Performance Objective

Task: Measure adult weight using a balance scale, and record measurement in pounds

Conditions: Balance scale, paper towel

Standards: Complete the procedure in 3 minutes, and achieve a satisfactory score on the procedure performance checklist

Scoring Key: (**S**)*atisfactory,* (**U**)*nsatisfactory,* (**NA**) *Not Applicable*
◆ *Denotes a critical element for a satisfactory score on the procedure*

Procedure Steps	1st trial	2nd trial	3rd trial
1. Wash hands.			
2. Identify patient.			
3. Explain procedure.			
4. Ask patient to remove his or her shoes.			
5. Place paper towel on scale.			
6. Balance scale if necessary.			
7. Ask patient to step on scale, facing scale.			
8. Move the 50-pound counterweight to the notch nearest but less than patient's weight.			
9. Slide the 1-pound counterweight along the top bar until the weight indicator "floats" at balance line.			
10. Determine weight by adding number on top bar (1-pound weight) to number on bottom bar (50-pound weight).			
11. Ask patient to step off scale.			
12. Discard paper towel.			
13. Return counterweights to zero.			
14. Wash hands.			
15. Record weight in patient medical record in pounds.			
16. The weight recorded is identical to that obtained by the evaluator. ◆			
17. Complete the procedure within 3 minutes. ◆			

Charting

DATE	

Evaluator Comments:

Score Calculation:

For each procedural step marked U (Unsatisfactory) deduct 6 points
For each procedural step (◆) marked U (Unsatisfactory) deduct 20 points

Score calculation 100 points

− ______ points missed

Total score

1st	2nd	3rd

Satisfactory score: 85 or above

Procedure 15-3: Measuring Oral Temperature Using a Glass-Mercury Thermometer

Performance Objective

Task: Take and record a patient's oral temperature using a glass mercury thermometer

Conditions: Glass thermometer, disposable plastic sheath, tissues, watch or clock, gloves, biohazard waste container

Standards: Complete the procedure in 7 minutes, and achieve a satisfactory score on the procedure performance checklist

Scoring Key: (**S**)*atisfactory,* (**U**)*nsatisfactory,* (**NA**) *Not Applicable*
◆ *Denotes a critical element for a satisfactory score on the procedure*

Procedure Steps	1st trial	2nd trial	3rd trial
1. Wash hands.			
2. Identify the patient.			
3. Explain procedure to patient.			
4. Ask if patient has had anything to eat, drink, or smoke in past 15 minutes.			
5. Select a clean dry glass thermometer.			
6. Read mercury level. If above 96°F, hold firmly in one hand and shake to get mercury below that level.			
7. Insert thermometer into the paper holder of a disposable plastic sheath.			
8. Grasp paper cuff at top of the sheath, twist, and remove paper.			
9. Put on gloves.			
10. Ask patient to open mouth.			
11. Place thermometer under patient's tongue.			
12. Instruct patient to hold the thermometer under the tongue and not to talk or bite down.			
13. After 3–5 minutes, remove thermometer.			
14. Holding thermometer at eye level, rotate until you can see mercury column.			
15. Read temperature (round up to next mark).			
16. Remove plastic sheath and dispose in biohazard waste container.			

Procedure Steps	1st trial	2nd trial	3rd trial
17. Wash thermometer with soap and cool water.			
18. Place thermometer in designated container for disinfection.			
19. Remove soiled gloves and discard in biohazard waste container.			
20. Wash hands.			
21. Record temperature, including location taken, in patient's chart.			
22. The temperature recorded is within ±0.2° of that obtained by the evaluator. ◆			
23. Complete the procedure within 7 minutes. ◆			

Charting

DATE	

Evaluator Comments:

Score Calculation:

For each procedural step marked U (Unsatisfactory) deduct 6 points
For each procedural step (◆) marked U (Unsatisfactory) deduct 20 points

Score calculation 100 points

− points missed

Total score

1st	2nd	3rd

Satisfactory score: 85 or above

Procedure 15-4: Measuring Oral Temperature Using an Electronic Thermometer

Performance Objective

Task: Take and record a patient's oral temperature using an electronic thermometer

Conditions: Electronic thermometer, disposable plastic probe cover, gloves, biohazard waste container

Standards: Complete the procedure in 5 minutes, and achieve a satisfactory score on the procedure performance checklist

Scoring Key: (**S**)*atisfactory,* (**U**)*nsatisfactory,* (**NA**) *Not Applicable*
◆ *Denotes a critical element for a satisfactory score on the procedure*

Procedure Steps	1st trial	2nd trial	3rd trial
1. Wash hands.			
2. Identify the patient.			
3. Explain procedure to patient.			
4. Ask if patient has had anything to eat, drink, or smoke in past 15 minutes.			
5. Remove thermometer from its rechargeable base.			
6. Put on gloves.			
7. Remove thermometer probe from holder.			
8. Insert probe firmly into disposable plastic probe cover.			
9. Turn the thermometer on.			
10. Wait for the display to signal that you may take temperature.			
11. Ask patient to open mouth and hold thermometer under tongue.			
12. Tell patient not to talk or bite down.			
13. When temperature is displayed, remove probe from mouth.			
14. Discard probe cover in a hazardous waste container.			
15. Return thermometer unit to base or storage.			
16. Discard soiled gloves.			
17. Wash hands.			

Procedure Steps	1st trial	2nd trial	3rd trial
18. Record temperature, including location taken, in patient chart.			
19. The temperature recorded is identical to that on the display screen. ◆			
20. Complete the procedure within 5 minutes. ◆			

Charting

DATE	

Evaluator Comments:

Score Calculation:

For each procedural step marked U (Unsatisfactory) deduct 6 points
For each procedural step (◆) marked U (Unsatisfactory) deduct 20 points

Score calculation 100 points

− points missed

Total score

1st	2nd	3rd

Satisfactory score: 85 or above

Procedure 15-5: Measuring Oral Temperature Using a Disposable Thermometer

Performance Objective

Task: Take and record a patient's temperature using a disposable thermometer

Conditions: Disposable thermometer, clock or watch, gloves, biohazard container

Standards: Complete the procedure in 7 minutes, and achieve a satisfactory score on the procedure performance checklist

Scoring Key: **(S)***atisfactory,* **(U)***nsatisfactory,* **(NA)** *Not Applicable*
◆ *Denotes a critical element for a satisfactory score on the procedure*

Procedure Steps	1st trial	2nd trial	3rd trial
1. Wash hands.			
2. Identify the patient.			
3. Explain procedure to patient.			
4. Ask if patient has had anything to eat, drink, or smoke in past 15 minutes.			
5. Select a disposable thermometer.			
6. Peel back wrapper to expose thermometer.			
7. Put on gloves.			
8. Pick up disposable thermometer.			
9. Ask patient to open mouth and hold thermometer under tongue.			
10. Instruct patient not to talk.			
11. Wait as long as directed by manufacturer.			
12. Remove thermometer, wait as long as directed by manufacturer, and read by looking at colored dots.			
13. Discard thermometer in a biohazard waste container.			
14. Remove soiled gloves and discard in biohazard waste container.			
15. Wash hands.			
16. Record temperature, including location taken, in patient chart.			
17. The temperature recorded is within $\pm 0.2°$ of that obtained by the evaluator. ◆			
18. Complete the procedure within 7 minutes. ◆			

Charting

DATE	

Evaluator Comments:

Score Calculation:

For each procedural step marked U (Unsatisfactory) deduct 6 points
For each procedural step (◆) marked U (Unsatisfactory) deduct 20 points

Score calculation 100 points

− points missed

Total score

1st	2nd	3rd

Satisfactory score: 85 or above

Procedure 15-6: Measuring Aural Temperature Using a Tympanic Thermometer

Performance Objective

Task: Take and record a patient's aural temperature using a tympanic thermometer

Conditions: Tympanic thermometer, disposable plastic probe cover, biohazard waste container

Standards: Complete the procedure in 5 minutes, and achieve a satisfactory score on the procedure performance checklist

Scoring Key: (**S**)*atisfactory,* (**U**)*nsatisfactory,* (**NA**) *Not Applicable*
◆ *Denotes a critical element for a satisfactory score on the procedure*

Procedure Steps	1st trial	2nd trial	3rd trial
1. Wash hands.			
2. Identify the patient.			
3. Explain procedure to patient.			
4. Remove thermometer unit from holder.			
5. Check the display screen to be sure the thermometer is set on the proper mode.			
6. Insert the probe firmly into a disposable plastic probe cover.			
7. Turn on the thermometer and wait until screen indicates that it is ready to take the temperature.			
8. Pull back on the patient's ear to straighten the ear canal.			
9. Insert the tip of the probe into the ear canal to form a tight seal but not cause the patient discomfort.			
10. Point the tip of the probe toward the opposite temple.			
11. Depress the activation button for one full second (or as directed by the manufacturer for the specific model of thermometer).			
12. Read the temperature from the display screen.			
13. Discard probe cover in biohazard waste container without touching it.			
14. Return the thermometer to the base.			
15. Wash hands.			

Procedure Steps	1st trial	2nd trial	3rd trial
16. Record temperature, including location taken, in patient's chart.			
17. The temperature recorded is identical to that on the display screen. ◆			
18. Complete the procedure within 5 minutes. ◆			

Charting

DATE	

Evaluator Comments:

Score Calculation:

For each procedural step marked U (Unsatisfactory) deduct 6 points
For each procedural step (◆) marked U (Unsatisfactory) deduct 20 points

Score calculation 100 points

− points missed

Total score

1st	2nd	3rd

Satisfactory score: 85 or above

Procedure 15-7: Measuring Rectal Temperature

Performance Objective

Task: Take and record a patient's rectal temperature

Conditions: Glass mercury or electronic thermometer with rectal probe, lubricant, disposable plastic sheath or probe cover, gauze square, tissue, gloves, biohazard waste container

Standards: Complete the procedure in 7 minutes, and achieve a satisfactory score on the procedure performance checklist

Scoring Key: (**S**)*atisfactory,* (**U**)*nsatisfactory,* (**NA**) *Not Applicable*
◆ *Denotes a critical element for a satisfactory score on the procedure*

Procedure Steps	**1st trial**	**2nd trial**	**3rd trial**
1. Wash hands.			
2. Identify the patient.			
3. Explain procedure to patient.			
4. Have patient get undressed from waist down (have parent undress infant).			
5. Prepare either a rectal mercury thermometer with plastic sheath or electronic thermometer with red probe and disposable plastic probe cover.			
6. Squeeze about an inch of lubricant on gauze square.			
7. Put on gloves.			
8. Lubricate first two inches of thermometer or probe cover.			
9. Position an adult patient on left side with right leg slightly forward (Sims' position). (Drape adult for privacy.) **or**			
9. Position infant on back or stomach, holding firmly.			
10. Gently insert thermometer or probe into rectum (about 1/2 inch for infant, 1–2 inches for adult).			
11. Instruct adult patient not to move. **or**			
11. Hold infant firmly.			
12. Leave mercury thermometer in place for 3–5 minutes.			
13. Remain with patient at all times and hold thermometer in place.			
14. Remove thermometer.			

Procedure Steps	1st trial	2nd trial	3rd trial
15. Remove plastic sheath or plastic probe cover.			
16. Discard plastic sheath or probe cover in biohazard container.			
17. Read temperature (gently wipe glass thermometer with tissue from shaft to bulb if necessary).			
18. Wipe anal area of infant with a tissue or give adult tissues to perform own wipe.			
19. Wash a glass thermometer using soap and water. Rinse and paper-towel dry.			
20. Place glass thermometer in designated container for disinfection. Place electronic thermometer in its base.			
21. Remove soiled gloves and discard in biohazard waste container.			
22. Wash hands.			
23. Assist adult to sit up. Offer privacy to get dressed.			
24. Record temperature, including location taken, in patient chart.			
25. The temperature recorded is within ±0.2°of that obtained by the evaluator (glass thermometer) or is identical to that on the display screen (electronic thermometer). ◆			
26. Complete the procedure within 7 minutes. ◆			

Charting

DATE	

Evaluator Comments:

Score Calculation:

For each procedural step marked U (Unsatisfactory) deduct 6 points
For each procedural step (◆) marked U (Unsatisfactory) deduct 20 points

Score calculation 100 points

− points missed

Total score

1st	2nd	3rd

Satisfactory score: 85 or above

Notes

Procedure 15-8: Measuring Axillary Temperature

Performance Objective

Task: Take and record a patient's axillary temperature

Conditions: Thermometer, disposable plastic sheath or probe cover, paper towel

Standards: Complete the procedure in 12 minutes, and achieve a satisfactory score on the procedure performance checklist

Scoring Key: (**S**)*atisfactory,* (**U**)*nsatisfactory,* (**NA**) *Not Applicable*
◆ *Denotes a critical element for a satisfactory score on the procedure*

Procedure Steps	1st trial	2nd trial	3rd trial
1. Wash hands.			
2. Identify the patient.			
3. Explain procedure to patient.			
4. Have patient undress so that underarm (axilla) is accessible. (Provide gown if patient desires.)			
5. Dry underarm with paper towel if necessary.			
6. Prepare either a mercury thermometer with a plastic sheath or an electronic thermometer with an oral probe and disposable probe cover.			
7. Place thermometer under patient's arm.			
8. Instruct patient to hold arm tight to side.			
9. Leave mercury thermometer 10 minutes. If using electronic thermometer, wait until the temperature is displayed.			
10. Remove thermometer.			
11. Dispose of plastic sheath or probe cover in a biohazard waste container.			
12. Read temperature.			
13. Wash glass thermometer with soap and water, rinse, and dry.			
14. Place glass thermometer in designated container for disinfection. Place electronic thermometer in its base.			
15. Wash hands.			
16. Offer privacy if desired for patient to dress.			

Procedure Steps	1st trial	2nd trial	3rd trial
17. Record temperature, including location taken, in patient chart.			
18. The temperature recorded is within ±0.2° of that obtained by the evaluator (glass thermometer) or is identical to that on the display screen (electronic thermometer). ◆			
19. Complete the procedure within 12 minutes. ◆			

Charting

DATE	

Evaluator Comments:

Score Calculation:

For each procedural step marked U (Unsatisfactory) deduct 6 points
For each procedural step (◆) marked U (Unsatisfactory) deduct 20 points

Score calculation 100 points

– points missed

Total score

1st	2nd	3rd

Satisfactory score: 85 or above

Procedure 15-9: Measuring the Radial Pulse

Performance Objective

Task: Measure and record the patient's radial pulse, and describe the rhythm and volume

Conditions: Watch with sweep second hand

Standards: Complete the procedure in 3 minutes, and achieve a satisfactory score on the procedure performance checklist

Scoring Key: (**S**)*atisfactory,* (**U**)*nsatisfactory,* (**NA**) *Not Applicable*
◆ *Denotes a critical element for a satisfactory score on the procedure*

Procedure Steps	1st trial	2nd trial	3rd trial
1. Wash hands.			
2. Identify the patient.			
3. Explain procedure to patient.			
4. Position patient so arm is supported and relaxed.			
5. Locate radial pulse with first three fingers.			
6. Begin to count heartbeats.			
7. Count heartbeats for 30 seconds and multiply by 2 to obtain heart rate. (If pulse is irregular, count for 1 full minute.)			
8. Note quality of pulse.			
9. If respirations are to be measured, proceed to Procedure 15-11 without removing hand from patient's wrist.			
10. Record pulse in patient's chart. Describe any variation from normal rhythm and/or rate.			
11. The pulse rate recorded is within ±2 of that obtained by the evaluator. ◆			
12. Complete the procedure within 3 minutes. ◆			

Charting

DATE	

Evaluator Comments:

Score Calculation:

For each procedural step marked U (Unsatisfactory) deduct 6 points
For each procedural step (◆) marked U (Unsatisfactory) deduct 20 points

Score calculation	100 points			
	− ___ points missed	1st	2nd	3rd
	Total score			

Satisfactory score: 85 or above

Procedure 15-10: Measuring the Apical Pulse

Performance Objective

Task: Measure and record a patient's apical pulse

Conditions: Stethoscope, alcohol wipes, watch with sweep second hand

Standards: Complete the procedure in 4 minutes, and achieve a satisfactory score on the performance procedure checklist

Scoring Key: (**S**)*atisfactory,* (**U**)*nsatisfactory,* (**NA**) *Not Applicable*
◆ *Denotes a critical element for a satisfactory score on the procedure*

Procedure Steps	1st trial	2nd trial	3rd trial
1. Wash hands.			
2. Identify the patient.			
3. Explain procedure to patient.			
4. Instruct the patient to remove clothing from the waist up. (Provide gown if desired.)			
5. Locate apex of the heart by palpating fifth intercostal space and moving laterally to midclavicular line.			
6. Clean stethoscope head and earpieces with alcohol wipe.			
7. Place stethoscope head over apex of heart.			
8. Insert earpieces of stethoscope into ears correctly.			
9. When pulse is located, count heartbeats for 1 full minute.			
10. Offer privacy if desired for patient to dress.			
11. Record as apical pulse in patient's chart. Describe any variation from normal rhythm and/or rate.			
12. The pulse rate recorded is within ±2 beats of that obtained by the evaluator. ◆			
13. Complete the procedure within 4 minutes. ◆			

Charting

DATE	

Evaluator Comments:

Score Calculation:

For each procedural step marked U (Unsatisfactory) deduct 6 points
For each procedural step (◆) marked U (Unsatisfactory) deduct 20 points

Score calculation 100 points

− points missed

Total score

1st	2nd	3rd

Satisfactory score: 85 or above

Procedure 15-11: Measuring Respirations

Performance Objective

Task: Measure and record a patient's respirations, and describe rhythm and depth of respirations

Conditions: Watch with sweep second hand

Standards: Complete procedure in 3 minutes, and achieve a satisfactory score on the procedure performance checklist

Scoring Key: (**S**)*atisfactory,* (**U**)*nsatisfactory,* (**NA**) *Not Applicable*
◆ *Denotes a critical element for a satisfactory score on the procedure*

Procedure Steps	1st trial	2nd trial	3rd trial
1. Observe patient while he or she is sitting or lying in comfortable position.			
2. Watch patient's chest rise and fall—each cycle is one respiration.			
3. If respiration rate is regular and strong, count for 30 seconds and multiply by 2. (If respiration rate is irregular, continue counting for 1 full minute.)			
4. Record respiration rate in patient's chart. Note irregularities in volume or rhythm.			
5. The respiratory rate recorded is within ±1 of that obtained by the evaluator. ◆			
6. Complete the procedure within 3 minutes. ◆			

Charting

DATE	

Evaluator Comments:

Score Calculation:

For each procedural step marked U (Unsatisfactory) deduct 6 points
For each procedural step (◆) marked U (Unsatisfactory) deduct 20 points

Score calculation   100 points

− points missed

Total score

1st	2nd	3rd

Satisfactory score: 85 or above

Procedure 15-12: Measuring Blood Pressure

Performance Objective

Task: Measure and record a patient's blood pressure

Conditions: Stethoscope, alcohol wipe, sphygmomanometer

Standards: Complete the procedure in 5 minutes, and achieve a satisfactory score on the procedure performance checklist

Scoring Key: (**S**)*atisfactory,* (**U**)*nsatisfactory,* (**NA**) *Not Applicable*
◆ *Denotes a critical element for a satisfactory score on the procedure*

Procedure Steps	1st trial	2nd trial	3rd trial
1. Wash hands.			
2. Identify the patient.			
3. Explain procedure to patient.			
4. Ask patient to roll up sleeve at least 4 inches above bend of arm (or remove shirt, offer gown if desired).			
5. Position patient so lower arm is supported on flat surface and relaxed, cuff and heart at same level.			
6. Place blood pressure cuff on arm with rubber bladder centered over brachial artery, 1 inch above bend in elbow.			
7. Wrap cuff snugly around arm and fasten.			
8. Palpate systolic pressure for a patient with no previously recorded blood pressure.			
8a. Hold bulb in your dominant hand with control valve between thumb and first finger.			
8b. Turn screw clockwise to tighten or counterclockwise to loosen if necessary.			
8c. Locate radial pulse with nondominant hand.			
8d. Inflate blood pressure cuff by squeezing bulb until just above the point where you stop feeling radial pulse.			
8e. Note reading (this is systolic pressure).			
8f. Deflate blood pressure cuff quickly by opening control valve.			
9. Clean stethoscope earpieces and head with alcohol.			

Procedure Steps	1st trial	2nd trial	3rd trial
10. Place head of stethoscope over brachial artery at bend of the elbow.			
11. Insert earpieces into ears correctly.			
12. Wait at least 1 minute before reinflating after previous attempt.			
13. Inflate cuff to 30 mm Hg higher than the palpated or previously recorded systolic pressure.			
14. Immediately, open the control valve slightly so the blood pressure indicator decreases about 2–4 mm Hg per second.			
15. Note the exact level where you hear the first sharp tapping sound. This is the systolic pressure.			
16. Continue deflating cuff at 2–4 mm Hg per second.			
17. Note exact level where the sound disappears. This is the diastolic pressure.			
18. Open control valve and allow cuff to deflate quickly.			
19. If you are satisfied, remove cuff. If you need to take pressure again, wait at least 1 minute before reinflating cuff.			
20. After removing cuff, wash hands.			
21. Record blood pressure in patient's chart. Note arm on which you took blood pressure.			
22. The blood pressure recorded is an even number and within ±2 mm Hg of that obtained by the evaluator. ◆			
23. Complete the procedure within 5 minutes. ◆			

Charting

DATE	

Evaluator Comments:

Score Calculation:

For each procedural step marked U (Unsatisfactory) deduct 6 points
For each procedural step (◆) marked U (Unsatisfactory) deduct 20 points

Score calculation	100 points			
	− ____ points missed	1st	2nd	3rd
	Total score			

Satisfactory score: 85 or above

SELF-EVALUATION

4. For what types of occupations are periodic physical examinations mandatory? Can this be seen as a violation of the rights of the employee? Why or why not?

PRACTICAL APPLICATIONS

1. After checking the following patients in and taking vital signs, exactly what instructions would you give to each of the following patients to prepare to be examined by the physician.

   a. Joseph Correira, a 46-year-old male, new patient who will undergo complete physical examination.

   b. Diane Russo, a 36-year-old female, established patient who has been ill with a cold, cough, and fears she may have bronchitis.

   c. Mary Stahl, a 19-year-old female, established patient for college physical with breast exam and her first pelvic examination.

d. Brian Meyers, a 26-year-old male, who injured his left knee and ankle playing basketball.

2. What examination technique(s) (palpation, percussion, auscultation, and/or inspection) is (are) used in each of the following situations:

   a. identifying the presence of skin lesions ____________

   b. estimating the position and size of the uterus ____________

   c. tapping the lower abdomen to determine if the bladder is full ____________

   d. performing a breast examination ____________

   e. listening for bruit in the carotid artery ____________

   f. measuring blood pressure ____________

   g. checking reflexes ____________

3. Identify each of the following positions for patient examination.

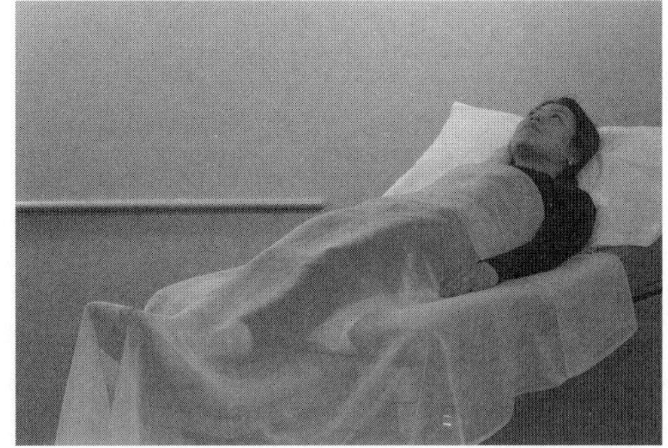

a. ____________

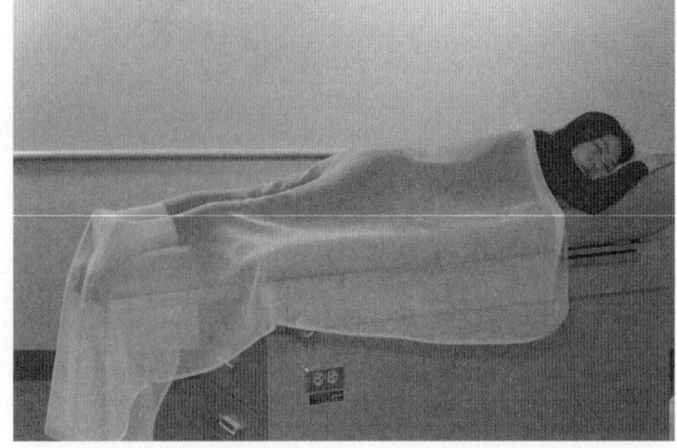

b. ____________

c.

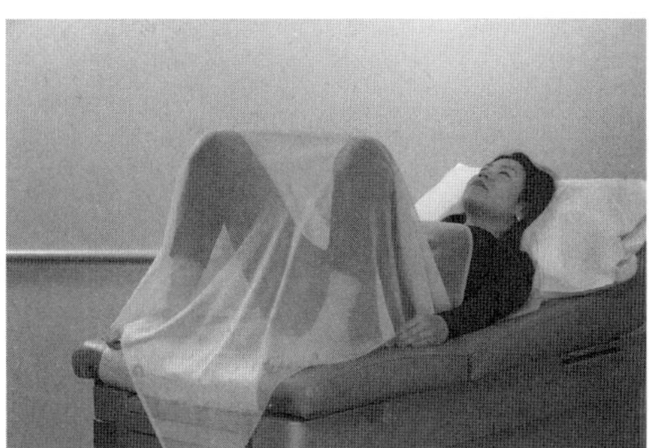

c. ______________________________

d.

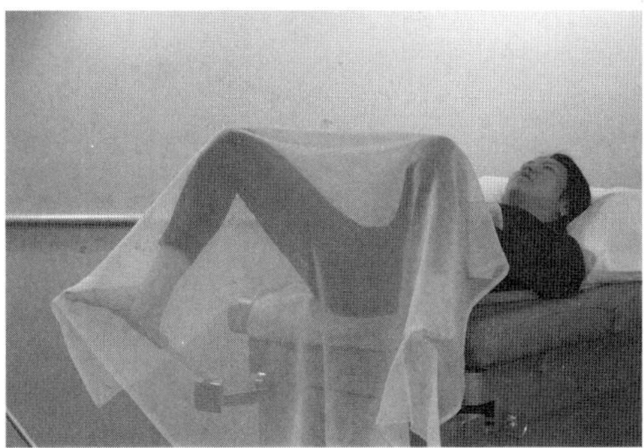

d. ______________________________

e.

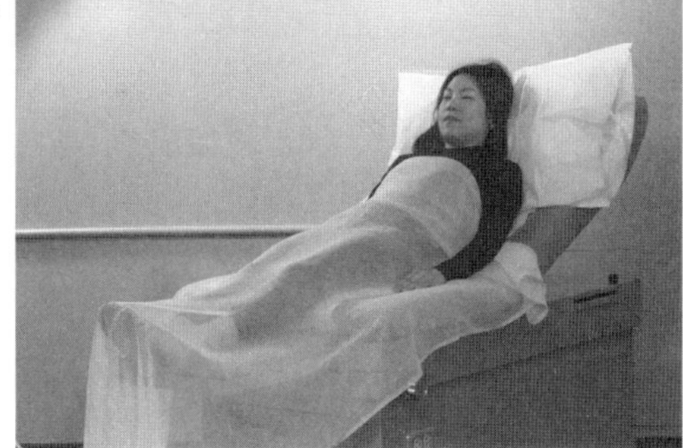

e. ______________________________

f.

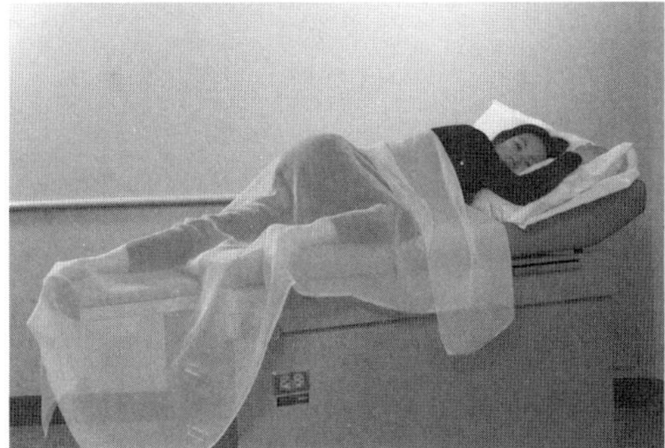

f. ______________________________

g. 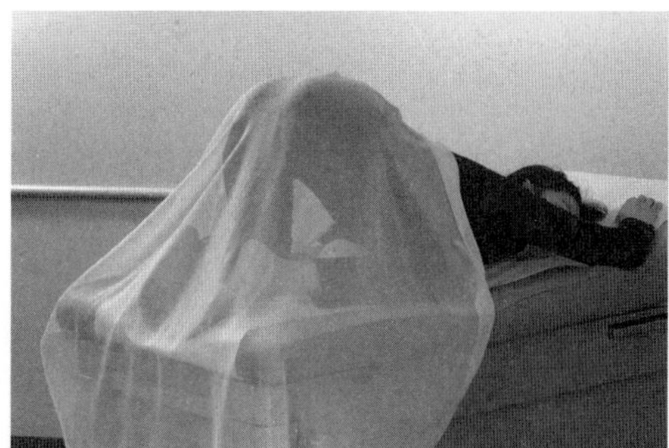

g. ______________________________

4. If a patient reads all the letters on the 20/20 line of the Snellen chart with the right eye and all the letters except one correctly on the 20/30 line with the left eye, how would you chart his or her vision?

____

____

____

5. If you are explaining the preparation for a proctosigmoidoscopy, how would you answer a patient who asks why this preparation is necessary?

____

____

____

6. Use the CD-ROM to complete the activities associated with positioning patients in the Clinical Skills section.

Procedure 16-1: Assisting with the Physical Examination

Performance Objective

Task: Prepare equipment and the patient for a physical exam, and assist with the exam

Conditions: Scale, thermometer, watch with sweep second hand, stethoscope, sphygmomanometer, gown, drape, ophthalmoscope, otoscope with new or clean ear speculum, tongue depressor, percussion hammer, gloves, lubricant, hemoccult test kit, gauze square, paper towels, and biohazard waste container

Standards: Complete the procedure in 20 minutes, and achieve a satisfactory score on the procedure performance checklist

Scoring Key: **(S)***atisfactory,* **(U)***nsatisfactory,* **(NA)** *Not Applicable*
◆ *Denotes a critical element for a satisfactory score on the procedure*

Procedure Steps	1st trial	2nd trial	3rd trial
1. Wash hands.			
2. Assemble supplies and equipment.			
3. Identify patient.			
4. Explain procedure to patient.			
5. Instruct patient to remove shoes and heavy clothing.			
6. Weigh patient.			
7. Measure new patient or child.			
8. Record height and weight in the medical record.			
9. Seat patient.			
10. Take vital signs.			
11. Record vital signs.			
12. Instruct patient how to obtain urine specimen.			
13. Label urine specimen cup.			
14. Instruct patient where to leave urine specimen.			
15. Bring patient back to exam room.			
16. Instruct patient to remove clothing and put on gown.			

Procedure Steps	1st trial	2nd trial	3rd trial
17. Instruct patient to sit on end of exam table when ready to be examined. (Leave room to provide privacy; or assist patient if necessary.)			
18. Notify doctor that patient is ready.			
19. Assist doctor during exam as requested.			
20. Assist patient to assume positions as needed during the examination.			
21. Position hazardous waste container for convenient disposal of used tongue blade, ear speculum, etc.			
22. Following exam, assist patient to sit up and get off the exam table if needed.			
23. Instruct patient to dress. (Provide privacy if desired, or assist if necessary.)			
24. When patient is dressed, provide any needed instructions.			
25. Discard disposable gown, drapes, and used table paper.			
26. Remove instruments to area where they will be cleaned and sterilized.			
27. Put on disposable gloves to clean any surfaces contaminated with blood or body fluids.			
28. Clean contaminated surfaces with 1:10 household bleach solution and allow to air-dry.			
29. Remove and dispose of soiled gloves.			
30. Wash hands.			
31. Cover exam table with clean paper and prepare exam room for the next patient.			
32. Accurate measurements for height, weight, and vital signs are documented below. ◆			
33. Complete the procedure within 20 minutes. ◆			

Charting

DATE	

Evaluator Comments:

Score Calculation:

For each procedural step marked U (Unsatisfactory) deduct 6 points
For each procedural step (◆) marked U (Unsatisfactory) deduct 20 points

Score calculation 100 points

− points missed

Total score

1st	2nd	3rd

Satisfactory score: 85 or above

Notes

Procedure 16-2: Assisting with Pap Test and Pelvic Examination

Performance Objective

Task: Prepare equipment and patient for a Pap test and pelvic examination, assist doctor with exam

Conditions: Gloves, water-soluble lubricant, tissues, gown, drape, vaginal speculum, slide and fixative or ThinPrep transport solution, cytobrush, vaginal spatula, and cotton-tipped applicator (or broom-type cervical sampling device for ThinPrep test), requisition form, and mailer

Standards: Complete the procedure in 20 minutes, and achieve a satisfactory score on the procedure performance checklist

Scoring Key: (**S**)*atisfactory,* (**U**)*nsatisfactory,* (**NA**) *Not Applicable*
◆ *Denotes a critical element for a satisfactory score on the procedure*

Procedure Steps	**1st trial**	**2nd trial**	**3rd trial**
1. Wash hands.			
2. Assemble supplies and equipment.			
3. Position light source so it can be adjusted.			
4. Position stirrups about 6–12 inches from the end of the exam table, and angled slightly outward if possible.			
5. Identify patient.			
6. Explain procedure to patient.			
7. Instruct patient to empty her bladder. Obtain a urine specimen if needed.			
8. Fill out lab slip for cytology lab.			
9. If breast exam will be performed, instruct patient to undress completely. For pelvic exam only, instruct patient to undress from waist down. Provide gown with back opening.			
10. Instruct patient to sit on end of exam table with drape over lower lap when ready.			
11. Provide privacy by leaving room, or assist patient if necessary.			
12. When doctor is ready, assist patient to lithotomy position.			
13. Assist doctor as requested.			
14. If breast exam is being performed, assist patient to untie and retie gown.			
15. At Pap test, assist doctor with instruments as requested.			
16. Mark slide(s) with patient's name or clinic number.			
17. Spray slides with fixative immediately or hold bottle of fixative solution for physician to place slides, or brush.			

Procedure Steps	1st trial	2nd trial	3rd trial
18. Be sure that a container for used metal speculum or biohazard waste container for plastic speculum is in doctor's easy reach.			
19. Apply water-soluble lubricant to doctor's gloved finger for bimanual exam.			
20. After exam, assist patient to remove feet from stirrups and to sit up.			
21. Offer tissues and a sanitary pad if needed.			
22. Instruct patient to dress. Provide privacy or assist if necessary.			
23. Put on disposable gloves to handle slides, culture tubes, and/or vials containing transport medium.			
24. Allow slides to air-dry for 10 to 15 minutes.			
25. Place any specimen in plastic container for transport to lab.			
26. Remove and discard soiled gloves in biohazard waste container.			
27. When patient is dressed, provide any needed instructions.			
28. Discard disposable gown, drape, used table paper and contaminated supplies or disposable equipment in appropriate biohazard container(s).			
29. Put on disposable gloves to handle soiled instruments or clean any surfaces contaminated with blood or body fluids.			
30. Remove instruments to where they will be cleaned and sterilized.			
31. Clean contaminated surfaces with 1:10 household bleach solution and allow to air-dry.			
32. Remove and dispose of soiled gloves in biohazard waste container.			
33. Wash hands.			
34. Cover exam table with clean paper and prepare exam room for the next patient.			
35. Complete all lab slips, including those for any cultures for vaginal infections.			
36. Place lab slip in transport bag and place in the appropriate place for pick up or mailing.			
37. Lab slip filled out completely and correctly. ◆			
38. Complete the procedure within 20 minutes. ◆			

Evaluator Comments:

Score Calculation:

For each procedural step marked U (Unsatisfactory) deduct 6 points
For each procedural step (◆) marked U (Unsatisfactory) deduct 20 points

Score calculation	100 points			
	− ____ points missed	1st	2nd	3rd
	Total score			

Satisfactory score: 85 or above

Notes

Procedure 16-3: Measuring Distance Visual Acuity Using a Snellen Chart

Performance Objective

Task: Measure visual acuity accurately using the Snellen eye chart

Conditions: Snellen chart, pointer, occluder or paper cup, alcohol wipes

Standards: Complete the procedure in 5 minutes, and achieve a satisfactory score on the procedure performance checklist

Scoring Key: (**S**)*atisfactory*, (**U**)*nsatisfactory*, (**NA**) *Not Applicable*
◆ *Denotes a critical element for a satisfactory score on the procedure*

Procedure Steps	1st trial	2nd trial	3rd trial
1. Wash hands.			
2. Assemble supplies and equipment.			
3. Identify patient.			
4. Explain procedure to patient.			
5. Position patient 20 feet from eye chart.			
6. Make sure room is well lighted.			
7. Patient should wear any glasses or contact lenses used for distance vision.			
8. Instruct patient to keep both eyes open and cover left eye with occluder or paper cup.			
9. Point to the 20/40 line and ask the patient to read each letter. (Ask a child to name the picture or point in the direction the E is facing.)			
10. If patient reads correctly, ask patient to read the line below until patient can no longer identify the letters.			
11. If patient cannot read 20/40 line, ask patient to read line above. Continue up until patient can read.			
12. When patient has read correctly to last line possible, ask him or her to cover the other eye and repeat process.			
13. Ask patient to read lowest line he or she can read with both eyes uncovered.			
14. Wipe occluder with alcohol and allow to dry before reusing (or discard paper cup).			
15. Wash hands.			

Procedure Steps	1st trial	2nd trial	3rd trial
16. Record the number of the smallest line patient was able to read with each eye, and with both eyes. Note up to two missed letters for each measurement.			
17. Document if the patient is wearing corrective lenses.			
18. The vision recorded is identical to that recorded by the evaluator. ◆			
19. Complete the procedure within 5 minutes. ◆			

Charting

DATE	

Evaluator Comments:

Score Calculation:

For each procedural step marked U (Unsatisfactory) deduct 6 points
For each procedural step (◆) marked U (Unsatisfactory) deduct 20 points

Score calculation 100 points
− points missed

Total score

1st	2nd	3rd

Satisfactory score: 85 or above

Procedure 16-4: Ishihara Test of Color Vision

Performance Objective

Task: Assess color vision using a book with Ischihara plates

Conditions: Book of Ishihara plates

Standards: Complete the procedure in 5 minutes, and achieve a satisfactory score on the procedure performance checklist

Scoring Key: (**S**)*atisfactory,* (**U**)*nsatisfactory,* (**NA**) *Not Applicable*
◆ *Denotes a critical element for a satisfactory score on the procedure*

Procedure Steps	1st trial	2nd trial	3rd trial
1. Wash hands.			
2. Assemble book of Ishihara plates.			
3. Identify patient.			
4. Explain procedure to patient.			
5. Seat patient and hold book of Ishihara plates approximately 30 inches from patient with the plate at right angle to the patient's line of vision.			
6. Make sure room is well lighted, and allow patient to wear glasses or contact lenses normally used.			
7. Instruct patient to tell you what number he or she sees in the first plate.			
8. Continue through the book until patient reads all plates.			
9. Record the plate number with an X for each plate the patient could not read.			
10. The results recorded are identical to those recorded by the evaluator. ◆			
11. Complete the procedure within 5 minutes. ◆			

Charting

DATE	

Evaluator Comments:

Score Calculation:

For each procedural step marked U (Unsatisfactory) deduct 6 points
For each procedural step (◆) marked U (Unsatisfactory) deduct 20 points

Score calculation 100 points

− ____ points missed

	1st	2nd	3rd
Total score			

Satisfactory score: 85 or above

Procedure 16-5: Measuring Hearing Using a Manual Audiometer

Performance Objective

Task: Measure hearing using a manual audiometer and record results accurately

Conditions: Manual audiometer with headphones, alcohol wipes

Standards: Complete the procedure in 5 minutes, and achieve a satisfactory score on the procedure performance checklist

Scoring Key: **(S)***atisfactory,* **(U)***nsatisfactory,* **(NA)** *Not Applicable*
◆ *Denotes a critical element for a satisfactory score on the procedure*

Procedure Steps	1st trial	2nd trial	3rd trial
1. Wash hands.			
2. Assemble audiometer and alcohol wipes.			
3. Identify patient.			
4. Explain procedure to patient.			
5. Seat patient in soundproof cubicle or quiet room.			
6. Instruct patient to raise hand every time a sound is heard, or to press button when tone is heard.			
7. Have patient put on earphones.			
8. Be sure patient cannot see you press buttons.			
9. Press correct button(s) to begin test and to change frequencies.			
10. Test each ear.			
11. Record how loud the tone needed to be for the patient to hear it at each pitch. (If machine records results, print the results at the end of the test.)			
12. Wash hands.			
13. Fill in a graph showing the loudness required for each frequency tested, or print results and label printout with patient's name and date of test.			
14. Complete the procedure within 5 minutes. ◆			

Evaluator Comments:

Score Calculation:

For each procedural step marked U (Unsatisfactory) deduct 6 points
For each procedural step (◆) marked U (Unsatisfactory) deduct 20 points

Score calculation 100 points

− points missed

Total score

1st	2nd	3rd

Satisfactory score: 85 or above

Procedure 16-6: Testing Stool for Occult Blood

Performance Objective

Task: Test a stool specimen for occult blood

Conditions: Stool specimen, wooden spatula or tongue depressor, gloves, test kit for occult blood including developer

Standards: Complete the procedure in 10 minutes, and achieve a satisfactory score on the procedure performance checklist

Scoring Key: **(S)***atisfactory,* **(U)***nsatisfactory,* **(NA)** *Not Applicable*
◆ *Denotes a critical element for a satisfactory score on the procedure*

Procedure Steps	1st trial	2nd trial	3rd trial
1. Wash hands.			
2. Assemble supplies and equipment.			
3. Put on disposable gloves.			
4. Open front of the card from an occult blood testing kit.			
5. Obtain stool from a container with stool, or from doctor's glove following rectal exam.			
6. Use wooden spatula, tongue depressor, or cotton-tipped applicator to apply a thin layer to paper in the first box on the card.			
7. Using stool from a second part of the sample, apply a thin layer to the paper in the second box.			
8. Wait 3–5 minutes before developing.			
9. Open box on rear of the test card and drop two drops of developer solution on each box to which stool was applied.			
10. Read results as directed by manufacturer.			
11. While wearing gloves, dispose of test card, applicators, and remainder of stool specimen in biohazard waste container.			
12. Clean any contaminated surfaces with 1:10 household bleach solution and allow to air-dry.			
13. Remove and dispose of soiled gloves in biohazard waste container.			
14. Wash hands.			
15. Record results in the medical record. If testing specimens obtained by patient at home, record the date specimens were collected.			
16. Results recorded are the same as those recorded by the evaluator. ◆			
17. Complete the procedure within 5 minutes. ◆			

Charting

DATE	

Evaluator Comments:

Score Calculation:

For each procedural step marked U (Unsatisfactory) deduct 6 points
For each procedural step (◆) marked U (Unsatisfactory) deduct 20 points

Score calculation 100 points

− ____ points missed

Total score

1st	2nd	3rd

Satisfactory score: 85 or above

Procedure 16-7: Assisting with Flexible Sigmoidoscopy

Performance Objective

Task: Set up for flexible sigmoidoscopy and assist doctor with exam

Conditions: Flexible sigmoidoscope with light source, insufflator, video monitor, suction machine, suction catheter, gloves, drape, patient gown, water-resistant lab coat for doctor, water-soluble lubricant, 12-inch sponge sticks, sterile biopsy forceps, specimen container with preservative solution, gauze sponges, tissues

Standards: Complete the procedure in 20 minutes, and achieve a satisfactory score on the procedure performance checklist

Scoring Key: (**S**)*atisfactory,* (**U**)*nsatisfactory,* (**NA**) *Not Applicable*
◆ *Denotes a critical element for a satisfactory score on the procedure*

Procedure Steps	1st trial	2nd trial	3rd trial
1. Wash hands.			
2. Assemble supplies and equipment.			
3. Hook up sigmoidoscope to light source, insufflator, and monitor.			
4. Prepare suction equipment and test.			
5. Place generous amount of lubricant on a gauze square.			
6. Identify patient.			
7. Explain procedure to patient.			
8. Have patient empty bladder before procedure. Collect urine specimen if needed.			
9. Tell patient to undress from waist down and put on a gown with a back opening. Provide privacy, or assist if necessary.			
10. Position patient in the Sims' position.			
11. Place drape over the patient's buttocks until exam begins.			
12. Assist doctor with fluid-resistant lab coat if requested.			
13. Put on disposable gloves.			
14. When doctor is ready, remove drape to expose anal area.			
15. Instruct patient to breathe deeply through mouth.			
16. Instruct patient to bear down slightly when sigmoidoscope is first introduced and take deep breaths.			

Procedure Steps	1st trial	2nd trial	3rd trial
17. Assist doctor as requested during exam.			
18. Offer support and encouragement to patient as needed.			
19. When exam is complete, offer tissues to patient.			
20. Remove and dispose of gloves, and assist patient to sit up.			
21. Instruct patient to remain sitting until any dizziness or lightheadedness passes.			
22. Instruct patient to dress. Provide privacy, or assist if necessary.			
23. Give patient any follow-up instructions.			
24. Fill out the correct lab slip for each specimen, including where the specimen was obtained.			
25. Place specimens in a plastic biohazard bag for transport to lab. Place lab slips in pocket of transport bag.			
26. Put on disposable gloves.			
27. Discard paper gown, drape, and used supplies in biohazard container. Place cloth gown or drape in contaminated laundry bag.			
28. Discard used table paper.			
29. Clean exam table with 1:10 household bleach, and allow to air-dry.			
30. Clean used equipment with soap and water, and place in soaking solution until ready to sterilize.			
31. Clean light attachment with alcohol swabs (do not soak).			
32. Rinse equipment and place in container with sterilizing solution. Use sterile syringes to push sterilizing solution into the interior chamber of the sigmoidoscope.			
33. Remove and discard soiled gloves in biohazard waste container.			
34. Wash hands.			
35. Complete the procedure within 20 minutes. ◆			

Evaluator Comments:

Score Calculation:

For each procedural step marked U (Unsatisfactory) deduct 6 points
For each procedural step (◆) marked U (Unsatisfactory) deduct 20 points

Score calculation 100 points

− ____ points missed

	1st	2nd	3rd
Total score			

Satisfactory score: 85 or above

SELF-EVALUATION

Chapter 17

Assisting with Surgical Procedures

CHAPTER FOCUS

In this chapter, you learned the principles of surgical asepsis, how to set up a sterile field and add items to the field, and how to assist with minor surgical procedures. Surgical aseptic techniques are used whenever the doctor is going to penetrate below the skin or enter a sterile body cavity. The medical assistant must be able to use proper technique to avoid introducing microorganisms that might cause disease in patients.

TERMINOLOGY REVIEW

Vocabulary Matching: Match each term with its definition.

___ 1. hemostasis

___ 2. ligate

___ 3. incision and drainage (I & D)

___ 4. bandage

___ 5. swaged

___ 6. abscess

___ 7. granulation

___ 8. cyst

A. Localized collection of pus, with inflammation of the surrounding tissue

B. When wound edges come together in a near-perfect fit

C. A covering that keeps a dressing in place and provides even pressure and support to the area around the wound

D. An examination of tissue under a microscope to determine if cancerous cells are present

E. Suture material with needle attached

F. An accumulation of sebum in a gland under the skin surrounding a clogged oil duct

G. Removal of dead tissue so proper healing can take place

H. A sterile covering that goes immediately over a closed surgical incision or laceration

___ 9. dressing	I. A type of surgical drape that has an opening to be placed over the area where a surgical incision will be made
___ 10. Mayo stand	J. Control of bleeding
___ 11. slough	K. When a wound heals by filling up with granulated tissue, from the bottom up
___ 12. approximated	L. A surgical procedure to cut into and drain an abscess or cyst
___ 13. debridement	M. Tie off so it does not bleed
___ 14. fenestrated	N. A small table with wheels designed to hold a doctor's necessary instruments and supplies
___ 15. biopsy	O. When dead tissue separates from healthy tissue

Instrument Matching: Match each instrument with its use or function.

____ 1. forceps	A. Scrape away tissue
____ 2. scalpel	B. Grasping, pulling, compressing, or holding tissue or other instruments
____ 3. curette	C. Hold suture needle during suturing
____ 4. retractor	D. Hold edge of incisions or wounds in place
____ 5. suture material	E. Hold an incision or cavity open so a doctor can view the area underneath
____ 6. needle holder	F. Making surgical incisions
____ 7. probe or sound	G. Control bleeding
____ 8. hemostat	H. Feel around inside an incision or measure the depth of a cavity before proceeding

Definitions: Insert the correct term to complete the definition.

1. A deliberate surgical cut through skin and tissue beneath is called an ____________________.
2. A cut made accidentally, which often must be sutured, is called ____________________.
3. A wound that heals by ____________________ ____________________ is one in which the place where the skin was open comes together in a near-perfect fit, with minimal scarring.
4. A wound that heals by ____________________ ____________________ is one that heals by filling in with granulated tissue, instead of the original type of tissue, from the bottom up.
5. Also called delayed primary intention, a wound that heals by ____________________ ____________________ is often purposely kept open until the wound is clean, then sutured.

CONTENT REVIEW QUESTIONS

1. What can touch a sterile object without contaminating it?

____

____

2. What part of a sterile field is considered sterile? What parts of a sterile gown are considered sterile?

3. Why is it poor technique to reach across a sterile field or to turn your back?

4. Identify three instruments used during minor surgery that are always placed in a rigid biohazard container after use.

a.

b.

c.

5. Why are instruments used for minor surgery soaked in solution until they can be sanitized?

6. Describe how each of the following supplies may be used for minor surgery:

a. gauze squares

b. povidone (Betadine) solution

c. Xylocaine (lidocaine)

d. drapes

7. When is absorbable suture material used? Nonabsorbable sutures? What is the difference?

8. Identify two ways to create a sterile field.

a.

b.

9. How can the medical assistant store a pair of sterile sponge forceps to use as sterile transfer forceps during a sterile procedure?

10. How can a sterile field be kept sterile between set up and use?

11. How is informed consent obtained from a patient for a surgical procedure?

12. Describe how the skin of a surgical area is prepared.

____

____

____

13. Identify six ways that the medical assistant may assist a physician during surgery without wearing sterile gloves.

a. ____

b. ____

c. ____

d. ____

e. ____

f. ____

14. Identify three ways that a medical assistant who is wearing sterile gloves may assist the physician during surgery.

a. ____

b. ____

c. ____

15. Identify five ways to control bleeding during surgery.

a. ____

b. ____

c. ____

d. ____

e. ____

16. How may a medical assistant assist with skin closure?

____

____

____

17. Describe how an abscess or cyst may be treated in the medical office.

____

____

____

18. When does a laceration usually require stitches?

a. ____

b. ____

c. ____

d. ____

19. Briefly describe the following techniques, and identify when they are used.

a. electrocautery ______________________________

____

b. cryosurgery ______________________________

____

c. laser surgery ______________________________

____

d. microsurgery ______________________________

____

20. What is the difference between a dressing and a bandage?

____

____

21. When are the following bandage turns used?

a. circular ______________________________

b. spiral ______________________________

c. spiral reverse ______________________________

d. recurrent ______________________________

e. figure-of-eight ______________________________

22. What are five areas of instruction that should be given to a patient following minor surgery?

a. ______________________________

b. ______________________________

c. ______________________________

d. ______________________________

e. ______________________________

CRITICAL THINKING QUESTIONS

1. Discuss advantages and disadvantages for the physician and patient of performing minor surgical procedures in the medical office, in a day surgery center, or in the hospital. What criteria do you think most physicians use when deciding where to perform surgical procedures?

____

____

____

____

____

____

2. Look up information to discuss the difference between inflammation and infection. Discuss how the medical assistant can identify possible infection in a wound for which she is changing the dressing. Why should the physician always be asked to look at a wound if infection is suspected?

____

____

____

____

____

____

3. Prepare procedure cards for any surgical procedure performed in your office, including equipment and supplies for the sterile pack, other supplies, patient position, equipment and supplies for the physician, and other information about the procedure.

PRACTICAL APPLICATIONS

1. Place the name of each of the following instruments in the space provided. In addition, describe what the instrument is used for.

   a. instrument ______________________________________

   use ______________________________________

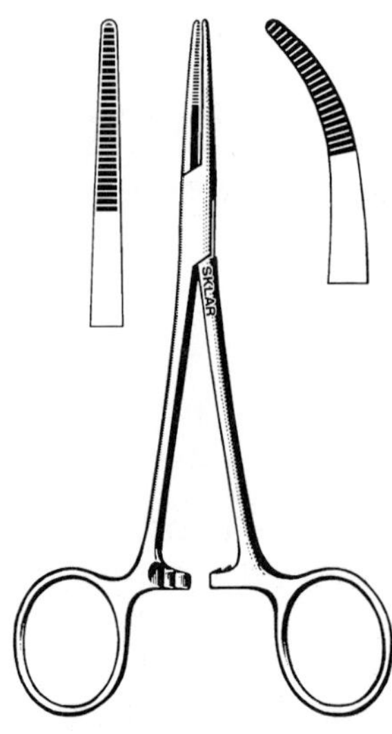

b. instrument ______________________________

use ______________________________

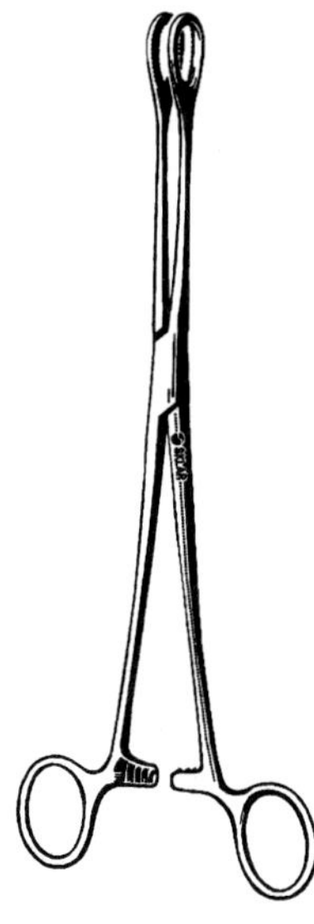

c. instrument ______________________________

use ______________________________

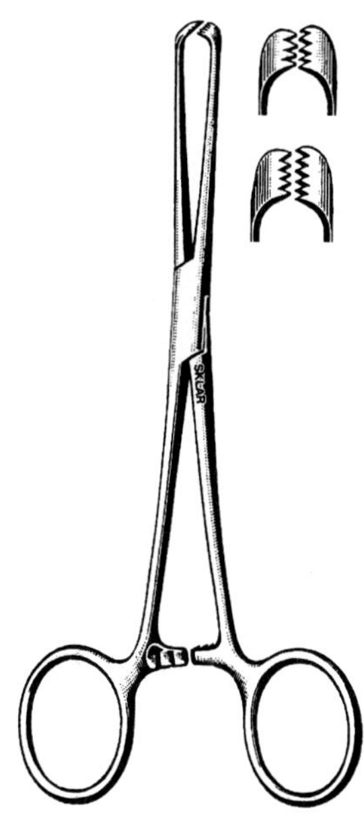

d. instrument ______________________________

use ______________________________

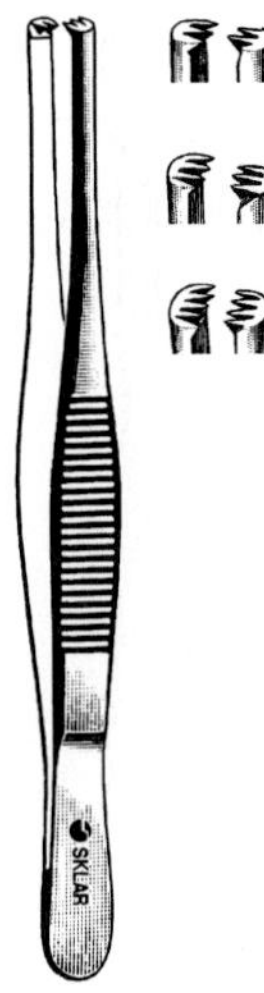

e. instrument ______________________________

use ______________________________

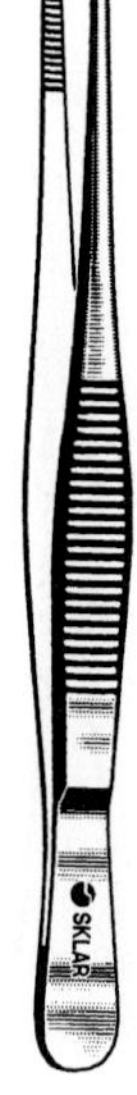

f. instrument ___

use ___

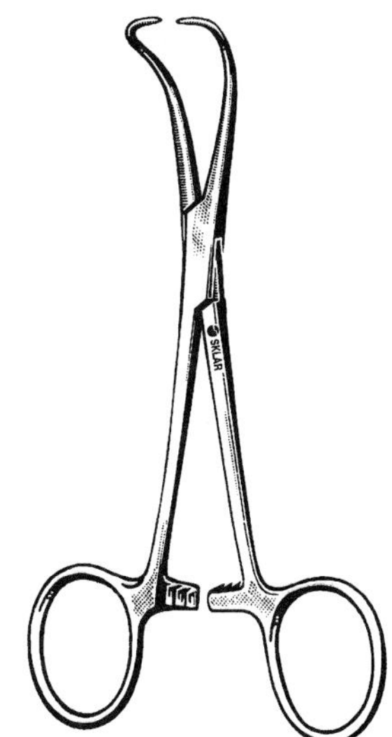

g. instrument ___

use ___

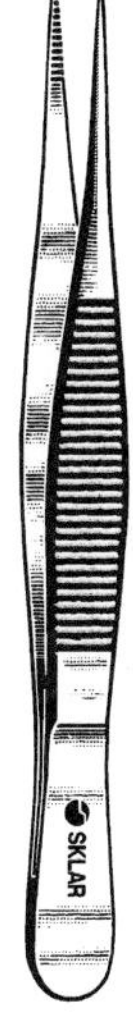

h. instrument ______________________________

use ______________________________

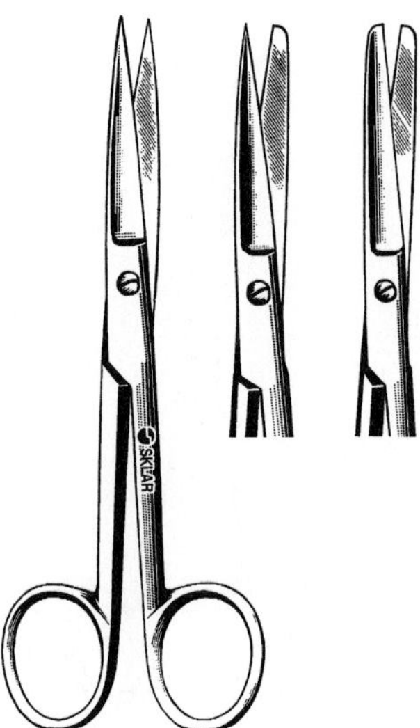

i. instrument ______________________________

use ______________________________

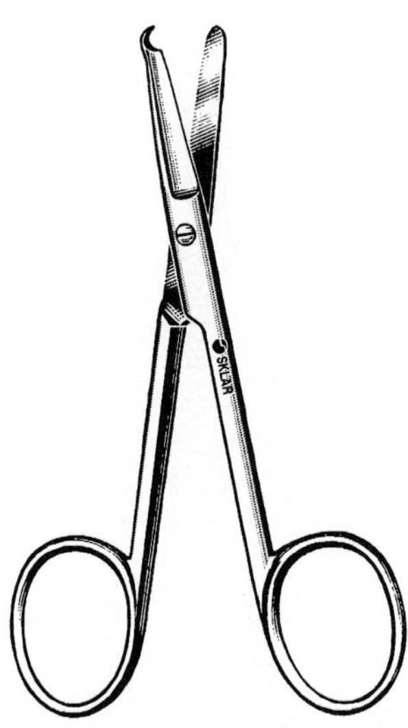

j. instrument ______________________________

use ______________________________

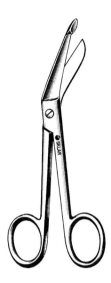

k. instrument ______________________________

use ______________________________

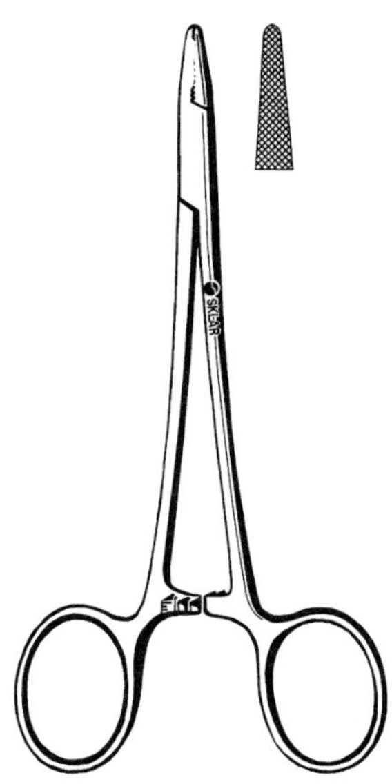

l. instrument ____________________

use ____________________

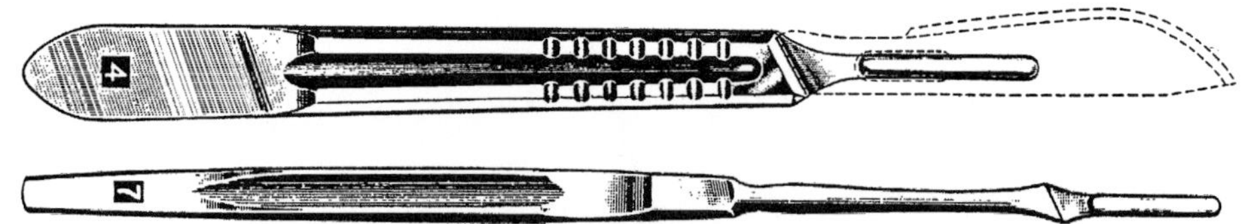

m. instrument ____________________

use ____________________

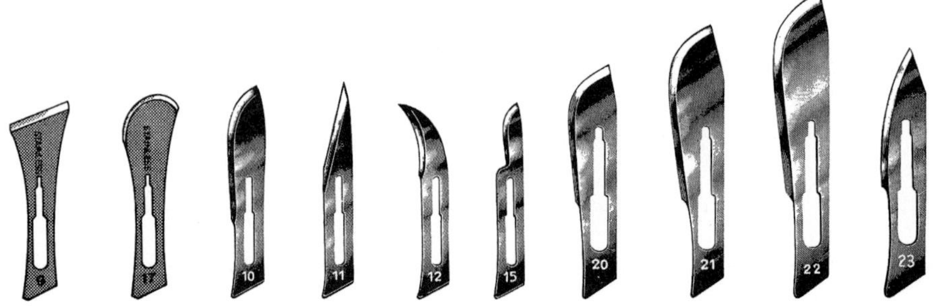

n. instrument ____________________

use ____________________

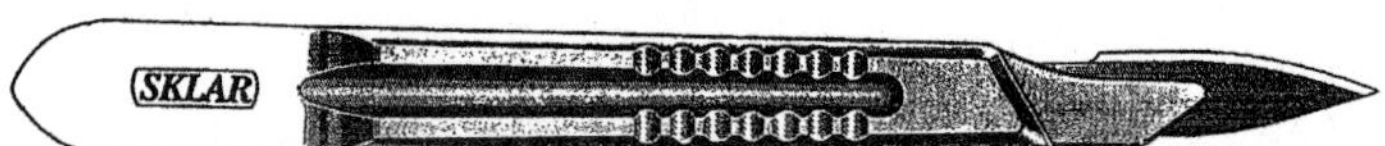

2. Prepare packs and supplies for the following, then open and set up a sterile field. When prepared, cover the sterile field with a sterile towel.

   a. Prepare a sterile field with two sterile bowls. Pour sterile water or normal saline into one bowl and povidone-iodine solution into the other. Add sterile gauze squares and sterile applicators to the sterile field.

   b. Prepare a sterile field for suture removal, including a sterile bowl, sterile gauze squares, suture removal scissors, and thumb (dressing) forceps. Pour hydrogen peroxide into the sterile bowl.

   c. Prepare a sterile field for a sterile dressing change, including a sterile bowl, gauze squares, thumb (dressing) forceps, and sterile dressing material. Pour antiseptic solution into the sterile bowl.

3. What bandage turn would be most appropriate for wrapping each of the following locations?

   a. the little finger ____________________

   b. the right ankle ____________________

   c. the head after suture of a scalp lesion ____________________

   d. a below-the-knee amputation ____________________

e. the left forearm ______________________________

f. the right calf when an elastic bandage is being applied to reduce swelling ____________

4. Complete exercises on Surgical Assisting in the Clinical Skills section of the CD-ROM.

PROCEDURE PERFORMANCE CHECKLISTS

Procedure 17-1: Surgical Aseptic Handwash

Performance Objective

Task: Perform a surgical aseptic handwash using correct technique

Conditions: Sink with foot or arm control for water and antimicrobial soap, sterile towels, disposable hand and nail brush

Standards: Complete the procedure in 10 minutes, and achieve a satisfactory score on the procedure performance checklist

Scoring Key: (**S**)*atisfactory,* (**U**)*nsatisfactory,* (**NA**) *Not Applicable*
◆ *Denotes a critical element for a satisfactory score on the procedure*

Procedure Steps	1st trial	2nd trial	3rd trial
1. Remove all jewelry and place for safekeeping.			
2. Open package of sterile towels.			
3. Using foot or arm controls, regulate water to comfortable warm temperature.			
4. Rinse hands and forearms, holding them with hands above forearms, above waist level.			
5. Clean under and around nails with brush or wooden orange stick.			
6. Apply soap to produce lather, scrub one hand and forearm, then the other, with brush, for at least 3 minutes each.			
7. Discard brush without touching sink or waste container.			
8. Rinse hands and forearms thoroughly, holding hands and arms up.			
9. Turn off water with foot or arm control or leave water running.			
10. Walk away from sink, holding hands above waist without touching any part of the sink.			
11. Pick up sterile towel without touching the package and dry one hand and arm.			
12. Drop towel.			
13. Use a second towel for the second hand and arm.			

Procedure Steps	1st trial	2nd trial	3rd trial
14. Drop towel.			
15. Continue to hold hands above the waist and in front of the body until sterile gloves can be put on.			
16. Complete the procedure within 10 minutes. ◆			

Evaluator Comments:

Score Calculation:

For each procedural step marked U (Unsatisfactory) deduct 6 points
For each procedural step (◆) marked U (Unsatisfactory) deduct 20 points

Score calculation 100 points

− points missed

	1st	2nd	3rd
Total score			

Satisfactory score: 85 or above

Procedure 17-2: Sterile Gloving

Performance Objective

Task: Put on sterile gloves using sterile technique

Conditions: Pair of sterile gloves in appropriate size

Standards: Complete the procedure in 3 minutes, and achieve a satisfactory score on the procedure performance checklist

Scoring Key: (**S**)*atisfactory,* (**U**)*nsatisfactory,* (**NA**) *Not Applicable*
◆ *Denotes a critical element for a satisfactory score on the procedure*

Procedure Steps	1st trial	2nd trial	3rd trial
1. Remove all jewelry, place for safekeeping, and perform surgical aseptic handwash. Dry hands with sterile towel.			
2. Place package of sterile gloves on clutter-free, flat surface that is at waist level.			
3. Open package, being careful not to touch sterile inner packaging.			
4. Grasp edge of inner packaging and pull paper open to expose both sterile gloves.			
5. With fingers and thumb of dominant hand, pick up the glove for the other hand by grasping the inside of the glove.			
6. Pick up the glove completely from the paper.			
7. Pull glove on without touching outside of glove.			
8. Using gloved hand, pick up the second glove by placing gloved fingers between folded cuff and fingers of second glove.			
9. Pick up the glove completely from the paper.			
10. Slide second hand into glove, being careful not to let gloved hand touch the skin of the hand you are gloving.			
11. Pull cuff away from arm as you slide hand into the glove, to prevent accidental contact between fingers of sterile glove and skin of your arm.			
12. Hold both gloved hands above waist.			
13. Adjust fingers for comfort.			
14. Do not touch anything unless it is sterile.			
15. Complete the procedure within 3 minutes. ◆			

Evaluator Comments:

Score Calculation:

For each procedural step marked U (Unsatisfactory) deduct 6 points
For each procedural step (◆) marked U (Unsatisfactory) deduct 20 points

Score calculation	100 points			
	– ___ points missed	1st	2nd	3rd
	Total score			

Satisfactory score: 85 or above

Procedure 17-3: Opening a Sterile Barrier Field

Performance Objective

Task: Drape a Mayo stand/tray with a sterile barrier field or cloth to create a sterile field

Conditions: Unopened package containing a sterile cloth or barrier field and Mayo stand or tray

Standards: Complete the procedure in 5 minutes, and achieve a successful score on the procedure performance checklist

Scoring Key: (**S**)*atisfactory,* (**U**)*nsatisfactory,* (**NA**) *Not Applicable*
◆ *Denotes a critical element for a satisfactory score on the procedure*

Procedure Steps	1st trial	2nd trial	3rd trial
1. Wash hands.			
2. Place the package containing the sterile drape on flat surface near Mayo stand or tray.			
3. Open package without touching drape.			
4. Pick up the barrier field as you move away from table and allow it to unfold without touching anything.			
5. Grasp corner of the long edge, and lay drape over Mayo stand/tray in one motion, without excess motion of the paper.			
6. Do not move drape once it touches stand/tray.			
7. Add sterile items to the sterile field without touching items.			
8. Never turn your back on the sterile field without covering with sterile towel.			
9. Complete the procedure within 5 minutes. ◆			

Evaluator Comments:

Score Calculation:

For each procedural step marked U (Unsatisfactory) deduct 6 points
For each procedural step (◆) marked U (Unsatisfactory) deduct 20 points

Score calculation	100 points			
	− ___ points missed	1st	2nd	3rd
	Total score			

Satisfactory score: 85 or above

Procedure 17-4: Opening a Sterile Surgical Pack

Performance Objective

Task: Open a sterile pack, using the inside of the pack as a sterile field

Conditions: Sterile pack containing sterile instrument(s) or supplies, package containing sterile gloves or sterile transfer forceps, Mayo stand or tray

Standards: Complete the procedure in 5 minutes, and achieve a satisfactory score on the procedure performance checklist

Scoring Key: (**S**)*atisfactory,* (**U**)*nsatisfactory,* (**NA**) *Not Applicable*
◆ *Denotes a critical element for a satisfactory score on the procedure*

Procedure Steps	**1st trial**	**2nd trial**	**3rd trial**
1. Wash hands.			
2. Place pack wrapped in paper or cloth that has been sterilized on the Mayo stand at waist level or higher.			
3. Check pack to be sure it has been sterilized within one month.			
4. Check tape to be sure it has changed color during sterilization.			
5. Remove tape that is holding pack closed.			
6. Grasp top flap by corner and pull first flap away from the pack. If needed, pick up the pack, unwrap, and rotate so that the first flap opens away from your body.			
7. Touching only corners, pull out one side flap and then the other, leaving last flap to open toward yourself.			
8. Touching only corners, pull final flap toward you.			
9. Fully extend corner and do not let any part of the wrap fall back toward the inside of the sterile field.			
10. Lay a package of sterile transfer forceps on a table beside the Mayo stand/tray and open the package.			
11. Touching only the forceps handles, arrange sterile items within the field if needed, OR			
11A. Put on sterile gloves, following steps of Procedure 17-2, and arrange sterile items within the sterile field.			

Procedure Steps	1st trial	2nd trial	3rd trial
12. Leave outer inch of sterile field free of objects.			
13. Add additional sterile items to the sterile field if necessary.			
14. Cover with sterile drape if the sterile field is not going to be used immediately.			
15. Complete the procedure within 3 minutes. ◆			

Evaluator Comments:

Score Calculation:

For each procedural step marked U (Unsatisfactory) deduct 6 points
For each procedural step (◆) marked U (Unsatisfactory) deduct 20 points

Score calculation	100 points			
	– points missed	1st	2nd	3rd
	Total score			

Satisfactory score: 85 or above

Procedure 17-5: Adding Sterile Solution to the Sterile Field

Performance Objective

Task: Pour a sterile solution into a container on a sterile field using sterile technique

Conditions: Bottle containing sterile solution, sterile field, with a sterile container already placed

Standards: Complete the procedure in 3 minutes, and achieve a satisfactory score on the procedure performance checklist

Scoring Key: (**S**)*atisfactory,* (**U**)*nsatisfactory,* (**NA**) *Not Applicable*
◆ *Denotes a critical element for a satisfactory score on the procedure*

Procedure Steps	1st trial	2nd trial	3rd trial
1. Wash hands.			
2. Obtain bottle of sterile solution and place beside the sterile field.			
3. Read label of sterile solution three times to ensure that what is to be poured is correct.			
4. Check expiration date.			
5. Place label of bottle toward palm of hand.			
6. Open bottle and place cap on counter with inside of cap facing up.			
7. Pour a small amount of liquid into the sink to cleanse the bottle lip.			
8. Approach sterile field, holding open bottle with label toward your hand.			
9. Pour desired amount into the sterile bowl or container on the field, holding the bottle 2 to 6 inches above the edge of the bowl.			
10. Avoid splashing or spilling.			
11. Do not touch any part of the sterile field.			
12. After pouring, replace cap on the bottle of sterile liquid.			
13. Complete the procedure within 3 minutes. ◆			

Evaluator Comments:

Score Calculation:

For each procedural step marked U (Unsatisfactory) deduct 6 points
For each procedural step (◆) marked U (Unsatisfactory) deduct 20 points

Score calculation 100 points

− ____ points missed

	1st	2nd	3rd
Total score			

Satisfactory score: 85 or above

Procedure 17-6: Preparing Skin for Minor Surgery

Performance Objective

Task: Prepare skin for a minor surgical procedure

Conditions: Antiseptic soap solution, gauze sponges, sterile gloves, razor, sterile basin, underpad with plastic backing (possibly second sterile basin for rinse)

Standards: Complete the procedure in 10 minutes, and achieve a satisfactory score on the procedure performance checklist

Scoring Key: (**S**)*atisfactory,* (**U**)*nsatisfactory,* (**NA**) *Not Applicable*
◆ *Denotes a critical element for a satisfactory score on the procedure*

Procedure Steps	1st trial	2nd trial	3rd trial
1. Wash hands.			
2. Assemble equipment.			
3. Identify patient.			
4. Check with patient and chart for any allergies to solution to be used, such as iodine or Betadine, and for shellfish allergy.			
5. Explain procedure and prep to patient.			
6. Open sterile basin(s) and pour solution(s).			
7. Open razor for surgical prep.			
8. Open gauze sponges and place underpad under area to be cleaned.			
9. Put on sterile gloves.			
10. Apply antiseptic soap with sterile gauze sponges, beginning at operative site, scrubbing for 2–5 minutes to ensure a thoroughly cleaned area.			
11. Do not break skin down with too much friction.			
12. Hold skin taut and shave hair in direction of hair growth if applicable.			
13. Scrub skin surface a second time after shaving, or at least twice if the area does not require shaving.			
14. If the doctor plans to clean the area again, wipe dry and cover with sterile towel.			

Procedure Steps	1st trial	2nd trial	3rd trial
15. If the doctor wishes the area to be rinsed, apply sterile solution from a separate sterile basin, using gauze sponges.			
16. Dry with gauze sponges or sterile towel and cover with sterile towel.			
17. Remove and discard sterile gloves.			
18. Replace soiled and/or wet underpad with clean, dry underpad.			
19. Wash hands.			
20. Complete the procedure within 10 minutes. ◆			

Evaluator Comments:

Score Calculation:

For each procedural step marked U (Unsatisfactory) deduct 6 points
For each procedural step (◆) marked U (Unsatisfactory) deduct 20 points

Score calculation 100 points

− points missed

Total score

1st	2nd	3rd

Satisfactory score: 85 or above

Procedure 17-7: Assisting with Minor Surgery

Performance Objective

Task: Assist in a minor surgical procedure

Conditions: Sterile pack, additional sterile items required for the procedure, sterile gown, sterile towels, sterile gloves for physician, sterile solution (if needed), sterile syringe and needle, local anesthetic, alcohol wipe, gooseneck lamp or other light source, specimen container with formalin

Standards: Complete the procedure in 30 minutes, and achieve a satisfactory score on the procedure performance checklist

Scoring Key: (**S**)*atisfactory,* (**U**)*nsatisfactory,* (**NA**) *Not Applicable*
◆ *Denotes a critical element for a satisfactory score on the procedure*

Procedure Steps	1st trial	2nd trial	3rd trial
1. Wash hands.			
2. Identify patient.			
3. Explain procedure to patient.			
4. Make sure patient has signed consent form.			
5. Adjust Mayo stand height for doctor and have additional stand or tray available for extra instruments.			
6. Assemble instruments and supplies.			
7. Set up sterile field and add any extra items needed using sterile technique.			
8. Use sterile gloves or transfer forceps to arrange items on the sterile field if needed.			
9. Cover sterile field with sterile towel.			
10. Beside sterile field, open outer package of sterile gloves, sterile towel, and sterile gown for physician.			
11. Set up next to surgical field additional wrapped sterile items and solutions (including local anesthetic) that may be needed during procedure.			
12. Position patient on examination or treatment table so the surgical site is accessible to the doctor.			
13. Position light so that there is adequate illumination.			
14. Prepare skin if necessary.			
15. Alert doctor that patient and equipment are ready.			

Procedure Steps	1st trial	2nd trial	3rd trial
16. Uncover field.			
17. Assist doctor to gown and glove.			
18. Wipe top of bottle of local anesthetic with alcohol and hold with label toward the doctor for doctor to draw up.			
19. Assist doctor as requested during procedure.			
20. Wearing sterile gloves, hand instruments to physician.			
21. Wearing sterile gloves, hold retractor if instructed.			
22. Wearing sterile gloves, sponge blood from operative site if necessary.			
23. Add items to the sterile field as directed.			
24. Provide comfort and encouragement to patient as needed.			
25. If tissue is removed, remove the lid from a specimen container and hold it so the doctor can drop the tissue specimen into it.			
26. Label any tissue specimen and complete the necessary requisition to an outside office for pathology/cytology.			
27. After suturing (if necessary), assist doctor with dressing and bandaging the wound.			
28. Be sure patient's condition is stable before he or she gets up.			
29. Check dressing for drainage.			
30. Instruct patient on home care of surgical site.			
31. Instruct patient when to return for follow-up if doctor has not already done so.			
32. Using appropriate PPE, clean room.			
33. Place disposable instruments and items contaminated with blood or body fluids in appropriate biohazard containers.			
34. Move reusable instruments to where they will be cleaned and sterilized.			
35. Use appropriate cleaning solution to ready room for next patient.			
36. Document any instructions you give to the patient on discharge.			
37. Document sending of any specimen to laboratory.			
38. Complete the procedure within 30 minutes. ◆			

Charting

DATE	

Evaluator Comments:

Score Calculation:

For each procedural step marked U (Unsatisfactory) deduct 6 points
For each procedural step (◆) marked U (Unsatisfactory) deduct 20 points

Score calculation 100 points

− points missed

Total score

1st	2nd	3rd

Satisfactory score: 85 or above

Notes

Procedure 17-8: Applying a Tubular Gauze Bandage

Performance Objective

Task: Apply a tubular gauze bandage

Conditions: Seamless tubular gauze bandage and applicator of appropriate size, dressing, tape, scissors

Standards: Complete the procedure in 5 minutes, and achieve a satisfactory score on the procedure performance checklist

Scoring Key: (**S**)*atisfactory,* (**U**)*nsatisfactory,* (**NA**) *Not Applicable*
◆ *Denotes a critical element for a satisfactory score on the procedure*

Procedure Steps	1st trial	2nd trial	3rd trial
1. Wash hands.			
2. Identify patient.			
3. Assemble applicator and tubular gauze bandage.			
4. Make sure tubular gauze is correct size for applicator.			
5. Cut a length of gauze that is 6 to 10 times longer than the extremity to be bandaged.			
6. Load applicator by stretching the gauze over it and feeding the length of gauze onto the applicator.			
7. Be sure that any open wound is covered by a sterile gauze dressing.			
8. Place applicator over extremity to be bandaged.			
9. Pull the first part of the tubular gauze from the applicator and hold with fingers at the proximal end of the extremity to be bandaged.			
10. Pull applicator away from the end you are holding until the entire extremity is covered with a layer of gauze and applicator is 1–2 inches beyond dressing.			
11. Rotate applicator one full turn to anchor bandage.			
12. Move applicator toward the extremity, adding a layer of gauze to the bandage.			
13. When applicator reaches the proximal end of the extremity, rotate one full turn to anchor.			

Procedure Steps	1st trial	2nd trial	3rd trial
14. Continue adding layers with a full turn at each proximal and distal end.			
15. Finish last layer at proximal end.			
16. Use tape to hold bandage in place or cut last part of tubular gauze into two sections and tie to hold bandage.			
17. Instruct patient when and how to remove or change bandage.			
18. Instruct patient when to return to office for follow-up.			
19. Document in the patient's medical record, including appearance of wound or skin under bandage.			
20. Complete the procedure within 5 minutes. ◆			

Charting

DATE	

Evaluator Comments:

Score Calculation:

For each procedural step marked U (Unsatisfactory) deduct 6 points
For each procedural step (◆) marked U (Unsatisfactory) deduct 20 points

Score calculation 100 points

− ______ points missed

Total score

1st	2nd	3rd

Satisfactory score: 85 or above

Procedure 17-9: Changing a Sterile Dressing

Performance Objective

Task: Change a sterile dressing maintaining aseptic technique

Conditions: Sterile dressing change kit that includes antiseptic solution, gauze sponges, thumb forceps or antiseptic swabs, disposable gloves, sterile gloves, small plastic bag, tape, and sterile dressing; culture tube with sterile swab

Standards: Complete the procedure in 10 minutes, and achieve a satisfactory score on the procedure performance checklist

Scoring Key: (**S**)*atisfactory,* (**U**)*nsatisfactory,* (**NA**) *Not Applicable*
◆ *Denotes a critical element for a satisfactory score on the procedure*

Procedure Steps	1st trial	2nd trial	3rd trial
1. Wash hands.			
2. Identify patient.			
3. Position patient for dressing change.			
4. Explain procedure to patient.			
5. Assemble supplies.			
6. Open disposable sterile kit.			
7. Remove plastic bag from top for use outside sterile field for disposal of items.			
8. Put on nonsterile gloves.			
9. Loosen tape on old dressing from edges to the middle.			
10. Remove dressing and place in plastic bag.			
11. If dressing is stuck to wound, use small amount of sterile water or hydrogen peroxide to loosen.			
12. Assess wound for signs of infection.			
13. If the wound is open and drainage is present, culture the wound using a sterile swab by running swab along the length of the wound and placing in a culture transfer tube.			
14. Squeeze tube to release formalin to preserve the specimen.			
15. If wound is open, with redness and/or drainage, ask doctor to check before re-dressing.			

Procedure Steps	1st trial	2nd trial	3rd trial
16. Remove nonsterile gloves and place in plastic bag.			
17. Wash hands.			
18. Set up sterile supplies; open or pour antiseptic solution.			
19. Put on sterile gloves.			
20. Clean wound using antiseptic solution with gauze and thumb forceps, or swabs, being careful not to irritate wound.			
21. Clean from center of wound to edge, using a new swab or gauze square each time you return to the center.			
22. Drop each used square or swab into the plastic bag.			
23. When all exudate is removed from wound, place sterile dressing material to completely cover the wound.			
24. Secure new dressing either with strips of tape or a bandage secured by tape or clips.			
25. Place culture container in plastic bag for transport to lab.			
26. Remove and discard sterile gloves in plastic bag.			
27. Dispose of all contaminated items in plastic bag.			
28. Dispose of plastic bag in biohazard waste container.			
29. Wash hands.			
30. Document observations, culture taken (if done), and dressing change in patient record.			
31. Complete requisition, place in pocket of transport bag, and place culture for lab pick-up.			
32. Complete the procedure within 10 minutes. ◆			

Charting

DATE	

Evaluator Comments:

Score Calculation:

For each procedural step marked U (Unsatisfactory) deduct 6 points
For each procedural step (◆) marked U (Unsatisfactory) deduct 20 points

Score calculation 100 points

− _____ points missed

	1st	2nd	3rd
Total score			

Satisfactory score: 85 or above

Notes

Procedure 17-10: Suture Removal

Performance Objective

Task: Remove sutures from a well-healed incision

Conditions: Sterile suture removal kit that includes thumb forceps, suture scissors, and gauze; antiseptic solution or antiseptic swabs; biohazard waste container; gloves

Standards: Complete the procedure in 10 minutes, and achieve a satisfactory score on the procedure performance checklist

Scoring Key: (**S**)*atisfactory,* (**U**)*nsatisfactory,* (**NA**) *Not Applicable*
◆ *Denotes a critical element for a satisfactory score on the procedure*

Procedure Steps	1st trial	2nd trial	3rd trial
1. Wash hands.			
2. Identify patient.			
3. Explain procedure to patient.			
4. Check medical record for number of sutures inserted.			
5. Position patient so incision is accessible.			
6. Assemble equipment.			
7. Open kit without touching contents.			
8. Pour solution into a sterile basin or open package of antiseptic swabs.			
9. Put on gloves.			
10. Clean area around sutures to dislodge any exudate buildup on suture material.			
11. Inspect incision to be sure that suture line is healed and clear.			
12. Using thumb forceps, gently find one knot of suture and lift upward.			
13. Slip scissor notch under knot and clip.			
14. Using thumb forceps, pull stitch straight up so the entire suture slips out of the incision.			
15. Lay suture on a gauze square.			
16. Repeat 11, 12, and 13 for each suture.			

Procedure Steps	1st trial	2nd trial	3rd trial
17. Count when all sutures are removed.			
18. Match number of sutures removed with number on chart.			
19. If any additional exudate or crusts are present, clean the wound again with more solution and dry.			
20. Apply dry dressing if necessary.			
21. Remove and discard gloves.			
22. Discard sutures, gauze, and disposable instruments in the appropriate biohazard waste containers.			
23. Instruct patient that the wound should be protected while it remains tender.			
24. Instruct patient on any further wound care.			
25. Document the procedure in the patient's medical record.			
26. Complete the procedure within 10 minutes. ◆			

Charting

DATE	

Evaluator Comments:

Score Calculation:

For each procedural step marked U (Unsatisfactory) deduct 6 points
For each procedural step (◆) marked U (Unsatisfactory) deduct 20 points

Score calculation 100 points
– points missed

	1st	2nd	3rd
Total score			

Satisfactory score: 85 or above

SELF-EVALUATION

Chapter 18

Taking Electrocardiograms

CHAPTER FOCUS

In this chapter you learned about the conduction system of electrical impulses through the heart and how electrical impulses are recorded. Without adequate circulation, the body cannot function properly. The electrocardiogram is a relatively simple test that provides valuable information to assess cardiac function, and medical assistants perform this test both as a screening test and when patients have symptoms of cardiac dysfunction. In addition this chapter provided information about other tests of cardiac function.

TERMINOLOGY REVIEW

Vocabulary Matching: Match each term with its definition.

___ 1. precordial
___ 2. ventricular fibrillation
___ 3. depolarize
___ 4. ischemia
___ 5. stylus
___ 6. somatic tremor
___ 7. baseline

A. The amount of electrical current going through an EKG machine reflected in the size of the complexes
B. Abnormality of the heart rate or heart rhythm
C. A change in EKG reading not caused by the heart's electrical impulse
D. Lack of heartbeat
E. A condition where deposits of cholesterol and lipids occur along the walls of arteries and arterioles, resulting in decreased flexibility of the blood vessels
F. A piece of pointed metal that moves to the right or left of the baseline on EKG tracing paper
G. The flat line that signifies no electrical activity

___ 8. plaque	H. Microscopic blood vessels whose walls are so thin that oxygen, carbon dioxide, glucose, and other substances can pass between them and the tissues
___ 9. stress testing	I. An electrocardiogram or cardiac monitoring done during exercise
___ 10. amplitude	J. To send electric current through the patient's chest in order to depolarize the entire heart so the SA node can reestablish a heartbeat
___ 11. atherosclerosis	K. When there is sudden change in the electrical charge of the cells, which allows an electrical impulse to begin flowing from one area to another
___ 12. artifact	L. Metal plates or metallic-coated paper tabs that conduct electricity
___ 13. electrode	M. Cream or solution used between the EKG electrodes and the skin to enhance electrical conduction
___ 14. intermittent	N. An erratic pulsation of cardiac cells that doesn't allow for sufficient blood to be pumped through the body
___ 15. lead	O. An area that undergoes necrosis due to interruption in blood supply
___ 16. arrhythmia	P. Not continuous, coming and going
___ 17. defibrillation	Q. Heart attack
___ 18. asystole	R. Combinations of electrodes used by an EKG machine to record the heart's electrical activity
___ 19. noninvasive	S. Not penetrating a body cavity
___ 20. electrolyte	T. Patches or deposits of cholesterol in arteries
___ 21. capillaries	U. EKG leads placed on the chest to view the activity of the heart in the horizontal plane
___ 22. repolarize	V. When the cells of the myocardium become able to contract again
___ 23. standardization	W. An unnatural baseline deflection caused by muscle tension or talking
___ 24. myocardial infarction	X. The action of making a mark on the EKG tracing to indicate which of three standard amplitudes is being used on the tracing

Definitions: Insert the correct word to complete the sentence.

1. The two upper chambers of the heart are called the ______________________________.
2. The ____________________ node is located in the inferior portion of the septum between the two atria.
3. The bundle of ____________________ is a group of specialized cardiac muscle fibers.
4. The heart muscle is called the ____________________.
5. The ____________________ fibers are nerve pathways that penetrate into both ventricles.

6. The partition that separates the sides of the heart is called the ____________________.

7. The ____________________ ____________________, or pacemaker, is located on the right atrial wall just below the entrance of the vena cava.

8. Membranous structures called ____________________ keep blood flowing in only one direction.

9. The two lower chambers of the heart are called ______________________________.

CONTENT REVIEW QUESTIONS

1. Describe the path of blood flow through the heart and body beginning from the left ventricle.

____

____

____

____

____

____

2. How is the pumping action of the heart regulated?

____

____

____

____

____

____

3. Trace the path of electrical impulses through the heart.

____

____

____

____

____

____

4. What is the purpose of electrocardiography?

____

____

____

____

____

____

5. What four pieces of equipment are necessary to take a standard 12-lead EKG?

   a. ______________________________

   b. ______________________________

   c. ______________________________

   d. ______________________________

6. What is the function of the electrode and electrolyte?

   ____

   ____

7. Identify the three standard leads (bipolar leads) and identify the electrical activity they record.

   a. ______________________________

   b. ______________________________

   c. ______________________________

8. How does the electrode on the right leg of the patient function?

   ____

   ____

   ____

9. Compare the appearance of the tracing of the augmented leads to the tracing of the bipolar leads.

   ____

   ____

   ____

10. Identify the three augmented leads (unipolar leads) and identify the electrical activity they record.

    a. ______________________________

    b. ______________________________

    c. ______________________________

11. Identify where the six precordial (chest) leads are placed.

    a. V_1 ______________________________

    b. V_2 ______________________________

    c. V_3 ______________________________

    d. V_4 ______________________________

    e. V_5 ______________________________

    f. V_6 ______________________________

12. What does standardization mean? How does standardization occur?

    ____

    ____

    ____

13. How does the speed of the paper correlate to the EKG tracing?

____

____

____

14. Draw a normal EKG heartbeat (lead II) in the space below and label each of the following: P wave, P-R interval, QRS complex, Q-T interval, ST segment, and T wave.

15. Identify what is happening in the heart during each of the following:

a. P wave ____

b. P-R interval ____

c. QRS complex ____

d. Q-T interval ____

e. ST segment ____

f. T wave ____

16. What information needs to be recorded when the medical assistant takes an EKG?

____

____

____

17. What are four types of artifact (unwanted deflection in the EKG tracing), and what can cause them?

a. ____

b. ____

c. ____

d. ____

18. Describe each of the following cardiac arrhythmias in terms of appearance and what is happening in the heart, and identify whether it is considered to be a serious arrhythmia.

a. PAC (premature atrial contraction) ____

____

b. PVC (premature ventricular contraction) ______

c. Third-degree heart block ______

d. Ventricular tachycardia ______

e. Ventricular fibrillation ______

19. When would Holter monitoring be ordered for a patient?

20. Why are Holter monitor electrodes larger and applied abrading the skin?

21. What instructions are given to a patient who is having a Holter monitor test?

22. What additional information does a stress test give a physician compared to a standard electrocardiogram?

CRITICAL THINKING QUESTIONS

1. Compare the advantages and disadvantages of single-channel and three-channel EKG machines for a medical office. What are some factors that may influence the type of machine used?

2. If the medical assistant identifies that artifact is present, what steps should be taken to correct the problem? Give specific examples.

3. When a patient is hooked up to cardiac monitoring, usually only two or three leads are used. Why would a smaller number of leads be adequate for monitoring when 10 leads are attached to take an electrocardiogram?

4. Find several resources to identify lead placement for Holter monitoring. What variations did you find? Why do you think there is more than one recommended system of placing leads?

5. A person can be taught to perform an EKG on the job in less than half an hour. What are the advantages to the medical assistant, the physician, and the patient if a medical assistant has had the additional training that you have received from studying the information in this chapter?

PRACTICAL APPLICATIONS

1. Write out how you would explain the electrocardiogram before beginning the test on a patient who had never had or seen one.

___
___
___
___
___
___

2. Describe how the medical assistant should adapt lead placement when taking an EKG for each of the following patients:

   a. a patient with a short leg cast (comes to the knee) ___
   ___

   b. a patient with an amputation of the left lower leg ___
   ___

   c. a patient with a large incision of the upper right arm covered by a bandage
   ___
   ___

   d. a patient with shortness of breath who states that he or she cannot lie flat ___
   ___

3. A patient wearing a Holter monitor calls the office and states that he or she is experiencing intense itching and discomfort around the electrodes. What would the medical assistant do?

___
___
___
___

4. Identify situations when you might want to do each of the following to improve the quality of an EKG tracing:

   a. decrease the standardization to one-half ___
   ___

   b. increase the standardization to double ___
   ___

   c. use an alcohol pad to clean the skin and reapply new electrodes ___
   ___

   d. move the patient to use a different plug or examination table ___
   ___

5. Working with the manual for the electrocardiograph machine that you are using for practice, determine how to do each of the following:

   a. increase and decrease the amplitude ______________________________

   ____

   b. adjust the standardization if it is more or less than 10 cm ______________________________

   ____

   c. run a single lead manually (on a single-channel machine) ______________________________

   ____

   d. change the speed at which the paper runs through the machine ______________________________

   ____

PROCEDURE PERFORMANCE CHECKLISTS

Procedure 18-1: Taking Electrocardiograms

Performance Objective

Task: Perform a 12-lead electrocardiogram

Conditions: Electrocardiograph machine with paper and patient cable, disposable tab electrodes (or metal limb electrodes with straps and suction cup chest electrodes, electrolyte pads, cream or liquid), alcohol prep pads, tissues, exam table, and gown/cape

Standards: Complete the procedure in 15 minutes, and achieve a satisfactory score on the procedure performance checklist

Scoring Key: (**S**)*atisfactory,* (**U**)*nsatisfactory,* (**NA**) *Not Applicable*
◆ *Denotes a critical element for a satisfactory score on the procedure*

Procedure Steps	1st trial	2nd trial	3rd trial
1. Wash hands.			
2. Identify patient.			
3. Explain procedure.			
4. Ask patient to remove clothing from waist up and instruct a female patient to put on gown or cape with opening in the front.			
5. Place patient in supine position.			
6. Assemble and prepare equipment. Plug in and turn on the machine.			
7. Place limb lead electrodes on nonbony areas.			
8. Remove paper backing of a disposable electrode and press tab firmly into position with the tab pointing upward on the legs and downward on the upper arms. **or**			
8A. If metal electrodes are used, place an electrolyte pad on the lower part of each leg and arm, position the metal electrode over it, and fasten the rubber strap.			
9. Be sure tab electrodes adhere completely. If there is difficulty, wipe the skin with an alcohol pad, allow to dry, then apply a new electrode.			

Procedure Steps	1st trial	2nd trial	3rd trial
10. For tab electrodes, remove backing without handling electrode and press firmly into place with tab pointing down. **or**			
10A. If Welch suction cup electrodes are used, apply a small amount of electrode cream or liquid where each electrode will be placed. **or**			
10B. Squeeze rubber bulb and place above the electrode cream to create suction.			
11. Attach all electrode wires from electrocardiograph to tabs (or electrodes).			
12. Enter any patient data your practice requires for identification.			
13. Make any needed adjustments to the machine.			
14. Instruct patient not to talk and to lie still.			
15. Press AUTO for automatic and the machine will perform the EKG tracing.			
16. Before disconnecting lead wires, check the tracing for artifacts, loose leads, and low voltage.			
17. If the tracing is not clear, baseline is deflected, or artifact appears, troubleshoot and repeat the tracing.			
18. Disconnect electrodes and wipe chest with tissue if bulbs and cream were used.			
19. Wash hands.			
20. Instruct the patient what to do next (either dress or wait to be examined).			
21. If necessary (e.g., single-channel tracing), mount the EKG. Fill in patient information on completed EKG.			
22. Place the completed EKG for the physician to review.			
23. Record that EKG was taken in patient record.			
24. Complete the procedure within 15 minutes. ◆			

Charting

DATE	

Evaluator Comments:

Score Calculation:

For each procedural step marked U (Unsatisfactory) deduct 6 points
For each procedural step (◆) marked U (Unsatisfactory) deduct 20 points

Score calculation 100 points

− ____ points missed

Total score

1st	2nd	3rd

Satisfactory score: 85 or above

Notes

Procedure 18-2: Applying a Holter Monitor

Performance Objective

Task: Apply a Holter monitor for 24-hour cardiac monitoring

Conditions: Holter monitor, replacement battery, magnetic or computer tape, patient diary, razor, alcohol swabs, disposable round electrodes with snap fasteners, skin-sensitive adhesive tape, carrying case with belt/shoulder strap

Standards: Complete the procedure in 20 minutes, and achieve a satisfactory score on the procedure performance checklist

Scoring Key: (**S**)*atisfactory,* (**U**)*nsatisfactory,* (**NA**) *Not Applicable*
◆ *Denotes a critical element for a satisfactory score on the procedure*

Procedure Steps	1st trial	2nd trial	3rd trial
1. Assemble and prepare equipment.			
2. Replace battery in monitor.			
3. Insert blank magnetic or computer tape into monitor.			
4. Wash hands.			
5. Identify patient.			
6. Ask patient to remove clothing from waist up and instruct a female patient to put on gown or cape with opening in the front.			
7. Wash hands.			
8. Explain procedure to patient.			
9. With patient in semi-Fowler or sitting position, identify lead locations on chest wall.			
10. Prepare skin by shaving any hair and, using an alcohol swab, abrading skin lightly.			
11. Let area dry.			
12. Place round electrodes with snap fastener in each prepared area by removing adhesive backing and firmly pressing electrode to skin surface.			
13. Attach lead wires to all electrodes.			
14. Attach lead wires to patient cable.			
15. Secure electrodes with adhesive, skin-sensitive tape.			
16. Plug monitor into EKG machine to test for baseline tracing.			

Procedure Steps	1st trial	2nd trial	3rd trial
17. Place electrode/patient cable so it comes out at waist level.			
18. Tape patient cable to patient's chest to allow movement but prevent lead wires from becoming disconnected.			
19. Place recorder in case.			
20. Attach case to belt or shoulder strap.			
21. Plug cable into Holter monitor.			
22. Make sure recorder is recording.			
23. Provide patient with verbal and written instructions about use, diary information to be kept, and when to return.			
24. Wash hands.			
25. Document in patient record.			
26. Complete the procedure within 20 minutes. ◆			

Charting

DATE	

Evaluator Comments:

Score Calculation:

For each procedural step marked U (Unsatisfactory) deduct 6 points
For each procedural step (◆) marked U (Unsatisfactory) deduct 20 points

Score calculation 100 points

– points missed

Total score

1st	2nd	3rd

Satisfactory score: 85 or above

SELF-EVALUATION

2. Discuss what additional knowledge a medical assistant who obtained a position working for a specialist such as a urologist, neurologist, or gynecologist might need to gain. How could he or she advance her learning and skills?

3. What personal feelings might the medical assistant have about artificial insemination that might make him or her reluctant to perform sperm testing and sperm washing? What should the medical assistant do if he or she does not approve of this procedure?

4. Why do you think the neurological examination is not usually performed in depth as part of the routine physical examination? What would be advantages and disadvantages of including it?

5. Patients with asthma often perform respiratory testing, called peak flow monitoring, at home. Find information about this test and describe how you would instruct the patient to perform it if ordered by the doctor.

6. Patients are sometimes referred to a testing facility for an electroencephalogram (EEG) to obtain a recording of brain waves. Find information about this test and its preparation in your area and describe how you would explain the test and instruct a patient to prepare for it.

PRACTICAL APPLICATIONS

1. Demonstrate and explain the steps in teaching a patient to perform an effective spirometry test. Identify specific ways to motivate the patient to breathe out completely and rapidly.

2. Write out how you would explain the reason and procedure for the following diagnostic tests in patient terms:

   a. catheterization

   b. colposcopy and/or LEEP procedure

   c. prostate-specific antigen test

   d. lumbar puncture

3. Prepare the sterile field and additional supplies for a lumbar puncture (if a lumbar puncture tray is available).
4. Prepare a pack and the sterile field for a colposcopy (if the supplies are available).
5. Prepare a sterile field for a catheterization and simulate the procedure on a mannikin.
6. Use the CD-ROM Case II (Raymond Johnson) to practice working with a patient with respiratory problems who will receive a spirometry test.

PROCEDURE PERFORMANCE CHECKLISTS

Procedure 19-1: Performing Spirometry to Measure Lung Volume

Performance Objective

Task: Perform spirometry to measure lung volume

Conditions: Spirometer, disposable mouthpiece and plastic tubing, nose clip, chair

Standards: Complete the procedure in 15 minutes, and achieve a satisfactory score on the procedure performance checklist

Scoring Key: (**S**)*atisfactory,* (**U**)*nsatisfactory,* (**NA**) *Not Applicable*
◆ *Denotes a critical element for a satisfactory score on the procedure*

Procedure Steps	1st trial	2nd trial	3rd trial
1. Wash hands.			
2. Identify patient.			
3. Explain procedure and purpose of test.			
4. Assemble equipment.			
5. Put new disposable mouthpiece and tubing on spirometer.			
6. Position patient in chair, sitting straight.			
7. Enter patient information using keypad.			
8. Apply nose clip if machine requires it.			
9. Instruct patient to take a deep breath and blow out as rapidly and forcefully as possible with lips around mouthpiece.			
10. Be sure machine is recording while patient is blowing out.			
11. Allow patient to rest for a few minutes.			
12. Repeat test until three good efforts have been recorded.			
13. Print results. Label with patient's name and date if not done by the machine.			
14. Place report in designated area for doctor to review.			
15. Record in medical record that spirometry was done and refer to report.			
16. Complete the procedure within 15 minutes. ◆			

Charting

DATE	

Evaluator Comments:

Score Calculation:

For each procedural step marked U (Unsatisfactory) deduct 6 points
For each procedural step (◆) marked U (Unsatisfactory) deduct 20 points

Score calculation 100 points

− points missed

Total score

1st	2nd	3rd

Satisfactory score: 85 or above

Procedure 19-2: Collecting a Sputum Sample

Performance Objective

Task: Instruct a patient on the proper collection of a sputum specimen, and assist in collection

Conditions: Sterile sputum specimen container, mask and goggles or face shield, lab coat or gown that is impervious to fluid, gloves

Standards: Complete the procedure in 10 minutes, and achieve a satisfactory score on the procedure performance checklist

Scoring Key: (**S**)*atisfactory*, (**U**)*nsatisfactory*, (**NA**) *Not Applicable*
◆ *Denotes a critical element for a satisfactory score on the procedure*

Procedure Steps	1st trial	2nd trial	3rd trial
1. Wash hands.			
2. Identify patient.			
3. Explain procedure to patient.			
4. Assemble equipment.			
5. Label specimen container.			
6. Put on mask, gown or lab coat, and gloves.			
7. Instruct patient on proper technique for collection.			
8. Encourage patient to cough deeply.			
9. Open specimen container and hold lid facing down but not touching anything.			
10. Hold container near patient's mouth, but avoid having anything touch the inside of the container.			
11. After specimen is collected, secure lid tightly.			
12. Place specimen in plastic laboratory transport bag.			
13. Clean and disinfect any surfaces that may have been contaminated by droplets while patient coughed.			
14. Dispose of gown and mask in biohazard bag.			
15. Remove soiled gloves, and discard in biohazard bag.			
16. Wash hands.			
17. Complete lab request and put in pocket of transport bag.			
18. Document that specimen obtained and sent to the laboratory.			
19. Complete the procedure within 10 minutes. ◆			

Charting

DATE	

Evaluator Comments:

Score Calculation:

For each procedural step marked U (Unsatisfactory) deduct 6 points
For each procedural step (◆) marked U (Unsatisfactory) deduct 20 points

Score calculation 100 points

− points missed

Total score

1st	2nd	3rd

Satisfactory score: 85 or above

Procedure 19-3: Performing Urinary Catheterization on a Female

Performance Objective

Task: Perform a urinary catheterization on a female patient

Conditions: Sterile, disposable urinary catheterization tray that includes sterile French catheter, sterile drapes, lubricant, sterile gloves, cotton balls, sterile forceps, Betadine or cleaning solution, specimen container with label, underpad

Standards: Complete the procedure in 20 minutes, and achieve a satisfactory score on the procedure performance checklist

Scoring Key: (**S**)*atisfactory,* (**U**)*nsatisfactory,* (**NA**) *Not Applicable*
◆ *Denotes a critical element for a satisfactory score on the procedure*

Procedure Steps	1st trial	2nd trial	3rd trial
1. Wash hands.			
2. Assemble equipment.			
3. Identify patient.			
4. Explain procedure to patient.			
5. Verify that the patient is not allergic to iodine or shellfish.			
6. Instruct the patient to undress from the waist down and provide a gown.			
7. Position the patient in the dorsal recumbent position on the examination table with an underpad under the patient's buttocks.			
8. Pull out the examination table extension to provide a work area.			
9. Open disposable sterile kit using aseptic technique.			
10. Touching only the edges, use the wrapping of the kit or a drape within the kit to form a sterile field directly beside the patient's buttocks.			
11. Holding fenestrated drape by corners, place it over exposed genital area.			
12. Put on sterile gloves.			
13. Open package of antiseptic solution and pour over cotton balls.			
14. Open lubricant and squeeze out a generous amount to lubricate the catheter tip for 2–3 inches.			
15. Place container near patient for urine collection. Remove lid of sterile specimen container.			

Procedure Steps	1st trial	2nd trial	3rd trial
16. Inform patient that you are beginning the procedure before you touch her.			
17. With nondominant hand, spread labia as far as possible and hold open without allowing to fall shut until catheter has been inserted. Reposition hand until you can visualize both the urethral opening and the vaginal opening.			
18. Using forceps in dominant hand, pick up one cotton ball that is saturated with antiseptic solution.			
19. In one motion, swipe down one side of labia and drop the cotton ball at the edge of the sterile field.			
20. Using two more cotton balls, clean the other side of the labia and the middle of the area between the labia.			
21. Drop the used forceps toward the edge of the sterile field.			
22. With dominant hand, pick up lubricated catheter, making sure the other end rests in the catheterization tray.			
23. Let patient know you are about to insert catheter.			
24. Insert catheter into urethral opening about 2–3 inches until urine begins to flow.			
25. Let some urine flow into the catheterization tray.			
26. Move sterile specimen container below urine flow.			
27. When sterile specimen container is full, let remaining urine flow into the catheterization tray.			
28. When urine stops flowing, gently remove catheter.			
29. Place lid on specimen container.			
30. Remove and discard all supplies in biohazard container. Measure the amount of urine in the tray before discarding.			
31. Before removing gloves, clean patient.			
32. If povidone (Betadine) solution has been used as an antiseptic, advise patient that genital area may be stained yellow for a few days.			
33. Place specimen in a plastic laboratory specimen bag and secure.			
34. Remove and discard gloves in biohazard waste container.			
35. Wash hands.			

Procedure Steps	1st trial	2nd trial	3rd trial
36. Complete lab request and place in pocket of specimen transport bag.			
37. Document procedure in the medical record. Indicate color and amount of urine removed and tests requested.			
38. Complete the procedure within 20 minutes. ◆			

Charting

DATE	

Evaluator Comments:

Score Calculation:

For each procedural step marked U (Unsatisfactory) deduct 6 points
For each procedural step (◆) marked U (Unsatisfactory) deduct 20 points

Score calculation 100 points
− ______ points missed

Total score

1st	2nd	3rd

Satisfactory score: 85 or above

Notes

Procedure 19-4: Performing Sperm Washing

Performance Objective

Task: Perform sperm washing techniques to prepare for intrauterine insemination

Conditions: 3 cc syringes with 18-gauge needles, microscope, slide marked with squares for counting sperm, centrifuge and two tubes, incubator, intrauterine catheters, sperm sample in sterile container, sperm washing medium, gloves, rigid biohazard container

Standards: Complete the procedure in 1 hour and 20 minutes, and achieve a satisfactory score on the procedure performance checklist

Scoring Key: (**S**)*atisfactory,* (**U**)*nsatisfactory,* (**NA**) *Not Applicable*
◆ *Denotes a critical element for a satisfactory score on the procedure*

Procedure Steps	1st trial	2nd trial	3rd trial
1. Wash hands.			
2. Obtain sperm sample in sterile container.			
3. Allow a frozen specimen to stand at room temperature for 10–15 minutes.			
4. Put on gloves.			
5. Open container and draw 2–3 cc of sperm into sterile 3 cc syringe using sterile 18-gauge needle.			
6. Place one drop of the sample on a slide marked with boxes for counting sperm.			
7. View under microscope for number of sperm and percent motility.			
8. Place sperm in a centrifuge tube.			
9. Add sperm washing medium in 3:1 ratio.			
10. Gently invert tube three times to mix.			
11. Centrifuge sperm at 15,000 RPM for 7 minutes. (If no pellet forms, another 2–3 minutes.)			
12. Hold tube with pellet facing up.			
13. Discard liquid (supernatant) in which pellet has been floating.			
14. Carefully add 1 cc fresh sperm washing medium to pellet.			
15. Allow to stand upright in 98.6°F incubator for 40–50 minutes.			
16. Draw up supernatant in IUI catheter attached to 3 cc syringe. Do not disturb pellet.			

Procedure Steps	1st trial	2nd trial	3rd trial
17. Place one drop of post-washed sperm on slide marked with boxes.			
18. View under microscope for number and motility.			
19. Inform doctor sample is ready for insertion.			
20. Clean area and dispose of used needles and syringes in a rigid biohazard container.			
21. Dispose of other materials contaminated with body fluid in biohazard bag.			
22. Remove and discard soiled gloves.			
23. Wash hands.			
24. Complete the procedure within 1 hour and 20 minutes. ◆			

Evaluator Comments:

Score Calculation:

For each procedural step marked U (Unsatisfactory) deduct 6 points
For each procedural step (◆) marked U (Unsatisfactory) deduct 20 points

Score calculation 100 points

− points missed

Total score

1st	2nd	3rd

Satisfactory score: 85 or above

Procedure 19-5: Assisting with the Neurological Exam

Performance Objective

Task: Assist a doctor with a neurological screening exam

Conditions: Percussion hammer, safety pin or neurological pinwheel, cotton balls, tuning fork, tongue blade, flashlight, ophthalmoscope, hot and cold water in test tubes, odorous substance

Standards: Complete the procedure in 30 minutes, and achieve a satisfactory score on the procedure performance checklist

Scoring Key: (**S**)*atisfactory,* (**U**)*nsatisfactory,* (**NA**) *Not Applicable*
◆ *Denotes a critical element for a satisfactory score on the procedure*

Procedure Steps	1st trial	2nd trial	3rd trial
1. Wash hands.			
2. Assemble equipment on a tray.			
3. Cover equipment.			
4. Identify patient.			
5. Explain purpose of exam and what doctor will be doing during exam.			
6. Perform mental status exam during history taking.			
7. Perform visual acuity test if applicable.			
8. Assist doctor as requested during exam by removing cover from the tray, handing instruments or supplies, and assisting the patient to move into different positions.			
9. When the physician tests heat and cold sensation, hold out test tubes containing hot and cold water.			
10. When the physician tests two-point discrimination, hold out an open safety pin or neurological pinwheel with the pointed end facing toward you.			
11. When the physician tests simple touch, hold out a cotton ball.			
12. Assist patient as needed during exam.			
13. Clean room and equipment after exam.			
14. Wash hands.			
15. Document vital signs and other findings in patient record as directed by doctor, or as noted during patient interview.			
16. Complete the procedure within 30 minutes. ◆			

Charting

DATE	

Evaluator Comments:

Score Calculation:

For each procedural step marked U (Unsatisfactory) deduct 6 points
For each procedural step (◆) marked U (Unsatisfactory) deduct 20 points

Score calculation 100 points

− ____ points missed

Total score

1st	2nd	3rd

Satisfactory score: 85 or above

Procedure 19-6: Assisting with Lumbar Puncture

Performance Objective

Task: Assist with a lumbar puncture

Conditions: Absorbent underpad, local anesthetic, disposable sterile lumbar puncture tray with all supplies, exam light, labels for specimen vials, plastic lab specimen bag, lab requisitions, rigid biohazard container

Standards: Complete the procedure in 30 minutes, and achieve a satisfactory score on the procedure performance checklist

Scoring Key: (**S**)*atisfactory,* (**U**)*nsatisfactory,* (**NA**) *Not Applicable*
◆ *Denotes a critical element for a satisfactory score on the procedure*

Procedure Steps	1st trial	2nd trial	3rd trial
1. Wash hands.			
2. Identify patient.			
3. Explain procedure to patient.			
4. Verify that patient (or parent) has signed consent form or obtain and witness signature on consent form.			
5. Verify that patient has emptied bladder and bowels (if possible).			
6. Assemble equipment.			
7. Instruct patient to undress completely and put on gown. (Provide privacy; assist if necessary.)			
8. Place Mayo stand or tray in position for equipment.			
9. Place absorbent pad under patient's buttocks.			
10. Position patient on side with knees drawn up to abdomen, grasping knees and flexing chin on chest.			
11. Cover patient leaving exposed area in lumbar region of the back.			
12. Reassure patient while doctor readies equipment for procedure.			
13. After the physician has prepared the area for insertion of the needle, assist the patient to arch the back as much as possible and hold the knees and neck.			
14. Reinforce to patient importance of maintaining position throughout procedure.			
15. Reinforce need for patient to breathe normally.			
16. Comfort patient as necessary.			

Procedure Steps	1st trial	2nd trial	3rd trial
17. When doctor directs, assist patient to straighten legs.			
18. Put on gloves to apply bandage to puncture site if directed by physician.			
19. Assist patient to a comfortable position to rest lying down for 2–3 hours. Provide comfort as necessary.			
20. Fill out laboratory requisition and labels.			
21. Put on nonsterile gloves.			
22. Label specimen tubes including order of filling (#1, #2, etc.).			
23. Place tubes and requisition forms into plastic laboratory transport bag.			
24. Clean up area and dispose of used supplies in appropriate biohazard containers.			
25. Remove soiled gloves and discard in biohazard waste container.			
26. Document procedure in patient record. Note specimens are being sent to laboratory.			
27. Complete the procedure within 30 minutes. ◆			

Charting

DATE	

Evaluator Comments:

Score Calculation:

For each procedural step marked U (Unsatisfactory) deduct 6 points
For each procedural step (◆) marked U (Unsatisfactory) deduct 20 points

Score calculation	100 points			
	− points missed	1st	2nd	3rd
	Total score			

Satisfactory score: 85 or above

SELF-EVALUATION

Chapter 20

Diagnostic Imaging

CHAPTER FOCUS

In this chapter you learned about diagnostic radiology and other types of diagnostic imaging. Although in most states medical assistants do not take radiographs, they often schedule procedures and instruct patients about proper preparation for various tests. The medical assistant must be able to provide accurate information about the ever-increasing number of diagnostic imaging procedures.

TERMINOLOGY REVIEW

Vocabulary Matching: Match each term with its definition.

___ 1. lateral projection

___ 2. positron emission tomography

___ 3. dosimetry

___ 4. transducer

___ 5. intravenous pyelogram

___ 6. radiologist

___ 7. contrast medium

___ 8. radiograph

A. The x-ray beam passes through the patient from front to back before striking the film

B. A substance that absorbs x-rays and highlights specific organs

C. The monitoring of an area and/or an individual to see how much radiation it has been exposed to over a period of time

D. Radiological study using continuous low-dose x-ray

E. An x-ray study of the urinary system that shows the kidneys, ureters, and bladder following injection of a contrast medium

F. The x-ray beam passes through the patient from one side to the other before striking the film

G. A diagnostic study that utilizes magnetic fields, in combination with radio waves and sophisticated computer technology, to create cross-sectional views of soft tissue

H. The x-ray beam passes through the patient at an angle to the body part being x-rayed.

___ 9. ultrasound	I.	A nuclear medicine scan that produces images in colors that vary, depending on how much of the radioactive material different cells absorb
___ 10. anteroposterior projection	J.	The x-ray beam passes through the patient from back to front before striking the film
___ 11. tomography	K.	An x-ray
___ 12. systemic	L.	A doctor who specializes in interpreting diagnostic radiology studies
___ 13. posteroanterior projection	M.	An instrument that sends and collects high-frequency sound waves during ultrasound examination or treatment
___ 14. magnetic resonance imaging	N.	A specialized radiological technique used to produce multiple images in selected planes of tissue
___ 15. oblique projection	O.	Affecting the entire body and not just a single area
___ 16. fluoroscopy	P.	Also called diagnostic medical sonography, it uses high-frequency sound waves to create images

Abbreviations: Expand each abbreviation to its complete form.

1. AP ______________________________
2. CT ______________________________
3. IVP ______________________________
4. lat ______________________________
5. MRI ______________________________
6. NPO ______________________________
7. PA ______________________________
8. PET ______________________________
9. SPECT ______________________________

CONTENT REVIEW QUESTIONS

1. Discuss why bones show up white on an x-ray, whereas other structures are gray or white.

____

____

____

2. When is a contrast medium used for x-ray?

____

____

____

3. Identify two common contrast media and describe the types of studies for which they are commonly used.

Contrast medium: Used for:

a. ______________________ ____

b. ______________________ ____

4. What is the advantage of performing procedures using fluoroscopy?

____

____

5. What material completely prevents penetration of x-ray?

____

6. What parts of the body are most likely to be damaged by exposure to x-ray?

____

____

7. What items are used to protect sensitive parts of the body from exposure to x-ray?

____

____

8. Describe how dosimetry is used to measure exposure to x-ray.

____

____

9. Why is a bowel preparation necessary for x-rays of the gastrointestinal tract, gallbladder, or urinary system?

____

____

____

10. What is the purpose of an upper GI series (barium swallow)?

____

____

____

11. What is the purpose of a barium enema?

____

____

____

12. What might be seen on a cholecystogram or cholangiogram (x-ray of the bile vessels)?

____

____

____

13. What allergies may indicate that a patient could be sensitive to the contrast medium used for an intravenous pyelogram or angiogram?

14. Describe how an intravenous pyelogram is done and what it shows.

15. What is the purpose of mammography? When are mammograms recommended?

16. Why is a consent form required before an angiogram?

17. When is a bone density study done?

18. Why is computed tomography a more useful test to detect tumors than ordinary x-rays?

19. What is the difference between tests done using x-ray and tests that are done by the nuclear medicine department?

20. What type of energy is used for ultrasound (diagnostic medical sonography)?

21. What is the advantage of using ultrasound to form diagnostic images?

22. What are some common tests using ultrasound?

23. What type of energy is used for magnetic resonance imaging?

24. Which patients cannot have an MRI because of possible danger to the patient?

25. What are some common reasons for the physician to order an MRI?

CRITICAL THINKING QUESTIONS

1. In many states, medical assistants are not allowed to perform diagnostic x-rays, but radiologic technologists often perform the duties of medical assistants when there are no patients who need x-rays. Discuss the fairness of this. Back up your opinions with facts and data if possible.

2. Do you think that the increased use of expensive diagnostic equipment has put excessive pressure on community hospitals and city hospitals serving low-income populations? Why or why not?

3. Find out where your own physician (or any local physician) would send you to have the following diagnostic tests: pelvic ultrasound, barium enema, thyroid scan, MRI of the knee, mammogram, PET scan, thallium scan. What factors determine where a patient ends up having a diagnostic test?

4. Locate specific information on the Internet about at least three diagnostic tests discussed in this chapter, and print a copy. Examine these resources carefully and give reasons why you think they are accurate and complete, or describe what should be added or changed.

5. It is recommended that women of childbearing age avoid x-rays unless they are sure that they are not pregnant and that such women should always be asked if there is any possibility that they are pregnant before an x-ray is scheduled or done. Find information about possible dangers of x-ray to a fetus, especially in early pregnancy, and discuss the possible legal liability of health care personnel if a pregnant woman receives x-rays.

PRACTICAL APPLICATIONS

1. Identify the patient positions and their abbreviations (if any) for each of the following x-rays:

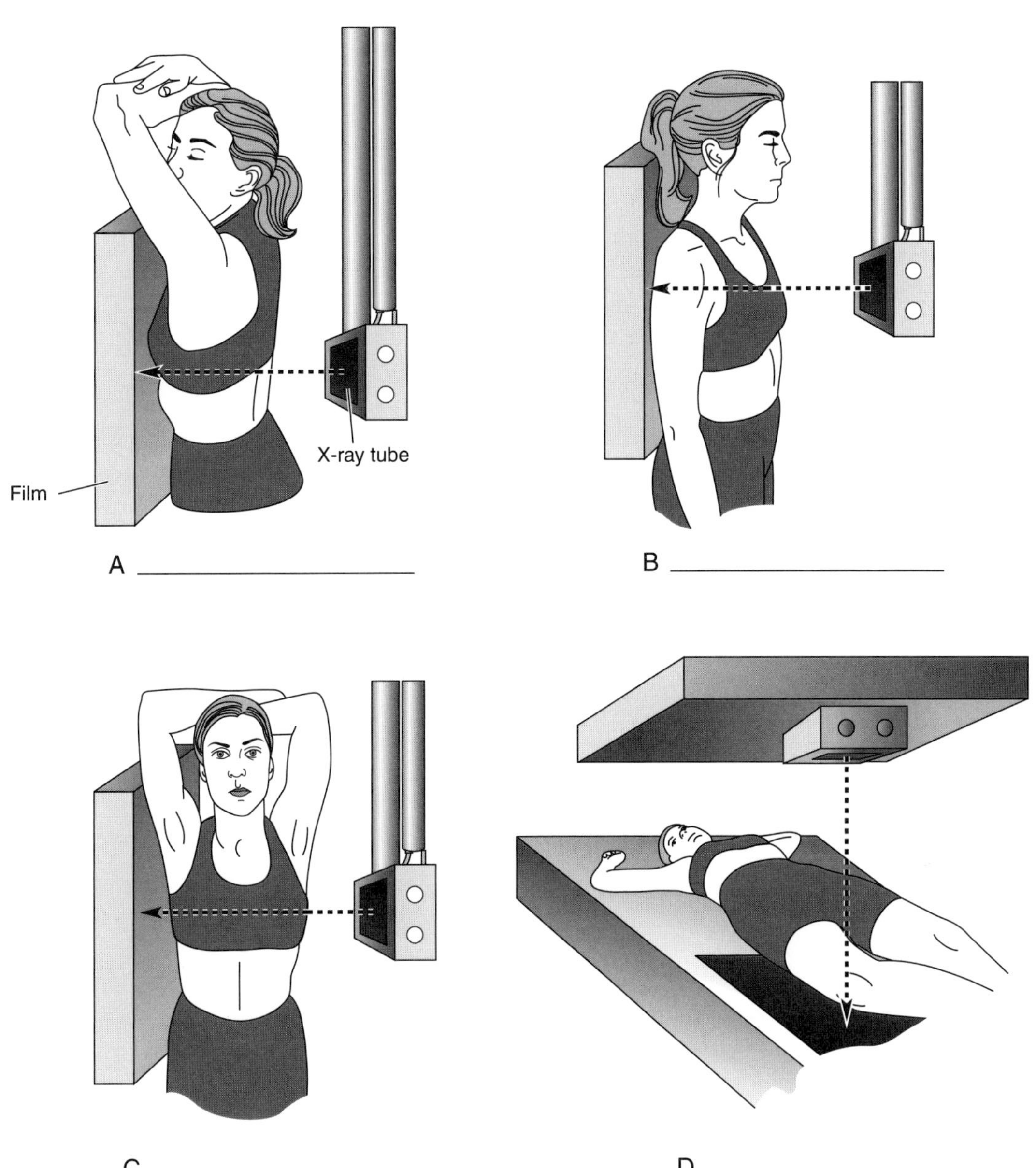

2. Describe how you would answer the following questions from patients regarding diagnostic tests:
   a. "Where should I get the magnesium citrate to prepare for my cholecystogram?"

      ___

      ___

   b. "What type of 'fat-free' meal should I eat the night before my test?"

      ___

      ___

   c. "Why do I have to take enemas on the morning of my barium enema?"

      ___

      ___

   d. "Am I going to be radioactive after my thyroid scan?"

      ___

      ___

   e. "I don't like being closed in. Will the MRI bother me? Will the CT scan bother me?"

      ___

      ___

   f. "I have already had x-rays several times this year. Am I getting too much radiation?"

      ___

      ___

   g. "Do I have to have my mammogram at Memorial Hospital? I live much closer to the university medical clinic."

      ___

      ___

3. Obtain information sheets from local hospitals or imaging facilities and instruct one of your classmates about preparation for the following diagnostic tests:
   a. upper GI series
   b. barium enema
   c. cholecystogram
   d. intravenous pyelogram
   e. pelvic ultrasound
   f. mammogram
   g. cardiac catheterization (coronary angiogram)
   h. CT scan of the abdomen

SELF-EVALUATION

Chapter 21

Assisting with Treatments

CHAPTER FOCUS

In this chapter you learned how to assist with treatments for patients during the office visit. These procedures are ordered by the physician in response to the patient's disease or condition. The medical assistant assists in treating the patient in the office and often instructs the patient how to follow up and/or continue similar treatments at home.

TERMINOLOGY REVIEW

Vocabulary Matching: Match each term with its definition.

___ 1. cast
___ 2. open reduction
___ 3. irrigation
___ 4. vasodilation
___ 5. hypotonic
___ 6. subluxation
___ 7. nebulizer
___ 8. traction
___ 9. vasoconstriction

A. A wet mist, the medium in which medicated fluid is delivered to the lungs from a nebulizer
B. Wasting of muscle that often occurs when an extremity is in a cast
C. Corner of the eye
D. A hard covering to hold a fracture in place during bone healing
E. Placing the bones into alignment without surgically opening the skin over the fracture
F. Treatment with cold
G. The injury that occurs when a bone is displaced from the articular surface of the joint
H. A break in the bone
I. A solution that contains fewer particles than another

__ 10. strain
__ 11. aerosol
__ 12. isotonic
__ 13. closed reduction
__ 14. fracture
__ 15. canthus
__ 16. atrophy
__ 17. cryotherapy
__ 18. pinna
__ 19. splint
__ 20. dislocation
__ 21. hypertonic solution

J. Application of a large amount of fluid to an area
K. Having the same concentration of electrolytes
L. Widening of the blood vessels
M. A device with a mouthpiece or mask through which a patient can receive an inhalation treatment
N. Aligning bones after surgical opening is made at the fracture site with the insertion of screws, rods, etc. to hold bone ends in place
O. Ear flap
P. A device to immobilize a suspected fracture during transport
Q. An injury to a muscle and the tendons that support the muscle, caused by overstretching
R. Partial dislocation
S. Using weight to pull on bone ends
T. Narrowing of the blood vessels
U. A solution that contains a greater concentration of particles than another

Abbreviations: Expand each abbreviation to its complete form.

1. UV __________
2. PT __________
3. MDI __________
4. ORIF __________
5. OT __________
6. POP cast __________
7. TENS __________
8. RICE __________

CONTENT REVIEW QUESTIONS

1. Identify four situations where an irrigation might be used.

   a. __________
   b. __________
   c. __________
   d. __________

2. Why is normal saline (0.9% sodium chloride solution) often used as an irrigating solution?

____

____

3. When irrigating the eye, how does the medical assistant prevent cross-contamination with the other eye?

____

____

4. Why should the medical assistant take special care to avoid touching the tip of the syringe for eye irrigation or an eye dropper to any part of the eye?

____

____

5. After instilling eye drops or ointment, why should the medical assistant instruct the patient to roll the eye around slowly?

____

____

6. How should the medical assistant straighten the ear canal before ear irrigation or instillation of an adult?

____

____

Of a child?

____

____

7. Why should irrigating solution for the ear be directed upward toward the top of the external auditory canal?

____

____

8. What are two methods for introducing medication into the lungs?

a. _______________

b. _______________

9. Why might the physician instruct the patient to use a plastic chamber or spacer with a metered-dose inhaler?

____

____

10. What are the advantages of applying moist heat or cold compared to dry heat or cold treatments?

____

____

11. What is the maximum heat that should actually be applied during heat treatments?

____

12. What does heat do and when is it used?

____

____

____

13. What does cold do and when is it used?

____

____

____

14. When should sterile supplies be used for moist compresses?

____

____

15. Why should heat and ice packs be wrapped in a layer of cloth?

____

____

16. What are four methods for delivering dry heat?

a. ____

b. ____

c. ____

d. ____

17. What are four ways to make an ice or cold pack?

a. ____

b. ____

c. ____

d. ____

18. What is the difference between a strain and a sprain? Will this show on x-ray?

____

____

19. Identify the following types of fractures:

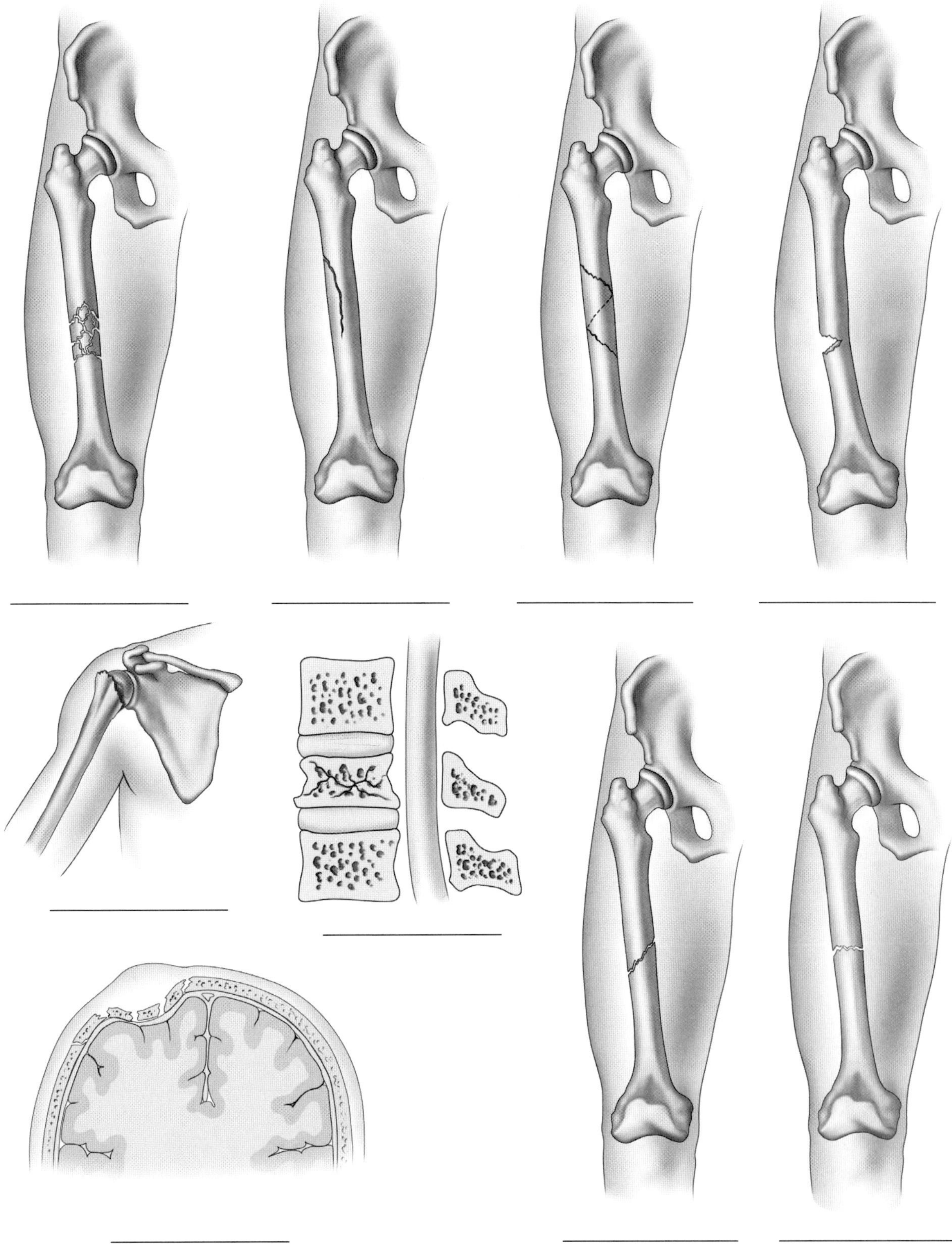

20. What is the usual treatment for strains and sprains?

____

____

21. If a patient sustains a fracture or fracture dislocation, what are two methods for reducing the fracture?

a. ____________________

b. ____________________

22. Differentiate between a cast and a splint.

____

____

____

23. What are four potential problems with casts?

a. ____________________

b. ____________________

c. ____________________

d. ____________________

24. What is a sling used for?

____

____

25. Describe briefly how each of the following is used as a treatment:

a. Ultraviolet light ____________________

____

b. Ultrasound ____________________

____

c. Electrical stimulation ____________________

____

d. Traction ____________________

____

e. Massage ____________________

____

CRITICAL THINKING QUESTIONS

1. Describe the advantages of using fiberglass as a casting material. List as many as you can think of. Try for at least six.

2. Do research about the therapeutic benefits and types of massage. Find out if there are educational programs for massage therapists in your area. Discuss the benefits of massage with your classmates.

3. What could happen if a person uses heat for an acute injury like a back sprain? How would you explain the rationale for using cold instead of heat for an acute injury?

PRACTICAL APPLICATIONS

1. Doctor Hughes has told a patient to use a heating pad at home on the lower back for 20 minutes three times a day. Write down the instructions you would give to the patient.

2. Write down what you would you tell a patient wearing a short arm cast who is about to have it removed. The doctor wants the patient to use a mild soap followed by a mild lotion on the arm and to perform arm exercises to flex, extend, and rotate the elbow, wrist, and fingers three times a day. Write down what you would tell the patient. You may refer to Chapter 33 for a description of normal range of motion of the arm.

____

____

____

____

____

____

____

3. Prepare a procedure card for assisting with application of a fiberglass cast based on Procedure 21-8.

4. What would you do if you accidentally touched a patient's eye with the dropper while instilling eye medication? If you accidentally touched the inside of the ear while instilling ear medication? What if the patient appears to be injured?

____

____

____

____

____

PROCEDURE PERFORMANCE CHECKLISTS

Procedure 21-1: Performing an Eye Irrigation

Performance Objective

Task: Cleanse an eye to remove a foreign substance or flush a harmful chemical

Conditions: Sterile irrigation solution and sterile container for solution, sterile bulb syringe, kidney-shaped basin, sterile gauze or cotton balls, draping towel, gloves, biohazard waste container

Standards: Complete the procedure in 10 minutes, and achieve a satisfactory score on the procedure performance checklist

*Scoring Key: (**S**)atisfactory, (**U**)nsatisfactory, (**NA**) Not Applicable*
◆ *Denotes a critical element for a satisfactory score on the procedure*

Procedure Steps	1st trial	2nd trial	3rd trial
1. Wash hands.			
2. Identify patient.			
3. Explain procedure to patient.			
4. Assemble equipment.			
5. Position patient with head turned toward affected side.			
6. Place a water-resistant draping towel over patient's shoulder to catch any drips.			
7. Check label of sterile solution bottle for correctly ordered medication.			
8. Warm solution by placing closed bottle under running hot water.			
9. Check expiration date.			
10. Open sterile container and place beside patient without touching inside.			
11. Open sterile solution bottle.			
12. Pour sterile solution into sterile container. (If using prepared eye irrigation solution, open bottle.)			
13. Open package of sterile bulb syringe.			
14. Put on disposable gloves.			
15. Ask patient to look up and fix gaze on object on wall.			

Procedure Steps	1st trial	2nd trial	3rd trial
16. Hold patient's eye open by pulling on lower eyelid with thumb of nondominant hand and top eyelid with forefinger.			
17. Fill syringe with irrigating solution.			
18. Instruct the patient to hold the kidney basin tightly against cheek.			
19. Irrigate affected eye with solution from inner canthus to outer canthus.			
20. Do not allow tip of syringe to touch the eye or eyelids.			
21. Continue irrigation for the length of time or amount of solution ordered by the physician.			
22. Dry eyelid and eyelashes with sterile gauze or cotton balls.			
23. Discard waste in biohazard container.			
24. Remove and discard gloves in biohazard container.			
25. Wash hands.			
26. Document procedure, including amount and type of solution using correct abbreviations for eye(s) irrigated.			
27. Complete the procedure within 10 minutes. ◆			

Charting

DATE	

Evaluator Comments:

Score Calculation:

For each procedural step marked U (Unsatisfactory) deduct 6 points
For each procedural step (◆) marked U (Unsatisfactory) deduct 20 points

Score calculation	100 points			
	– points missed	1st	2nd	3rd
	Total score			

Satisfactory score: 85 or above

Notes

Procedure 21-2: Instilling Eye Medication

Performance Objective

Task: Instill medication into a patient's eye as ordered by doctor

Conditions: Non-sterile gloves, bottle of eye drops or tube of eye ointment, gauze pads

Standards: Complete procedure in 5 minutes, and achieve a satisfactory score on the procedure performance checklist

Scoring Key: (**S**)*atisfactory*, (**U**)*nsatisfactory*, (**NA**) *Not Applicable*
◆ *Denotes a critical element for a satisfactory score on the procedure*

Procedure Steps	1st trial	2nd trial	3rd trial
1. Obtain chart with doctor's medication order.			
2. Obtain correct medication and compare to medication order.			
3. Check expiration date.			
4. Identify patient.			
5. Explain procedure to patient.			
6. Place patient in sitting or supine position.			
7. Wash hands.			
8. Put on gloves.			
9. Ask patient to look up.			
10. Using sterile 2 x 2 gauze pad with nondominant hand, gently pull lower eyelid down to expose conjunctiva.			
11. Discard first bead of ointment or drop of medication.			
12. Place drop of medication in center of lower conjunctiva or ointment along lower conjunctiva from inner to outer canthus.			
13. Do not touch tip of dropper or tube to the eye or lashes.			
14. Ask patient to close eye and roll eyeball to distribute medication.			
15. Blot excess with another sterile gauze square from inner to outer canthus.			
16. Assess patient for any adverse reaction.			
17. Throw away supplies in biohazard waste container.			

Procedure Steps

Procedure Steps	1st trial	2nd trial	3rd trial
18. Remove and discard soiled gloves in biohazard waste container.			
19. Give patient verbal and written instructions about future care.			
20. Document administration and instructions in chart using correct abbreviation for eye(s) treated.			
21. Complete the procedure within 5 minutes. ◆			

Charting

DATE	

Evaluator Comments:

Score Calculation:

For each procedural step marked U (Unsatisfactory) deduct 6 points
For each procedural step (◆) marked U (Unsatisfactory) deduct 20 points

Score calculation 100 points

− points missed

Total score

1st	2nd	3rd

Satisfactory score: 85 or above

Procedure 21-3: Performing an Ear Irrigation

Performance Objective

Task: Irrigate ear to remove foreign matter

Conditions: Irrigation solution, container for irrigation solution, bulb syringe or 10 cc syringe, ear basin for returned solution, plastic drape, gauze or cotton balls, gloves, biohazard waste container

Standards: Complete the procedure in 10 minutes, and achieve a satisfactory score on the procedure performance checklist

Scoring Key: (**S**)*atisfactory,* (**U**)*nsatisfactory,* (**NA**) *Not Applicable*
◆ *Denotes a critical element for a satisfactory score on the procedure*

Procedure Steps	1st trial	2nd trial	3rd trial
1. Wash hands.			
2. Identify patient.			
3. Explain procedure to patient.			
4. Assemble equipment.			
5. Position patient in sitting or supine position with head turned toward affected ear.			
6. Apply waterproof drape under ear and cover patient's shoulder.			
7. Place ear basin under ear to catch irrigation fluid.			
8. Check label on solution to be sure it is solution ordered.			
9. Check expiration date.			
10. Put on gloves and apron.			
11. Pour solution into container.			
12. Fill syringe with solution.			
13. Place cotton balls and gauze squares near filled syringe and basin.			
14. Straighten adult auditory canal by gently pulling pinna up and back. (For a child pull out and straight back.)			
15. Gently insert tip of bulb or syringe.			
16. Direct solution upward with mild force.			
17. Continue irrigation as ordered by doctor.			
18. Discard waste in appropriate biohazard containers.			

Procedure Steps	1st trial	2nd trial	3rd trial
19. Remove and discard gloves in biohazard container.			
20. Wash hands.			
21. Document in patient record identifying ear(s) irrigated. Estimate amount of cerumen or other matter that was removed.			
22. Complete the procedure within 10 minutes. ◆			

Charting

DATE	

Evaluator Comments:

Score Calculation:

For each procedural step marked U (Unsatisfactory) deduct 6 points
For each procedural step (◆) marked U (Unsatisfactory) deduct 20 points

Score calculation 100 points

– ___ points missed

Total score

1st	2nd	3rd

Satisfactory score: 85 or above

Procedure 21-4: Instilling Ear Medication

Performance Objective

Task: Instill drops into ear as ordered by doctor

Conditions: Ear drops in self-dropper bottle or separate sterile ear dropper, gauze pads, gloves

Standards: Complete the procedure in 5 minutes, and achieve a satisfactory score on the procedure performance checklist

Scoring Key: (**S**)*atisfactory,* (**U**)*nsatisfactory,* (**NA**) *Not Applicable*
◆ *Denotes a critical element for a satisfactory score on the procedure*

Procedure Steps	1st trial	2nd trial	3rd trial
1. Obtain chart with doctor's medication order.			
2. Obtain correct medication and compare to medication order.			
3. Check expiration date.			
4. Assemble supplies.			
5. Identify patient.			
6. Explain procedure to patient.			
7. Place patient in sitting or supine position with affected ear tilted up.			
8. Wash hands.			
9. Put on gloves and apron.			
10. Using nondominant hand, gently pull pinna up and back. (For a child, pull out and straight back.)			
11. Place ordered amount of medication in ear.			
12. Do not touch tip of dropper to any part of the ear.			
13. Instruct the patient to remain in position for 2–3 minutes.			
14. Insert an ear plug or portion of a cotton ball in ear if directed by physician.			
15. Discard waste in biohazard container.			
16. Remove and discard gloves in biohazard container.			

Procedure Steps	1st trial	2nd trial	3rd trial
17. Assess patient for any adverse reaction.			
18. Provide verbal and written instructions for continued treatment.			
19. Document administration and instructions in patient chart including ear(s) treated.			
20. Complete the procedure within 5 minutes. ◆			

Charting

DATE	

Evaluator Comments:

Score Calculation:

For each procedural step marked U (Unsatisfactory) deduct 6 points
For each procedural step (◆) marked U (Unsatisfactory) deduct 20 points

Score calculation 100 points

− points missed

Total score

1st	2nd	3rd

Satisfactory score: 85 or above

Procedure 21-5: Instructing a Patient to Use a Metered-Dose Inhaler

Performance Objective

Task: Instruct a patient to use a metered-dose inhaler properly to deliver aerosol medication

Conditions: Placebo inhaler or patient's inhaler with plastic holder, medication canister, and extended-delivery chamber/spacer (optional)

Standards: Complete the procedure in 10 minutes, and achieve a satisfactory score on the procedure performance checklist

Scoring Key: (**S**)*atisfactory,* (**U**)*nsatisfactory,* (**NA**) *Not Applicable*
◆ *Denotes a critical element for a satisfactory score on the procedure*

Procedure Steps	**1st trial**	**2nd trial**	**3rd trial**
1. Wash hands.			
2. Identify patient.			
3. Open inhaler package.			
4. Explain and ask patient to demonstrate each step.			
5. Place placebo medication canister upside down into the plastic holder. If spacer is used, remove cap from plastic holder and insert into spacer.			
6. Shake holder, spacer (if used), and medication canister.			
7. Remove cap from plastic holder or spacer.			
8. Exhale fully.			
9. Close lips around the mouthpiece of the holder or spacer.			
10. Push down on the canister and inhale deeply. Take deep breath, inhale medication into lungs. If using a spacer, inhale as slowly as possible.			
11. Exhale slowly.			
12. Repeat as ordered by doctor.			
13. Explain reactions of many inhaled medications.			
14. Wash hands.			
15. Document teaching.			
16. Complete the procedure within 10 minutes. ◆			

Charting

DATE	

Evaluator Comments:

Score Calculation:

For each procedural step marked U (Unsatisfactory) deduct 6 points
For each procedural step (◆) marked U (Unsatisfactory) deduct 20 points

Score calculation 100 points

− points missed

Total score

1st	2nd	3rd

Satisfactory score: 85 or above

Procedure 21-6: Applying Warm Moist Compresses

Performance Objective

Task: Apply heat therapy in the form of a warm moist compress

Conditions: 4 x 4 gauze pads, gloves, basin, thermometer, warm water

Standards: Complete the procedure in 10 minutes, and achieve a satisfactory score on the procedure performance checklist

Scoring Key: (**S**)*atisfactory,* (**U**)*nsatisfactory,* (**NA**) *Not Applicable*
◆ *Denotes a critical element for a satisfactory score on the procedure*

Procedure Steps	**1st trial**	**2nd trial**	**3rd trial**
1. Wash hands.			
2. Identify patient.			
3. Explain heat therapy to patient.			
4. Place absorbent pad with plastic backing under area to be treated.			
5. Pour warm water into basin.			
6. Measure water temperature with thermometer (not to exceed 125°F).			
7. Put on gloves.			
8. Immerse gauze squares in water.			
9. Squeeze to remove excess water.			
10. Apply compress to area as ordered.			
11. Ask patient if temperature is too warm.			
12. Change for new warm compresses every 2–3 minutes for length of time as ordered. Add hot water as needed.			
13. Dry skin thoroughly.			
14. Document appearance of area and response to treatment in patient record.			
15. Complete the procedure within 10 minutes. ◆			

Charting

DATE	

Evaluator Comments:

Score Calculation:

For each procedural step marked U (Unsatisfactory) deduct 6 points
For each procedural step (◆) marked U (Unsatisfactory) deduct 20 points

Score calculation	100 points			
	– ___ points missed	1st	2nd	3rd
	Total score			

Satisfactory score: 85 or above

Procedure 21-7: Applying an Ice Pack

Performance Objective

Task: Perform cold therapy treatment using an ice pack

Conditions: Commercially prepared ice pack or ice bag and ice, cloth to cover bag/pack

Standards: Complete the procedure in 10 minutes, and achieve a satisfactory score on the procedure performance checklist

Scoring Key: (**S**)*atisfactory,* (**U**)*nsatisfactory,* (**NA**) *Not Applicable*
◆ *Denotes a critical element for a satisfactory score on the procedure*

Procedure Steps	1st trial	2nd trial	3rd trial
1. Wash hands.			
2. Identify patient.			
3. Explain therapy to patient and reason for applying pack.			
4. Place ice cubes in disposable glove or bag and secure, or open chemical pack and apply enough pressure to activate chemicals.			
5. Wrap in cloth before applying to skin.			
6. Apply pack to area for length of time ordered by doctor.			
7. Check skin periodically.			
8. Wash hands.			
9. Document therapy in patient record.			
10. Complete the procedure within 10 minutes. ◆			

Charting

DATE	

Evaluator Comments:

Score Calculation:

For each procedural step marked U (Unsatisfactory) deduct 6 points
For each procedural step (◆) marked U (Unsatisfactory) deduct 20 points

Score calculation	100 points			
	− ____ points missed	1st	2nd	3rd
	Total score			

Satisfactory score: 85 or above

Procedure 21-8: Assisting with Cast Application

Performance Objective

Task: Assist a doctor to apply a fiberglass cast

Conditions: Rolls of fiberglass casting material, stockinette, sheet wadding and/or spongy padding, tape, water basin, bandage scissors, gloves, stand to support lower extremity (if necessary)

Standards: Complete the procedure in 20 minutes, and achieve a satisfactory score on the procedure performance checklist

Scoring Key: (**S**)*atisfactory,* (**U**)*nsatisfactory,* (**NA**) *Not Applicable*
◆ *Denotes a critical element for a satisfactory score on the procedure*

Procedure Steps	1st trial	2nd trial	3rd trial
1. Wash hands.			
2. Identify patient.			
3. Explain procedure.			
4. Assemble equipment.			
5. Seat patient comfortably, as directed by doctor. Support extremity on a stand if necessary.			
6. Cleanse and dry area cast will cover.			
7. Note any objective signs.			
8. Ask about subjective symptoms.			
9. Cut stockinette to fit area cast will cover.			
10. Apply stockinette smoothly to area and be sure there are no wrinkles.			
11. Apply sheet wadding along length of cast, using spiral bandage turns. Apply extra padding to bony protrusions such as elbow or ankle.			
12. Put on gloves.			
13. Pour warm water into basin.			
14. Wet fiberglass tape.			
15. Assist doctor as requested.			
16. Discard water and excess materials.			
17. Remove and discard gloves.			

Procedure Steps	1st trial	2nd trial	3rd trial
18. Reassure patient.			
19. Wash hands.			
20. Assist patient as needed. Provide sling or crutches and instruction as needed.			
21. Review cast-care instruction verbally.			
22. Provide written cast-care instructions.			
23. Document observations and procedure in patient record.			
24. Complete the procedure within 20 minutes. ◆			

Charting

DATE	

Evaluator Comments:

Score Calculation:

For each procedural step marked U (Unsatisfactory) deduct 6 points
For each procedural step (◆) marked U (Unsatisfactory) deduct 20 points

Score calculation 100 points
− points missed

Total score

1st	2nd	3rd

Satisfactory score: 85 or above

Procedure 21-9: Applying a Sling Using a Triangular Bandage

Performance Objective

Task: Apply a sling using a triangular bandage

Conditions: Large cloth triangular bandage, tape or safety pin

Standards: Complete the procedure in 5 minutes, and achieve a satisfactory score on the procedure performance checklist

Scoring Key: (**S**)*atisfactory,* (**U**)*nsatisfactory,* (**NA**) *Not Applicable*
◆ *Denotes a critical element for a satisfactory score on the procedure*

Procedure Steps	1st trial	2nd trial	3rd trial
1. Wash hands.			
2. Identify patient.			
3. Explain procedure.			
4. Assemble equipment.			
5. Seat patient comfortably.			
6. Support arm while placing triangular material on chest with point facing axilla.			
7. Place half material under arm on chest, let other half hang below arm.			
8. While continuing arm support, bring up bottom half of triangle in front of lower arm and tie knot behind neck to one side of the midline avoiding vertebral bump.			
9. Fold point to support elbow and tape or pin in place.			
10. Check for comfort and support.			
11. Wash hands.			
12. Document in patient record.			
13. Complete the procedure within 5 minutes. ◆			

Charting

DATE	

Evaluator Comments:

Score Calculation:

For each procedural step marked U (Unsatisfactory) deduct 6 points
For each procedural step (◆) marked U (Unsatisfactory) deduct 20 points

Score calculation	100 points			
	– ___ points missed	1st	2nd	3rd
	Total score			

Satisfactory score: 85 or above

SELF-EVALUATION

CRITICAL THINKING QUESTIONS

1. What are some measures that should be implemented by the medical office to prevent patients from obtaining medications and/or supplies to support a drug habit? Why is this important?

2. Discuss the use of the metric system in pharmacology and medicine. Why do you think the metric system has replaced the more traditional systems in this field for the United States as a whole? Should the United States switch to the metric system completely? Why or why not? Be sure to discuss both sides of the question in your answer.

3. Develop a plan for a medical assistant to learn about pharmacology in a systematic way and discuss why this is an important part of the medical assistant's knowledge base.

4. Discuss the advantages and disadvantages of ampules as packaging for parenteral medication.

5. Discuss the advantages of the air-lock and Z-track injection methods and describe when it would be appropriate to use either or both.

____

____

____

____

____

____

PRACTICAL APPLICATIONS

1. Write the following amounts using correct abbreviations and standard notation for the metric system.

   a. sixteen micrograms ____________

   b. five-hundredths of a liter ____________

   c. eight-tenths of a milligram ____________

   d. six and one-half grams ____________

   e. two hundred fifty micrograms ____________

2. Write the following amounts using correct abbreviations and standard notation for the apothecaries and household systems.

   a. five grains ____________

   b. two and one half ounces ____________

   c. two teaspoons ____________

   d. three drops ____________

   e. eight minims ____________

3. Convert the following metric measurements. Remember to include a zero before the decimal point of a number less than one.

   a. 4.15 kg = ______ g

   b. 12.5 μg = ______ mg

   c. 62 mL = ______ L

   d. 834 mg = ______ g

   e. 300 mcg = ______ mg

   f. 291 mL = ______ cc

   g. 2.5 mg = ______ mcg

   h. 80 L = ______ mL

   i. 0.25 g = ______ mg

   j. 1,622 mg = ______ g

4. Use the appropriate conversion equation to convert between the apothecary and metric system.

1 teaspoon = 5 mL	1 fluid ounce = 30 mL
1 tablespoon = 15 mL	1 grain = 60 mg

a. tsp III = ______ mL

b. 30 mg = gr ______

c. Tbsp IV = ______ mL

d. 240 mL = fl oz ______

e. 15 mL = tsp ______ or Tbsp ______

5. Calculate the following doses of solid medication using the simulated medication labels to the right. Then write the correct method for charting the medication.

a. Physician order: Coumadin 6 mg po

Coumadin 2 mg tablets
(crystalline warfarin sodium USP)

How many tablets? ____________________

Charting ____

b. Physician order: Tagamet 1.6 g po

800 mg
Tagamet
cimetidine tablets

How many tablets? ____________________

Charting ____

c. Physician order: phenobarbital 60 mg po

PHENOBARBITAL
TABLETS, USP
15 mg

How many tablets? ____________________

Charting ____

d. Physician order: verapamil 120 mg po

Verapamil tablets
40 mg

How many tablets? ____________________

Charting ____

e. Physician order: Zithromax 500 mg po

250 mg
Zithromax
azithromycin capsules

How many capsules? ____________________

Charting ____

f. Physician order: Lanoxin 0.25 mg po

Lanoxin 0.125 mg
(digoxin tablets)

How many tablets? ____________________

Charting ____

g. Physician order: Lasix 60 mg po

40 mg Lasix furosemide tablets

How many tablets? ____________________

Charting ____

h. Physician order: DiaBeta 5 mg po

DiaBeta *glyburide* 1.25 mg tablets

How many tablets? ____________________

Charting ____

i. Physician order: alprazolam 1.5 mg po

0.5 mg alprazolam tablets

How many tablets? ____________________

Charting ____

j. Physician order: atenolol 75 mg po

ATENOLOL 25 mg tablets

How many tablets? ____________________

Charting ____

6. Calculate the following doses of oral liquid medication using the simulated medication labels to the right. Then look up each medication and identify what it is used for.

a. Physician order: Proventil syrup 8 mg po

Proventil (albuterol sulfate) Syrup 2 mg/5mL

How many mL? ____________________

Used for ____

b. Physician order: Amoxicillin oral suspension 0.75 g po

AMOXICILLIN ORAL SUSPENSION 125 mg/5mL

How many mL? ____________________

Used for ____

c. Physician order: Prozac liquid 40 mg po

PROZAC LIQUID fluoxetine hydrochloride oral solution 20 mg per 5 mL

How many mL? ____________________

Used for ____

d. Physician order: Robitussin A-C Syrup tsp Iss po

Robitussin A-C Syrup
(codeine 10 mg
guaifenesin 100 mg
in each teaspoon)

How many mg codeine? ________ How many mg guaifenesin? ________

Used for ____

7. Calculate the following doses of liquid medication for injection using the simulated medication labels to the right. Then mark the correct dose on the syringe below each question.

   a. Physician order: Heparin sodium 4000 units sc

   HEPARIN SODIUM
   INJECTION, USP
   5000 USP units/mL

   How many mL? ____________________

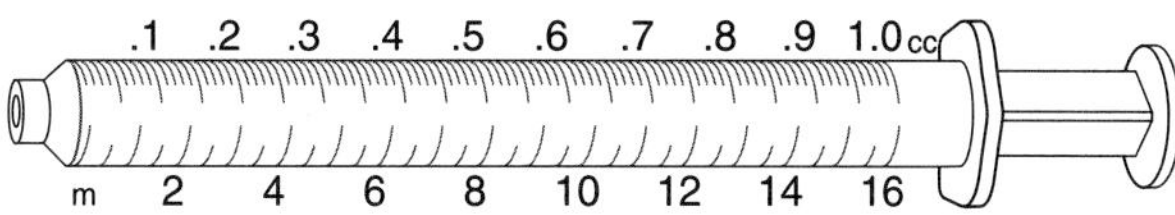

   b. Physician order: Furosemide 15 mg IM

   FUROSEMIDE
   INJECTION, USP
   20 mg/2 mL

   How many mL? ____________________

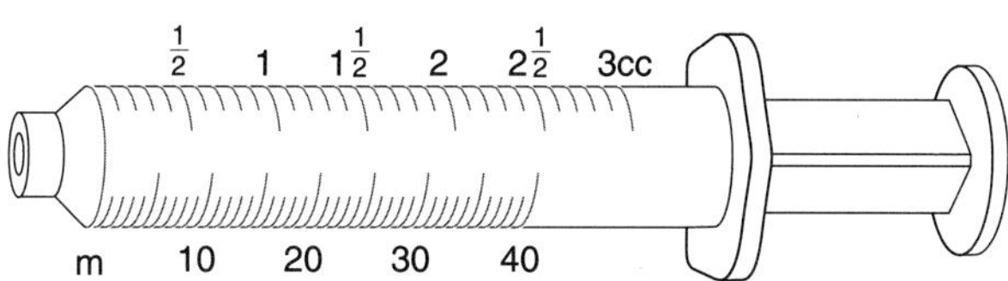

   c. Physician order: Vitamin B_{12} (cyanocobalamin) 200 mcg IM

   CYANOCOBALAMIN
   INJECTION, USP
   (crystalline Vitamin B_{12})
   1 mg/mL

   How many mL? ____________________

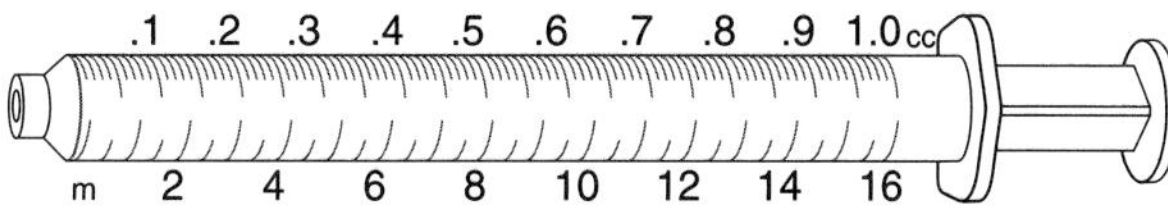

d. Physician order: Depo-Provera 800 mg IM

Depo-Provera
sterile medroxyprogesterone
acetate suspension, USP
400 mg/mL

How many mL? ____________________

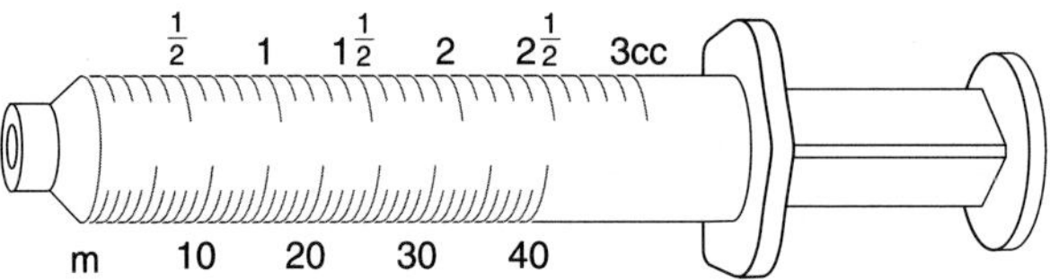

e. Physician order: Diazepam 8 mg IM

Diazepam
injection, USP
5 mg/mL

How many mL? ____________________

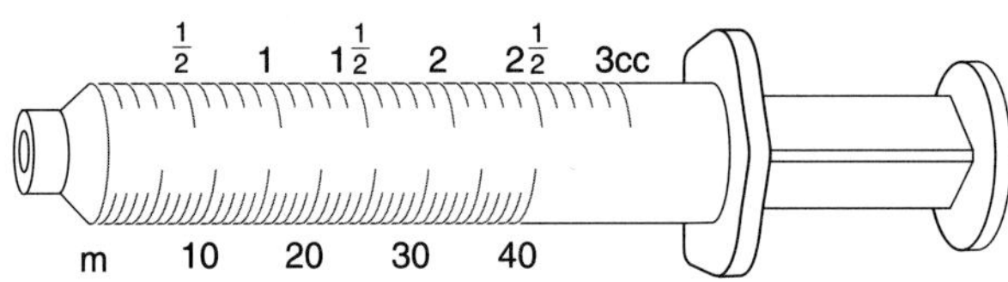

f. Physician order: Kanamycin sulfate 45 mg IM

KANAMYCIN
SULFATE INJECTION, USP
75 mg/2 mL

How many mL? ____________________

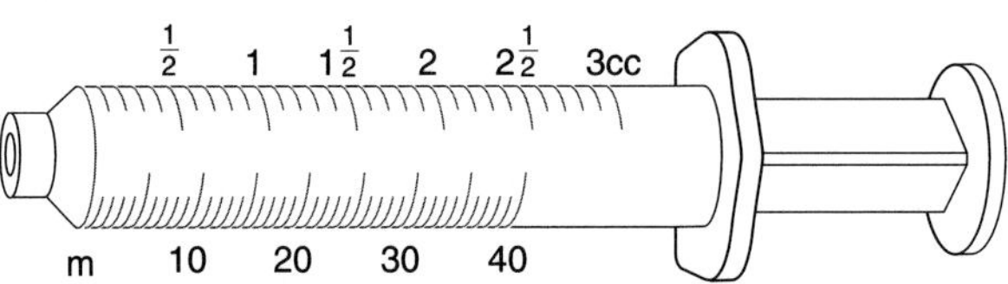

g. Physician order: chlorpromazine HCl injection 20 mg IM

CHLORPROMAZINE
HYDROCHLORIDE INJECTION, USP
25 mg/mL

How many mL? ____________________

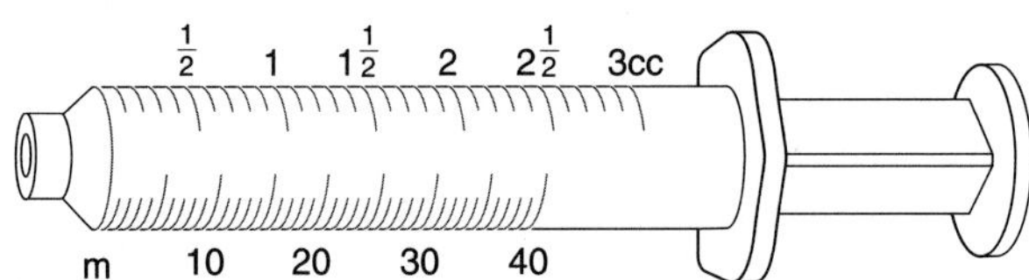

h. Physician order: Atropine sulfate 0.2 mg IM

ATROPINE SULFATE
INJECTION, USP
0.4 mg/mL

How many mL? ____________________

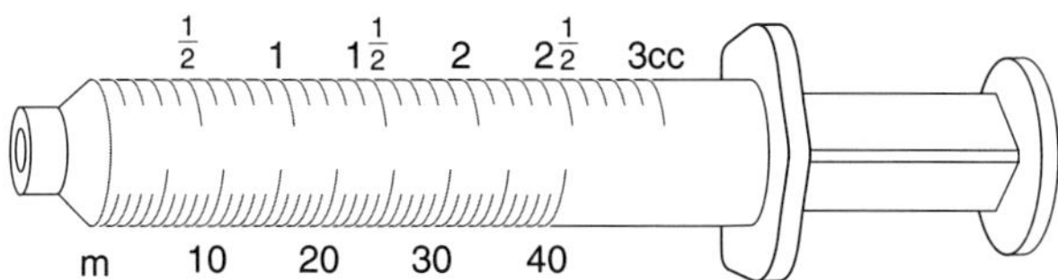

i. Physician order: Naloxone Hcl 0.4 mg IM

NALOXONE
HCL INJECTION, USP
400 mcg/mL

How many mL? ____________________

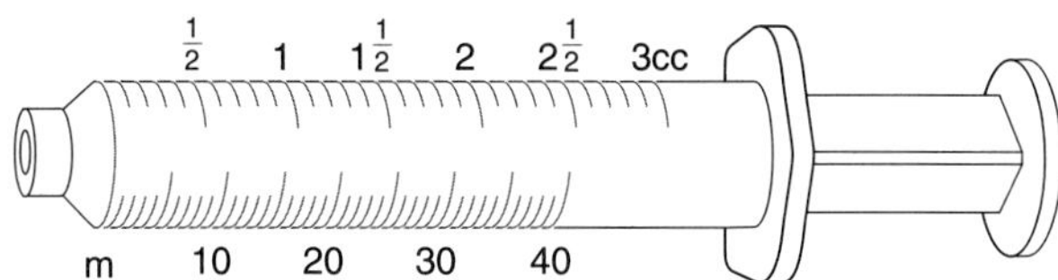

j. Physician order: Gentamicin sulfate 24 mg IM

GENTAMICIN
SULFATE INJECTION, USP
40 mg/mL

How many mL? ____________________

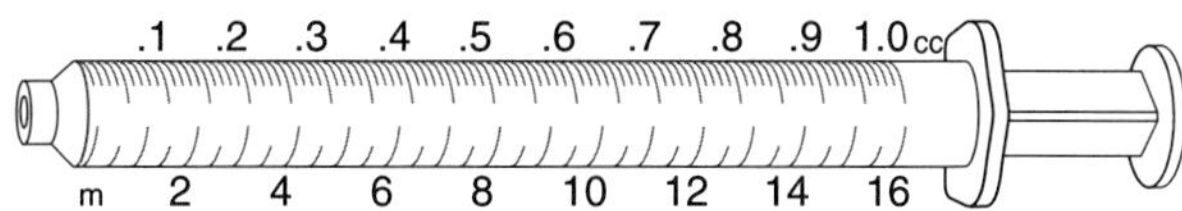

8. What should the medical assistant do if the following situations occur when administering an intramuscular injection?

a. If blood appears during aspiration? ____________________

____

b. If the patient complains of severe pain or numbness during the injection? ____________________

____

c. If the needle breaks? ____________________

____

d. If the patient faints? ____________________

____

9. Write the exact instructions you would give to a patient following a Mantoux test.

____

____

____

10. Change the following statements using abbreviations to words:

a. Digoxin gr 1/60 po qam _______________

b. Penicillin G 1,000,000 U IM stat _______________

c. Mylanta 30 cc po qid ac & hs _______________

d. Diphenhydramine HCl elixir fl oz IV, Sig tsp I q 4 h prn _______________

____

e. Lasix 20 mg po tid _______________

11. Using Table 22-2 from your textbook, prepare drug cards for 10 of the 50 most commonly prescribed prescriptions of 1999. Use the format of the drug card that accompanies the box "Learning About Medications" including both brand and generic names, group, action, use, common side effects, severe side effects, patient teaching needs, contraindications, precautions, and safety in pregnancy and children.

12. For each of the following medications, add the generic name, identify the medication group(s) that it belongs to and its major use(s).

	Generic name	Group	Uses
a. Coumadin			
b. Solganol			
c. Solu-Medrol			
d. Rocephin			
e. Lasix			
f. Mevacor			
g. Cardizem			
h. Paxil			
i. Prilosec			
j. Xylocaine			

PROCEDURE PERFORMANCE CHECKLISTS

Procedure 22-1: Administering Oral Medication

Performance Objective

Task: Prepare and administer oral medication in tablet or liquid form following a doctor's order

Conditions: Medication ordered by doctor, medicine cup, cup of water, written medication order

Standards: Complete the procedure in 10 minutes, and achieve a satisfactory score on the procedure performance checklist

Scoring Key: (**S**)*atisfactory,* (**U**)*nsatisfactory,* (**NA**) *Not Applicable*
◆ *Denotes a critical element for a satisfactory score on the procedure*

Procedure Steps	1st trial	2nd trial	3rd trial
1. Obtain chart with medication order.			
2. Wash hands.			
3. Assemble medication and supplies.			
4. Check label when taking the medication from storage shelf.			
5. Calculate dosage if necessary. ◆			
6. Check label before pouring to make sure it is correct medication.			
7. Check expiration date on medication label.			
8. If liquid medication, shake well.			
9. If solid medication, pour correct number of capsules or tablets into bottle cap. ◆			
9A. If liquid medication, place thumbnail at level of correct amount on medication cup.			
10. If solid medication, pour correct number of capsules or tablets from bottle cap into medicine cup.			
10A. If liquid medication, pour correct amount from bottle into medicine cup, holding medicine cup at eye level and label toward palm. Read correct dose at lowest level of the meniscus. ◆			
11. Discard excess liquid medication or dropped tablets.			
12. Place medication cup on counter and recap bottle.			
13. Check medication label to be sure it is the correct medication.			
14. Take medication and medical record to the patient.			

Procedure Steps	1st trial	2nd trial	3rd trial
15. Identify patient.			
16. Assess patient and take vital signs if needed.			
17. Seat patient in chair for comfort.			
18. Explain purpose of medication administration.			
19. Hand medicine cup to patient followed by cup of water (if solid medication).			
20. Observe patient swallow medication.			
21. Wash hands.			
22. Document medication administration in patient record.			
23. Complete the procedure within 10 minutes. ◆			

Charting

DATE	

Evaluator Comments:

Score Calculation:

For each procedural step marked U (Unsatisfactory) deduct 6 points
For each procedural step (◆) marked U (Unsatisfactory) deduct 20 points

Score calculation 100 points

− points missed

Total score	1st	2nd	3rd

Satisfactory score: 85 or above

Procedure 22-2: Drawing Up Medication from an Ampule

Performance Objective

Task: Prepare an injectable medication from an ampule

Conditions: Syringe with needle, ampule of medication, alcohol swab, gauze, rigid biohazard container

Standards: Complete the procedure in 5 minutes, and achieve a satisfactory score on the procedure performance checklist

Scoring Key: (S)atisfactory, (U)nsatisfactory, (NA) Not Applicable
◆ *Denotes a critical element for a satisfactory score on the procedure*

Procedure Steps	1st trial	2nd trial	3rd trial
1. Obtain chart with medication order.			
2. Calculate dosage if necessary. ◆			
3. Wash hands.			
4. Assemble medication and supplies.			
5. Check label of ampule as you remove it from storage shelf.			
6. Check expiration date.			
7. Tap top of ampule until all medication falls to bottom.			
8. Check label of ampule against medication order to be sure it is the correct medication.			
9. Wipe ampule neck with alcohol swab.			
10. Wrap gauze square around ampule neck.			
11. Holding top and bottom firmly, push top away from yourself to break completely off.			
12. Discard upper part of ampule in rigid biohazard container.			
13. Place opened ampule on flat surface.			
14. Open syringe with needle attached.			
15. Remove needle cover.			
16. Insert needle into ampule, being careful not to touch inside surface of ampule.			
17. Draw up ordered amount of medication. If necessary, tilt ampule or invert ampule so that needle tip stays within fluid.			

Procedure Steps	1st trial	2nd trial	3rd trial
18. Withdraw needle from ampule.			
19. With needle pointing up, tap syringe until all bubbles rise toward the needle.			
20. Push plunger toward syringe gently to expel air.			
21. If there is excess medication in syringe, hold over a sink and gently push plunger to measure correct dose. ◆			
22. Recap needle, using method to avoid needlestick.			
23. Check ampule label again against medication order.			
24. Discard ampule in rigid biohazard container.			
25. Wash hands.			
26. Complete the procedure within 5 minutes. ◆			

Evaluator Comments:

Score Calculation:

For each procedural step marked U (Unsatisfactory) deduct 6 points
For each procedural step (◆) marked U (Unsatisfactory) deduct 20 points

Score calculation 100 points

− points missed

Total score

1st	2nd	3rd

Satisfactory score: 85 or above

Procedure 22-3: Drawing Up Medication from a Vial

Performance Objective

Task: Prepare an injectable medication using a medication vial

Conditions: Syringe with needle, vial of medication, alcohol pads, rigid biohazard container

Standards: Complete the procedure in 5 minutes, and achieve a satisfactory score on the procedure performance checklist

Scoring Key: (S)atisfactory, (U)nsatisfactory, (NA) Not Applicable
◆ *Denotes a critical element for a satisfactory score on the procedure*

Procedure Steps	1st trial	2nd trial	3rd trial
1. Obtain chart with medication order.			
2. Calculate dosage if necessary. ◆			
3. Wash hands.			
4. Assemble medication and supplies.			
5. Check the label of the vial as you remove it from storage shelf.			
6. Check expiration date on medication label.			
7. Wipe off vial top with alcohol wipe.			
8. Check label against medication order to make sure it is correct medication.			
9. Open syringe with needle attached and draw up air into the syringe equal to the amount of medication to be removed from the vial.			
10. Place vial on flat surface.			
11. Remove needle cover.			
12. Insert needle into vial without holding vial in your hand until tip of needle has safely entered the rubber stopper.			
13. Do not touch any part of the needle with your fingers.			
14. Inject air into the vial above the fluid line to avoid bubbles.			
15. Invert the vial so the tip of the needle is below fluid line.			
16. Pull back on the plunger of the syringe to withdraw medication.			
17. If air bubbles appear in syringe, tap syringe to allow bubbles to rise to top.			

Procedure Steps	1st trial	2nd trial	3rd trial
18. Holding syringe vertically, push air through needle.			
19. Adjust medication to exact medication dosage. ◆			
20. Remove needle from vial.			
21. Recap needle using method to avoid needle stick.			
22. Check label of vial against medication order again before you put vial back in medicine cabinet.			
23. Wash hands.			
24. Complete the procedure within 5 minutes.◆			

Evaluator Comments:

Score Calculation:

For each procedural step marked U (Unsatisfactory) deduct 6 points
For each procedural step (◆) marked U (Unsatisfactory) deduct 20 points

Score calculation 100 points

− points missed

	1st	2nd	3rd
Total score			

Satisfactory score: 85 or above

Procedure 22-4: Reconstituting a Powdered Medication

Performance Objective

Task: Prepare an injectable medication by reconstituting the powdered form to a liquid, using a diluent

Conditions: Syringe with needle, vial of powdered medication, vial of diluent as specified, additional needle, alcohol pads, rigid biohazard container

Standards: Complete the procedure in 10 minutes, and achieve a satisfactory score on the procedure performance checklist

Scoring Key: (**S**)*atisfactory,* (**U**)*nsatisfactory,* (**NA**) *Not Applicable*
◆ *Denotes a critical element for a satisfactory score on the procedure*

Procedure Steps	1st trial	2nd trial	3rd trial
1. Obtain chart with medication order.			
2. Calculate dosage if necessary. ◆			
3. Wash hands.			
4. Assemble medication and supplies.			
5. Check the medication label as you remove it from storage shelf.			
6. Check the expiration date on the medication label.			
7. Read the label of the powdered medication to identify the amount and type of diluent needed.			
8. Wipe off the top of the vial of powdered medication with an alcohol pad.			
9. Wipe off the top of the vial of diluent with an alcohol pad.			
10. Open the syringe with needle attached and draw up air into it equal to the amount of diluent to be removed from the bottle.			
11. Place vial of diluent on flat surface.			
12. Remove needle cover.			
13. Insert needle into vial without holding vial in your hand until tip of needle has safely entered the rubber stopper.			
14. Withdraw correct amount of diluent. ◆			
15. Place vial of powdered medication on flat surface.			
16. Insert needle into vial without holding vial in your hand until tip of needle has safely entered the rubber stopper.			

Procedure Steps	1st trial	2nd trial	3rd trial
17. Inject diluent into vial of powdered medication.			
18. Remove needle and recap using method to avoid needle stick.			
19. Roll the vial between your hands until the medication is completely mixed.			
20. Label the vial of reconstituted medication with the date, time, your initials, and the concentration of the reconstituted medication. ◆			
21. Draw up the correct dose of reconstituted medication following Procedure 22-3. ◆			
22. Check medication label to be sure it is the correct medication before refrigerating any unused medication or storing according to manufacturer's directions.			
23. Discard needle in a rigid biohazard container and place a new needle on the syringe for administration.			
24. Wash hands.			
25. Complete the procedure within 10 minutes. ◆			

Evaluator Comments:

Score Calculation:

For each procedural step marked U (Unsatisfactory) deduct 6 points
For each procedural step (◆) marked U (Unsatisfactory) deduct 20 points

Score calculation 100 points

− ___ points missed

	1st	2nd	3rd
Total score			

Satisfactory score: 85 or above

Procedure 22-5: Administering a Subcutaneous Injection

Performance Objective

Task: Administer a subcutaneous injection

Conditions: Syringe and needle containing medication, alcohol pad, gauze pad, gloves, bandage, rigid biohazard container, patient medical record

Standards: Complete the procedure in 5 minutes, and achieve a satisfactory score on the procedure performance checklist

*Scoring Key: (**S**)atisfactory, (**U**)nsatisfactory, (**NA**) Not Applicable*
◆ *Denotes a critical element for a satisfactory score on the procedure*

Procedure Steps	1st trial	2nd trial	3rd trial
1. Wash hands.			
2. Using the medical record, identify patient.			
3. Explain the procedure.			
4. Tell patient the reason for the injection.			
5. Ask patient if he or she has any allergies to the medication.			
6. Put on gloves.			
7. Select an appropriate injection site for subcutaneous injection.			
8. Clean the site with an alcohol pad.			
9. Remove needle cover.			
10. With thumb and first two fingers of nondominant hand, form a skin fold.			
11. Grasp syringe between thumb and first two fingers of dominant hand.			
12. Insert the needle up with a quick, smooth motion at a 45-degree angle into the subcutaneous tissue.			
13. Without moving needle, pull back on plunger slightly and observe to be sure no blood enters syringe. ◆			
13A. If blood appears, withdraw needle, apply pressure to site, and prepare a new injection.			
14. If no blood appears, push in the plunger slowly and steadily until all the medication has been administered.			
15. Withdraw needle swiftly at same angle it was inserted.			

Procedure Steps	1st trial	2nd trial	3rd trial
16. Apply pressure to the site using a gauze pad or alcohol pad.			
17. Gently massage the injection site (except for heparin or insulin).			
18. Dispose of syringe and needle in a rigid biohazard container without recapping needle.			
19. Remove and discard gloves.			
20. Wash hands.			
21. Ask patient to remain in office for 10–15 minutes.			
22. Document the medication, dose, injection site, and any reaction or adverse effect in the patient medical record.			
23. Complete the procedure within 5 minutes. ◆			

Charting

DATE	

Evaluator Comments:

Score Calculation:

For each procedural step marked U (Unsatisfactory) deduct 6 points
For each procedural step (◆) marked U (Unsatisfactory) deduct 20 points

Score calculation 100 points
− points missed

Total score

1st	2nd	3rd

Satisfactory score: 85 or above

Procedure 22-6: Selecting a Site for an Intramuscular Injection

Performance Objective

Task: Identify landmarks and appropriate intramuscular injection sites

Conditions: Manikin or student to locate the following injection sites: deltoid, ventrogluteal, dorsogluteal, vastus lateralis (for infants)

Standards: Complete the procedure in 10 minutes, and achieve a satisfactory score on the procedure performance checklist

Scoring Key: (**S**)*atisfactory,* (**U**)*nsatisfactory,* (**NA**) *Not Applicable*
◆ *Denotes a critical element for a satisfactory score on the procedure*

Procedure Steps	1st trial	2nd trial	3rd trial
Deltoid			
1. Place patient in sitting, prone, supine, or lateral position.			
2. Locate the borders of the deltoid muscle.			
3. Palpate the acromion process of the scapula.			
4. Drop straight down to the middle of the muscle for injection site.			
Ventrogluteal			
1. Place patient in supine or lateral position.			
2. Palpate the greater trochanter, anterior superior iliac spine, and bony ridge of the iliac crest.			
3. Placing the palm against the greater trochanter, with the tip of index finger on the anterior superior iliac spine, spread middle finger as far away from index finger as possible.			
4. Locate center of area between index and middle finger for injection site.			
Dorsogluteal			
1. Place patient in prone position, with appropriate draping of lower buttocks area.			
2. Palpate posterior iliac spine and greater trochanter of the femur.			
3. Draw an imaginary diagonal line between the two landmarks.			
4. Locate injection site above this line two inches below the iliac crest in the upper outer quadrant of the buttock.			

Procedure Steps	1st trial	2nd trial	3rd trial
Vastus Lateralis (Infants)			
1. Place child in supine or lateral position, with parent holding child still.			
2. Locate vastus lateralis muscle below the greater trochanter of the femur, within lateral quadrant of thigh.			
3. Visually divide thigh into thirds, down to the kneecap.			
4. Locate injection side in middle third area.			
5. Complete the procedure within 10 minutes. ◆			

Evaluator Comments:

Score Calculation:

For each procedural step marked U (Unsatisfactory) deduct 6 points
For each procedural step (◆) marked U (Unsatisfactory) deduct 20 points

Score calculation 100 points
− points missed

	1st	2nd	3rd
Total score			

Satisfactory score: 85 or above

Procedure 22-7: Administering an Intramuscular Injection

Performance Objective

Task: Administer an intramuscular injection

Conditions: Syringe and needle containing ordered medication, alcohol pad, gauze pad, gloves, bandage, rigid biohazard container, patient medical record

Standards: Complete the procedure in 5 minutes, and achieve a satisfactory score on the procedure performance checklist

*Scoring Key: (**S**)atisfactory, (**U**)nsatisfactory, (**NA**) Not Applicable*
◆ *Denotes a critical element for a satisfactory score on the procedure*

Procedure Steps	1st trial	2nd trial	3rd trial
1. Wash hands.			
2. Using medical record, identify patient.			
3. Explain procedure.			
4. Tell patient reason for injection.			
5. Ask patient if he or she has any allergies to the medication.			
6. Put on gloves.			
7. Select an appropriate intramuscular injection site.			
8. Clean area with alcohol pad using circular motion.			
9. Remove needle cover.			
10. With thumb and first two fingers of nondominant hand, spread skin around injection site.			
11. Grasp syringe between thumb and first two fingers of dominant hand.			
12. Insert needle using a quick, smooth motion at a 90-degree angle to the muscle.			
13. Without moving needle, pull back on plunger slightly and observe to be sure no blood enters syringe. ◆			
13A. If blood appears, withdraw needle, apply pressure, and prepare a new injection.			
14. If no blood appears, push in the plunger slowly and steadily until all medication has been administered.			
15. Withdraw needle quickly at the same angle it was inserted.			

Procedure Steps	1st trial	2nd trial	3rd trial
16. Apply pressure to the site using a gauze pad or alcohol pad.			
17. Gently massage the injection site (except for heparin or insulin).			
18. Dispose of syringe and needle in rigid biohazard container.			
19. Continue applying pressure until bleeding subsides.			
20. Apply bandage to injection site.			
21. Remove and discard gloves.			
22. Wash hands.			
23. Ask patient to remain in office for 10–15 minutes.			
24. Document the medication, dose, injection site, and any reaction in medical record.			
25. Complete the procedure within 5 minutes. ◆			

Charting

DATE	

Evaluator Comments:

Score Calculation:

For each procedural step marked U (Unsatisfactory) deduct 6 points
For each procedural step (◆) marked U (Unsatisfactory) deduct 20 points

Score calculation 100 points

– points missed

Total score

1st	2nd	3rd

Satisfactory score: 85 or above

Procedure 22-8: Administering a Z-Track Injection

Performance Objective

Task: Administer a Z-track injection

Conditions: Syringe and needle containing medication ordered, alcohol pad, gauze pad, gloves, bandage, rigid biohazard container, patient medical record

Standards: Complete the procedure in 5 minutes, and achieve a satisfactory score on the procedure performance checklist

Scoring Key: (**S**)*atisfactory,* (**U**)*nsatisfactory,* (**NA**) *Not Applicable*
◆ *Denotes a critical element for a satisfactory score on the procedure*

Procedure Steps	1st trial	2nd trial	3rd trial
1. Wash hands.			
2. Using medical record, identify patient.			
3. Explain procedure.			
4. Tell patient the reason for injection.			
5. Ask patient if he or she has any allergies to medication.			
6. Put on gloves.			
7. Locate the dorsogluteal injection site.			
8. Be sure the needle was changed after drawing up the medication to prevent tissue irritation.			
9. Clean injection site using alcohol pad.			
10. Remove needle cover.			
11. Before injecting, draw 0.2–0.5 mL of air into the syringe.			
12. With your fingers, pull the skin at injection site to the left of its usual position about 2 to 3 inches.			
13. Hold the tissue to the side while you insert needle with a quick, smooth motion at a 90-degree angle.			
14. Without moving the needle in the tissue, pull back on the plunger slightly and observe to be sure that no blood enters the syringe. ◆			
15. Continue holding skin 2 to 3 inches to left of normal position while aspirating.			
16. If no blood appears, push in the plunger slowly and steadily until all medication has been administered.			

Procedure Steps	1st trial	2nd trial	3rd trial
17. Withdraw needle swiftly at same angle as insertion, and release tissue being held by non-dominant hand at same time.			
18. Apply pressure to the site using a gauze pad or alcohol pad.			
19. Do not massage injection site.			
20. Dispose of syringe and needle in rigid biohazard container without recapping needle.			
21. Apply bandage after bleeding has stopped.			
22. Remove and discard gloves.			
23. Wash hands.			
24. Ask patient to remain in office for 10–15 minutes.			
25. Document medication, dose, injection site, that Z-track method was used, and any reaction.			
26. Complete the procedure within 5 minutes. ◆			

Charting

DATE	

Evaluator Comments:

Score Calculation:

For each procedural step marked U (Unsatisfactory) deduct 6 points
For each procedural step (◆) marked U (Unsatisfactory) deduct 20 points

Score calculation 100 points

– points missed

Total score

1st	2nd	3rd

Satisfactory score: 85 or above

Procedure 22-9: Administering an Intradermal Injection

Performance Objective

Task: Administer an intradermal injection

Conditions: Syringe and needle containing ordered medication, alcohol pad, gauze pad, gloves, bandage, rigid biohazard container, patient medical record

Standards: Complete the procedure in 5 minutes, and achieve a satisfactory score on the procedure performance checklist

Scoring Key: (**S**)*atisfactory,* (**U**)*nsatisfactory,* (**NA**) *Not Applicable*
◆ *Denotes a critical element for a satisfactory score on the procedure*

Procedure Steps	1st trial	2nd trial	3rd trial
1. Wash hands.			
2. Using medical record, identify patient.			
3. Explain procedure.			
4. Tell patient reason for injection.			
5. Ask patient if he or she has any allergies to the medication.			
6. Put on gloves.			
7. Select an appropriate intradermal injection site.			
8. Clean site with alcohol pad.			
9. Remove needle cover.			
10. With thumb and index finger of non-dominant hand, pull skin taut.			
11. Holding the syringe bevel up, insert needle at 10–15 degree angle.			
12. Insert until bevel has penetrated the skin but not further.			
13. Do not aspirate.			
14. Slowly inject medication to form a bubble, or wheal, at skin surface.			
15. Remove needle quickly at the same angle as insertion.			
16. Place gauze or alcohol wipe over site, but do not apply pressure or massage.			
17. Dispose of syringe and needle in rigid biohazard container without recapping needle.			
18. Discard soiled supplies in biohazard bag.			

Procedure Steps	1st trial	2nd trial	3rd trial
19. Remove and discard gloves.			
20. Instruct patient when reaction, if any, will occur. If necessary, instruct the patient when to return to the office to have the injection site observed or how to report test results.			
21. Document injection, site, and patient instructions in medical record.			
22. Complete the procedure within 5 minutes. ◆			

Charting

DATE	

Evaluator Comments:

Score Calculation:

For each procedural step marked U (Unsatisfactory) deduct 6 points
For each procedural step (◆) marked U (Unsatisfactory) deduct 20 points

Score calculation 100 points
– points missed

	1st	2nd	3rd
Total score			

Satisfactory score: 85 or above

Procedure 22-10: Administering a Tine or Mantoux Test

Performance Objective

Task: Perform a Tine or Mantoux injection to test for tuberculosis

Conditions: Tuberculin syringe with 3/8 to 1/2 inch needle containing PPD (Purified Protein Derivative) or four-pronged multiple-puncture unit for Tine test, gloves, alcohol swab, gauze pad, rigid biohazard container

Standards: Complete the procedure in 5 minutes, and achieve a satisfactory score on the procedure performance checklist

Scoring Key: (**S**)*atisfactory,* (**U**)*nsatisfactory,* (**NA**) *Not Applicable*
◆ *Denotes a critical element for a satisfactory score on the procedure*

Procedure Steps	1st trial	2nd trial	3rd trial
1. Wash hands.			
2. Using medical record, identify patient.			
3. Explain procedure.			
4. Tell patient reason for injection.			
5. Ask patient if he or she has ever had a reaction to a test for tuberculosis, or ever been immunized for tuberculosis.			
6. If patient answers in affirmative, consult doctor.			
7. Put on gloves.			
8. Select a site on the anterior aspect of the lower arm, free from moles, lesions, or skin discoloration.			
9. Remove needle cover or plastic protector on four-prong test.			
10. With thumb and index of nondominant hand, pull skin taut.			
11. If administering Tine test, press firmly into designated forearm area.			
11A.Press, hold, and release to distribute medication on the prongs.			
12. If administering the Mantoux test, hold syringe with bevel up and insert needle at a 10–15-degree angle until bevel has penetrated the skin.			
13. Do not aspirate.			
14. For the Mantoux test, inject the medication slowly to form a wheal.			

Procedure Steps	1st trial	2nd trial	3rd trial
15. Withdraw needle quickly at the same angle as insertion.			
16. Place gauze or alcohol wipe over site, but do not apply pressure or massage.			
17. Dispose of syringe and needle or Tine applicator in rigid biohazard container without recapping needle.			
18. Discard other soiled supplies in biohazard bag.			
19. Remove and discard gloves.			
20. Instruct patient to return to have test read in 48–72 hours, or to call in with description of any reaction.			
21. Document the type of TB test, location, and instructions given.			
22. Complete the procedure within 5 minutes. ◆			
23. When patient returns to have the test read, observe site.			
24. Measure diameter of any induration (raised, hard, and reddened area) in millimeters. (For Tine test, measure the largest single reaction.)			
25. Record if no reaction noted or exact size of any reaction.			

Charting

DATE	

Evaluator Comments:

Score Calculation:

For each procedural step marked U (Unsatisfactory) deduct 6 points
For each procedural step (◆) marked U (Unsatisfactory) deduct 20 points

Score calculation	100 points			
	– points missed	1st	2nd	3rd
	Total score			

Satisfactory score: 85 or above

SELF-EVALUATION

UNIT 5

The Laboratory and Laboratory Tests

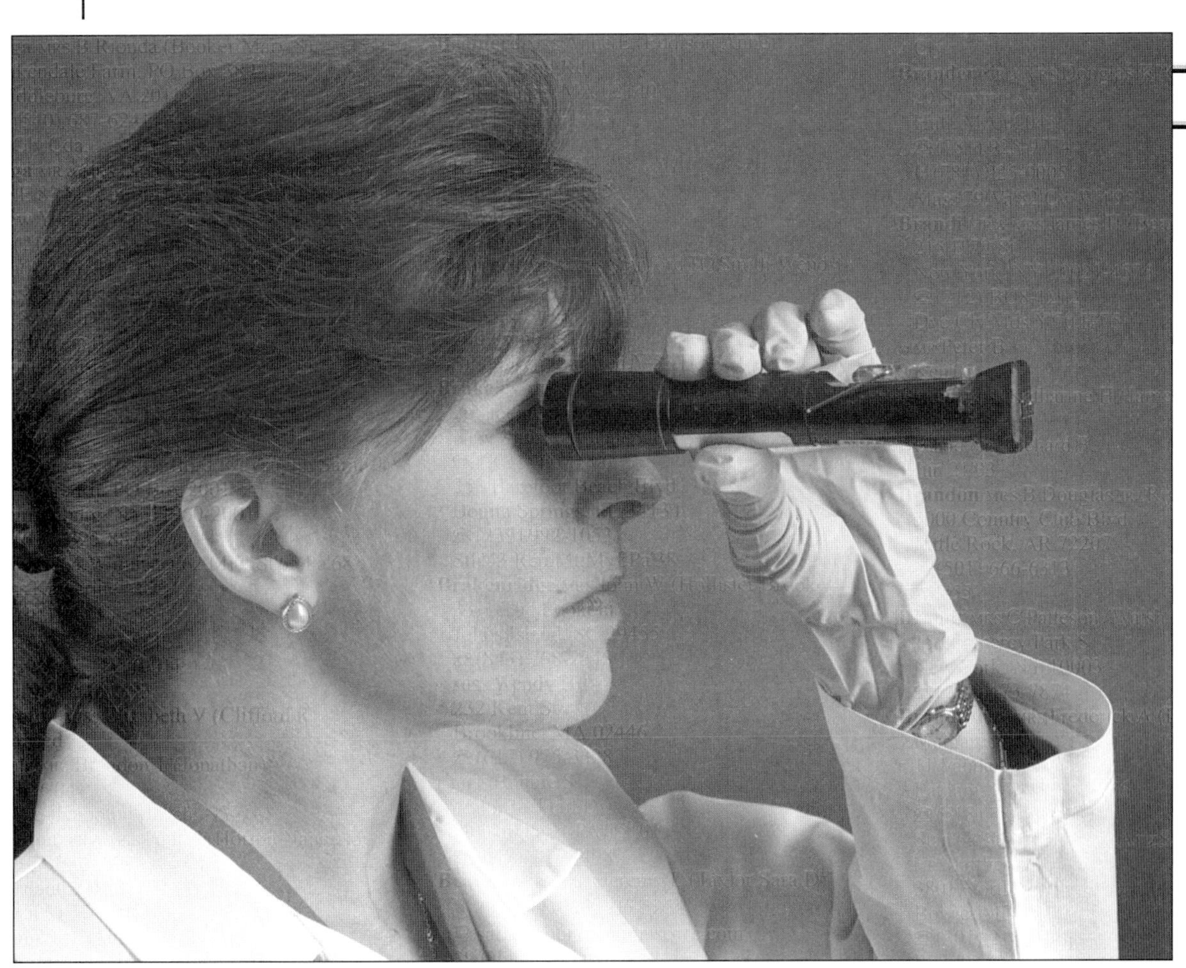

Chapter 23

The Physician's Office Laboratory

CHAPTER FOCUS

This chapter introduced you to the clinical laboratory and described how laboratories are regulated by different government agencies. In addition, you learned about laboratory safety and how to care for laboratory equipment and specimens. The following chapters in this section describe how to obtain specimens and perform specific laboratory tests.

TERMINOLOGY REVIEW

Vocabulary Matching: Match each term with its definition.

__ 1. pathologist

__ 2. reference laboratory

__ 3. calibration

__ 4. pathology

__ 5. fluorescence

__ 6. centrifuge

__ 7. pipette

__ 8. accuracy

__ 9. quality control

__ 10. oil-immersion

A. A measure of how close a laboratory measurement is to the true value

B. The testing and adjustment of test equipment

C. A device used to separate the components of a liquid by rapid rotation

D. Use of an ultraviolet light source to illuminate an object

E. Use of oil on a microscope lens to enhance magnification

F. A physician who specializes in the study of disease processes

G. The scientific analysis of the cause and effects of disease

H. A small glass or plastic vessel used to transfer fluid from one place to another

I. A process used to insure the validity or accuracy of test results

J. Large laboratories, either privately owned or run by universities or research centers

Abbreviations: Expand each abbreviation to its complete form.

1. CLIA '88 ______
2. POL ______
3. QA ______
4. QC ______
5. RPM ______

CONTENT REVIEW QUESTIONS

1. Describe each of the following four types of laboratories briefly.

   a. Hospital-based laboratories ______

   b. Reference laboratories ______

   c. Clinical laboratories ______

   d. Other laboratories ______

2. If a laboratory has a Certificate of Waiver, what kinds of tests can be performed?

3. If the physician looks at slides under a microscope and medical assistants perform "waived" laboratory tests, what kind of certificate must the physician's office laboratory have?

4. What is the purpose of a quality assurance and quality control program for a POL?

5. How are control reagents used in the POL? How often should controls be run?

6. Why must laboratory equipment be calibrated regularly?

____

____

____

7. Identify the five categories of activities that will be monitored during a physical inspection of a laboratory that is applying for a certificate of accreditation.

a. ____

b. ____

c. ____

d. ____

e. ____

8. Give examples for each of the following categories of hazards in a POL.

a. physical hazards ____

____

b. chemical hazards ____

____

c. biological hazards ____

____

9. What measures are used to respond to the increased fire hazard in a POL?

____

____

10. What measures are used to respond to the presence of hazardous chemicals in a POL?

____

____

11. How should blood, body fluids, and items contaminated with blood or body fluids be handled?

____

____

____

12. Identify at least four types of equipment that may be found in a POL and give the use of each.

a. ____

b. ____

c. ____

d. ____

13. What kind of records must be kept for laboratory equipment?

____

____

____

14. What is a microscope used for in the POL?

____

____

____

15. Identify the parts of a microscope seen below.

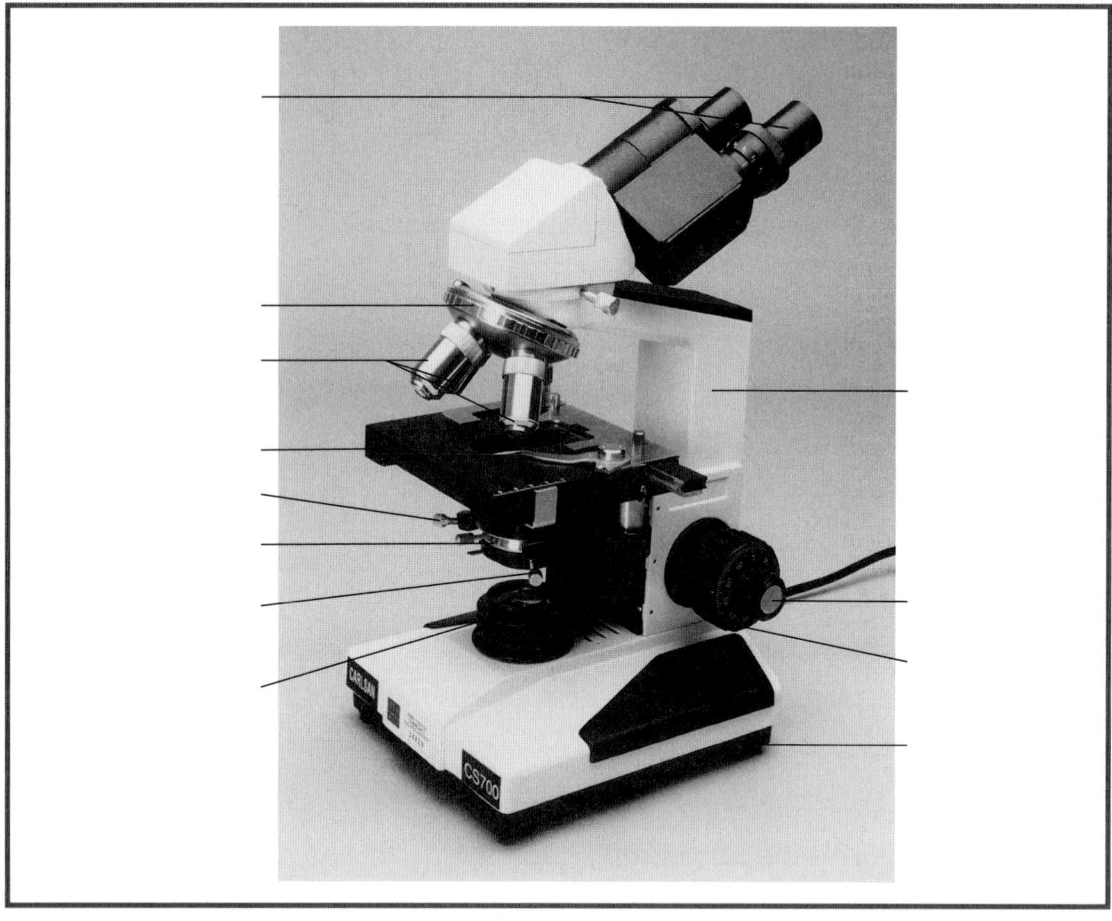

16. When is a pipette used to transfer specimens?

____

____

____

17. What information must usually be provided on a laboratory requisition?

18. What general guidelines are used when collecting and handling specimens of blood or body fluid?

CRITICAL THINKING QUESTIONS

1. Discuss the medical assistant's responsibility when receiving laboratory results by mail, by computer, or when recording laboratory results after performing procedures.

2. Discuss the implications for patients if quality assurance and quality control measures are not implemented correctly.

3. Some physicians' offices have stopped performing laboratory tests because they feel that there are too many regulations to comply with. Take a survey of offices in your area (working together with your classmates) to find out what laboratory tests are performed in the 15 medical offices that are closest to your school. Discuss your findings with your classmates.

PRACTICAL APPLICATIONS

1. In the clinical laboratory for your medical assisting program, find the MSDS sheet for at least three of the following and determine what safety precautions should be followed if these substances are spilled.

   a. isopropyl alcohol ______________________________

   ____

   b. mercury (such as from a broken sphygmomanometer) ______________________________

   ____

   c. test kits such as Clinitest, rapid strep test, mono test, etc. ______________________________

   d. reagents used for blood typing ______________________________

   ____

   e. Wright's stain or other stains ______________________________

   ____

   f. chemical disinfectant used in the lab. ______________________________

   ____

2. Examine slides given to you by your instructor under a microscope using low, moderate, and high magnification following Procedure 23-1. You may also examine one of your own hairs, a flake of skin, a drop of saliva, and/or a thin piece of the transparent layer that lies beneath the outer layers of onion skin. Draw what you see at different magnifications.

3. List all warning signs found in your medical assisting lab and/or science laboratories at your school. Are there any areas that should have additional signs? In addition, identify all fire safety equipment present and the location of eyewash stations and showers.

   ____

   ____

   ____

   ____

   ____

   ____

Procedure 23-1: Using a Microscope

Performance Objective

Task: Use a microscope to view slides under all magnifications

Conditions: Compound light microscope with dust cover, oil-immersion lens paper, prepared microscope slides, lens cleaner

Standards: Complete the procedure in 15 minutes, and achieve a satisfactory score on the procedure performance checklist

Scoring Key: (**S**)*atisfactory,* (**U**)*nsatisfactory,* (**NA**) *Not Applicable*
◆ *Denotes a critical element for a satisfactory score on the procedure*

Procedure Steps	1st trial	2nd trial	3rd trial
1. Using both hands (one on arm and one under base), carry microscope to work area.			
2. Set microscope on secure, flat surface.			
3. Remove dust cover.			
4. Unwind cord.			
5. Plug microscope into grounded outlet.			
6. Place excess cord on table.			
7. Clean lenses and oculars with lens cleaning solution and lens paper.			
8. Clean oil immersion objective last.			
9. Turn on light at rheostat control, keeping light intensity low.			
10. Place a prepared slide–coverslip up–or a prepared smear on the center hole of the mechanical stage.			
11. Secure slide with clips or slide holder.			
12. Swing low-power or scan objective into place.			
13. Adjust width of oculars until a single image appears.			
14. Adjust iris diaphragm if more light is needed.			
15. Observe slide with naked eye while raising the stage, using the coarse adjustment.			
16. Look into the oculars.			

Procedure Steps	1st trial	2nd trial	3rd trial
17. Begin to focus by lowering the stage with the coarse adjustment.			
18. Bring the object into focus with fine adjustment.			
19. Switch to the high-power objective.			
20. Use fine adjustment to focus.			
21. To observe an object on a prepared slide with the oil-immersion objective, place a drop of immersion oil on the slide and click the oil-immersion objective into place.			
22. Use fine adjustment to bring objective down until it touches oil but not slide.			
23. Adjust light if necessary.			
24. When finished, turn the oil-immersion objective to the side before removing the slide.			
25. Record or report results of identification as appropriate for specimen types.			
26. Clean the slide and the oil-immersion objective with lens paper before storing microscope.			
27. Turn off the microscope.			
28. Grasp plug to remove.			
29. Wrap cord around microscope.			
30. Replace dust cover.			
31. Store microscope.			
32. Complete the procedure within 60 minutes. ◆			

Evaluator Comments:

Score Calculation:

For each procedural step marked U (Unsatisfactory) deduct 6 points
For each procedural step (◆) marked U (Unsatisfactory) deduct 20 points

Score calculation	100 points		1st	2nd	3rd
	– points missed				
	Total score				

Satisfactory score: 85 or above

SELF-EVALUATION

Chapter 24

Urinalysis

CHAPTER FOCUS

One of the most common laboratory tests performed in the physician's office is the urinalysis. In this chapter you learned how urine is formed, how urine specimens are collected, how to perform a dipstick urinalysis, how to perform other urine tests to confirm results, and how to prepare urine for a microscopic examination.

TERMINOLOGY REVIEW

Vocabulary Matching: Match each term with its definition.

___ 1. sediment	A. A breakdown product of hemoglobin
___ 2. oxidation	B. Formed when protein accumulates in the kidney tubules, and is deposited in the urine as it passes through the tubules
___ 3. urinary meatus	C. Solid components of urine sediment with a regular shape
___ 4. urobilinogen	D. A small glass tube that floats in a container of urine
___ 5. glomerulus	E. Cells from the outer layer of skin or mucous membranes
___ 6. casts	F. The act of retaining large particles as smaller particles pass through
___ 7. bilirubin	G. A tuft of very small capillaries that filter blood
___ 8. ketones	H. The products of incomplete fatty acid metabolism
___ 9. ureter	I. Form of bilirubin that is excreted in urine and feces
___ 10. nitrites	J. The kidney's microscopic filtration unit

___ 11. turbid	K. Their presence in fresh urine indicates bacterial growth
___ 12. urethra	L. A chemical reaction in which a compound unites with oxygen, forming a new compound
___ 13. epithelial cells	M. Measure of hydrogen ion concentration (acidity)
___ 14. urea	N. Also known as a dipstick
___ 15. refractometer	O. An instrument that measures the refractive index of a solution
___ 16. urinometer	P. Material left at the bottom of a test tube after centrifuging
___ 17. solute	Q. Substance that dissolves in a solution
___ 18. reagent strip	R. Very cloudy
___ 19. pH	S. Organic compound derived from the breakdown of protein metabolism
___ 20. nephron	T. A long, cylindrical tube attached to each kidney allow urine to pass to the bladder
___ 21. crystals	U. Tube that carries urine from the bladder to the outside of the body
___ 22. filtration	V. The external opening of the urethra

CONTENT REVIEW QUESTIONS

1. Identify the five major functions of the urinary system.

   a. ____________________

   b. ____________________

   c. ____________________

   d. ____________________

   e. ____________________

2. Describe briefly how the filtrate is formed that eventually becomes urine. What does this filtrate contain?

   ____

   ____

   ____

   ____

3. Name the three sections of the renal tubule and describe what happens in each.

   a. ____________________

   b. ____________________

   c. ____________________

4. Identify at least eight substances that are found in urine.

a. ______________________ e. ______________________

b. ______________________ f. ______________________

c. ______________________ g. ______________________

d. ______________________ h. ______________________

5. What minimum information should the medical assistant place on the label of any urine specimen?

____

____

____

6. What is the difference between a random urine specimen and a clean-catch midstream urine specimen?

____

____

____

7. When might a urine specimen be collected for a drug screen?

____

____

____

8. Why is it important to validate the "chain of custody" for a drug-screen urine specimen?

____

____

____

9. Describe how urine is tested for three physical properties.

a. ______________________

b. ______________________

c. ______________________

10. Why is the specific gravity reading important? What might it mean if it is low? High?

____

____

____

11. What is the difference between qualitative and quantitative tests of urine?

____

____

____

12. Identify five general measures that the medical assistant should take when using urine dipsticks to produce accurate test results.

a. ______

b. ______

c. ______

d. ______

e. ______

13. Identify each of the following and discuss what it might mean if each is found in the urine.

a. Blood ______

b. Leukocytes ______

c. Nitrites ______

d. Protein ______

e. Glucose ______

f. Ketones ______

g. Bilirubin ______

h. Urobilogen ______

14. Describe the confirmatory test for sugar. Why is it used?

______

______

______

______

15. Describe the confirmatory test for ketones. Why is it used?

______

______

______

______

16. Describe the confirmatory test for bilirubin. Why is it used?

______

______

______

______

17. Identify five types of substances that might be observed during a microscopic examination of urine.

a. ______

b. ______

c. ______

d. ______________________________

e. ______________________________

18. Describe how a urine specimen is prepared for microscopic analysis.

____

____

____

____

19. How should the medical assistant report the results of a routine urinalysis?

____

____

____

____

CRITICAL THINKING QUESTIONS

1. At your externship, you are asked to prepare a microscopic urine sample, perform the microscopic examination, and report results. Would you feel qualified to do this? Why or why not?

____

____

____

____

____

____

2. Discuss what urine controls show and why it is important to perform urine controls on a regular basis. What could happen if controls are not performed and/or records of controls are not kept?

____

____

____

____

____

____

3. Discuss the ethics of requiring urine testing for drugs for employment or participation in athletic events. When do you think it is justified? When do you think it might be an invasion of a person's right to privacy?

____

____

____

4. Do research on the following kidney diseases, describe each briefly, and identify specific abnormal findings that might be found in the urinalysis.
   a. glomerulonephritis
   b. pyelonephritis
   c. renal calculi
   d. renal failure
   e. cystitis

PRACTICAL APPLICATIONS

1. What type of urine specimen should be collected for each of the following tests?
   a. urine glucose
   b. pregnancy test
   c. urine for culture and sensitivity
   d. urine pH
   e. test of kidney's ability to produce urine
   f. methadone maintenance program
2. Prepare written instruction sheets for the following urine tests in terms a patient can understand:
   a. first morning urine specimen
   b. clean-catch midstream urine specimen (male)
   c. clean-catch midstream urine specimen (female)
   d. 24-hour urine for creatinine clearance (collection bottle contains a preservative)

PROCEDURE PERFORMANCE CHECKLISTS

Procedure 24-1: Collecting a Clean-Catch Midstream Urine Specimen

Performance Objective

Task: Explain to patient the correct procedure for collecting a clean-catch midstream urine specimen

Conditions: Sterile urine specimen kit, including two aseptic cleaning towels and a sterile specimen container

Standards: Complete the procedure in 5 minutes, and achieve a satisfactory score on the procedure performance checklist

Scoring Key: (**S**)*atisfactory,* (**U**)*nsatisfactory,* (**NA**) *Not Applicable*
◆ *Denotes a critical element for a satisfactory score on the procedure*

Procedure Steps	1st trial	2nd trial	3rd trial
1. Assemble supplies or prepackaged kit.			
2. Identify patient.			
3. Explain procedure to patient.			
4. Label specimen container with patient's name (and date if specimen is to be collected in office).			
5. Give patient kit or supplies and specific instructions.			
Instruct patient to:			
6. Wash hands before collecting the urine specimen.			
7. Loosen the lid of urine container without touching the inside.			
Collection procedure for females:			
8. Spread the labia and clean the genital area from front to back using each cleansing towel only once.			
9. Continue to hold the labia apart and void a small amount into the toilet. Then void into the specimen cup until it is about half full and void any remaining urine into the toilet.			
Collection procedure for males:			
8. Retract the foreskin of the penis (if uncircumcised) and cleanse the glans using each cleansing towel once.			
9. Holding the foreskin retracted, void a small amount into the toilet. Then void into the specimen cup until it is about half full and void any remaining urine into the toilet.			

Procedure Steps	1st trial	2nd trial	3rd trial
Instruct patient to:			
10. Replace the cover without touching the inside of the cover or the specimen cup.			
11. Wash hands after collection is complete.			
12. Place the specimen in (or take it to) a designated location.			
13. Complete the procedure within 5 minutes. ◆			

Evaluator Comments:

Score Calculation:

For each procedural step marked U (Unsatisfactory) deduct 6 points
For each procedural step (◆) marked U (Unsatisfactory) deduct 20 points

Score calculation 100 points

− ____ points missed

Total score

1st	2nd	3rd

Satisfactory score: 85 or above

Procedure 24-2: Collecting a 24-Hour Urine Specimen

Performance Objective

Task: Explain to patient the correct procedure for collecting a 24-hour urine specimen

Conditions: Collection container(s) for test(s) ordered, preservatives to be added to container(s), urinal or toilet inserts for urine collection, a funnel for transfer into collection container(s)

Standards: Complete the procedure in 5 minutes, and achieve a satisfactory score on the procedure performance checklist

Scoring Key: **(S)***atisfactory,* **(U)***nsatisfactory,* **(NA)** *Not Applicable*
◆ *Denotes a critical element for a satisfactory score on the procedure*

Procedure Steps	1st trial	2nd trial	3rd trial
1. Consult procedure manual to identify type of container, amount and type of preservative to add.			
2. Add preservative to container(s).			
3. Label each container with type and amount of preservative.			
4. Label container(s) with patient name and other identifying information required by lab.			
5. Identify patient.			
6. Inform patient that test requires all urine to be collected in a 24-hour time period.			
7. Give patient the container(s).			
8. Instruct patient both verbally and in writing about the correct procedure for collecting the specimen(s).			
Instruct the patient to:			
9. Avoid alcoholic beverages, vitamins, and over-the-counter medications for at least 24 hours before and during specimen collection.			
10. Refrain from emptying the bottle before starting the test and avoid contact with any chemical in the bottle.			
11. Keep the container out of the reach of children.			
12. Keep the collection bottle in a cool place, preferably in the refrigerator.			
13. Collect the urine on a day that you will be able to collect all urine (each time you void) and bring it to the collection facility promptly when specimen collection is complete.			

Procedure Steps	1st trial	2nd trial	3rd trial
14. Begin this test in the morning. Do not collect the first morning specimen. Void the first time that day into the toilet and flush. Note the time and date of this void on the container.			
15. Collect all urine specimens for the next 24 hours. Collect the specimens in a urinal (males) or toilet insert (females) and pour into the collection bottle using a funnel. Make the final collection include the first morning void the next morning.			
16. Do not put anything except urine into the container (avoid putting in toilet paper, stool, tampons, etc.)			
17. Do not dip urine from the toilet bowl because it will be diluted with water.			
18. Call the office if you have questions or concerns.			
19. Return the specimen to the laboratory the morning the test is completed.			
20. Complete the procedure within 5 minutes. ◆			

Evaluator Comments:

Score Calculation:

For each procedural step marked U (Unsatisfactory) deduct 6 points
For each procedural step (◆) marked U (Unsatisfactory) deduct 20 points

Score calculation 100 points

− points missed

Total score

1st	2nd	3rd

Satisfactory score: 85 or above

Procedure 24-3: Measuring Urine Specific Gravity Using a Refractometer

Performance Objective

Task: Measure the specific gravity of a urine specimen, using a refractometer

Conditions: Gloves, urine specimen, distilled water, disposable pipette, refractometer, lint-free tissues, biohazard waste container

Standards: Complete the procedure in 5 minutes, and achieve a satisfactory score on the procedure performance checklist

Scoring Key: (**S**)*atisfactory,* (**U**)*nsatisfactory,* (**NA**) *Not Applicable*
◆ *Denotes a critical element for a satisfactory score on the procedure*

Procedure Steps	1st trial	2nd trial	3rd trial
1. Wash hands.			
2. Assemble supplies and equipment.			
3. Urine specimen should be at room temperature.			
4. Put on gloves.			
5. Check to make sure that refractometer is clean and free of debris.			
6. Use lint-free tissue to wipe instrument if necessary.			
7. Do not scratch lens.			
8. Calibrate refractometer daily using distilled water.			
9. Be sure controls have been run for the day.			
10. Using disposable pipette, stir urine to mix it.			
11. Draw urine from specimen.			
12. Drop one or two drops into chamber entrance of the refractometer.			
13. Allow specimen to be drawn into chamber by capillary action.			
14. Hold refractometer to a light source.			
15. Rotate eyepiece until the calibrated scale is clear.			
16. Read specific gravity from the urine scale at the boundary between the light area and the dark area.			
17. Clean the prism by dropping a few drops of distilled water and wiping with a lint-free tissue.			
18. Discard used supplies in biohazard waste container.			

Procedure Steps	1st trial	2nd trial	3rd trial
19. Remove and discard gloves in biohazard waste container.			
20. Wash hands.			
21. Document results, including date, time, and specific gravity reading.			
22. The reading recorded is within 0.002 of the evaluator's reading. ◆			
23. Complete the procedure within 5 minutes. ◆			

Charting

DATE	

Evaluator Comments:

Score Calculation:

For each procedural step marked U (Unsatisfactory) deduct 6 points
For each procedural step (◆) marked U (Unsatisfactory) deduct 20 points

Score calculation 100 points

− points missed

Total score

1st	2nd	3rd

Satisfactory score: 85 or above

Procedure 24-4: Chemical Testing of Urine Using Reagent Strip Method

Performance Objective

Task: Perform a urinalysis using the reagent strip method

Conditions: Gloves, vial of urine reagent dipsticks (e.g. Multistix 10 SG or Chemstix), clean dry gauze pads, timer that measures seconds and minutes, fresh and well-mixed urine specimen

Standards: Complete the procedure in 5 minutes, and achieve a satisfactory score on the procedure performance checklist

Scoring Key: (**S**)*atisfactory,* (**U**)*nsatisfactory,* (**NA**) *Not Applicable*
◆ *Denotes a critical element for a satisfactory score on the procedure*

Procedure Steps	1st trial	2nd trial	3rd trial
1. Wash hands.			
2. Assemble supplies and equipment.			
3. Put on gloves.			
4. Be sure controls have been run that day for bottles of reagent strips you are using.			
5. Open bottle of reagent strips.			
6. Remove one strip.			
7. Immediately close bottle.			
8. Quickly dip urine strip into urine sample, insuring that strip is completely immersed in sample.			
9. Remove strip.			
10. Hold in a horizontal position so urine does not run from one test pad to another.			
11. Blot strip sideways into clean gauze, careful not to touch reagent test pads onto gauze.			
12. Begin timing procedure.			
13. Read each urine chemical result at the appropriate time by the indicated by manufacturer.			
14. Match color of each pad on strip to color chart on back of bottle.			
15. Make a mental note of each abnormal result.			
16. Dispose of reagent strip and used supplies in biohazard waste container.			

Procedure Steps	1st trial	2nd trial	3rd trial
17. Remove and discard gloves in biohazard waste container.			
18. Wash hands.			
19. Record results correctly.			
20. The results recorded are the same as those recorded by the evaluator. ◆			
21. Complete the procedure within 5 minutes. ◆			

Record Results:

Leukocytes ____________________

Nitrite ____________________

Urobilinogen ____________________

Protein ____________________

pH ____________________

Blood ____________________

Specific gravity ____________________

Ketones ____________________

Bilirubin ____________________

Glucose ____________________

Evaluator Comments:

Score Calculation:

For each procedural step marked U (Unsatisfactory) deduct 6 points
For each procedural step (◆) marked U (Unsatisfactory) deduct 20 points

Score calculation 100 points

− points missed

Total score

1st	2nd	3rd

Satisfactory score: 85 or above

Procedure 24-5: Urine Testing Using Clinitest 5-Drop Method

Performance Objective

Task: Test urine for sugars using Clinitest 5-drop method

Conditions: Gloves, freshly voided urine specimen, Clinitest kit that contains thick glass test tube, dropper, and holding rack; bottle of Clinitest tablets, distilled water, clean pair of thumb forceps, timer that measures seconds and minutes, biohazard waste container

Standards: Complete the procedure in 5 minutes, and achieve a satisfactory score on the procedure performance checklist

Scoring Key: (**S**)*atisfactory,* (**U**)*nsatisfactory,* (**NA**) *Not Applicable*
◆ *Denotes a critical element for a satisfactory score on the procedure*

Procedure Steps	1st trial	2nd trial	3rd trial
1. Wash hands.			
2. Assemble supplies and equipment.			
3. Place test tube in rack.			
4. Do not hold test tube in hands while performing test.			
5. Do not place face close to the test tube during the test.			
6. Put on gloves.			
7. Using dropper from kit, place five drops of urine into test tube.			
8. Rinse dropper with distilled water.			
9. Add 10 drops distilled water to test tube.			
10. Using forceps to pick up Clinitest tablet, drop tablet into test tube.			
11. Do not handle tablet with hands.			
12. Do not shake test tube as the mixture boils or for 15 seconds after boiling has stopped.			
13. At the end of 15-second period, shake test tube gently.			
14. Compare color of liquid to color chart provided by manufacturer.			
15. Discard contents of test tube and rinse with water.			
16. Discard other supplies in biohazard waste container.			
17. Remove and discard gloves in biohazard waste container.			
18. Wash hands.			

Procedure Steps

Procedure Steps	1st trial	2nd trial	3rd trial
19. Record date, time, and results in patient medical record.			
20. The results recorded are the same as those of the evaluator. ◆			
21. Complete the procedure within 5 minutes. ◆			

Charting

DATE	

Evaluator Comments:

Score Calculation:

For each procedural step marked U (Unsatisfactory) deduct 6 points
For each procedural step (◆) marked U (Unsatisfactory) deduct 20 points

Score calculation 100 points

− points missed

Total score

1st	2nd	3rd

Satisfactory score: 85 or above

Procedure 24-6: Urine Testing Using Acetest Method

Performance Objective

Task: Perform urine testing using the Acetest method

Conditions: Gloves, freshly voided urine specimen, bottle of Acetest tablets, clean white paper towel, clean pair of thumb forceps, dropper, timer that measures seconds and minutes, biohazard waste bag

Standards: Complete procedure in 5 minutes, and achieve a satisfactory score on the procedure performance checklist

Scoring Key: (**S**)*atisfactory,* (**U**)*nsatisfactory,* (**NA**) *Not Applicable*
◆ *Denotes a critical element for a satisfactory score on the procedure*

Procedure Steps	1st trial	2nd trial	3rd trial
1. Wash hands.			
2. Assemble supplies and equipment.			
3. Place clean white test paper on table.			
4. Put on gloves.			
5. Remove one tablet from bottle using forceps and place on test paper.			
6. Recap bottle.			
7. Using dropper, place one drop of urine directly on top of the tablet.			
8. Compare color of the tablet to the color chart provided by manufacturer at 30 seconds after application.			
9. Discard tablet and test paper in biohazard waste container.			
10. Remove and discard gloves in biohazard waste container.			
11. Wash hands.			
12. Record date, time, and test results in patient medical record.			
13. The results recorded are the same as those of the evaluator. ◆			
14. Complete the procedure within 5 minutes. ◆			

Charting

DATE	

Evaluator Comments:

Score Calculation:

For each procedural step marked U (Unsatisfactory) deduct 6 points
For each procedural step (◆) marked U (Unsatisfactory) deduct 20 points

Score calculation   100 points

− ____ points missed

Total score

1st	2nd	3rd

Satisfactory score: 85 or above

Procedure 24-7: Urine Testing Using Ictotest Procedure

Performance Objective

Task: Perform a urine test using the Ictotest procedure

Conditions: Gloves, freshly voided urine specimen (or one protected from light if more than eight hours old), Ictotest kit including tablets and test pads, distilled water, clean paper towel, clean pair of thumb forceps, dropper, timer that measures seconds and minutes, biohazard waste container

Standards: Complete procedure in 5 minutes, and achieve a satisfactory score on the procedure performance checklist

Scoring Key: (**S**)*atisfactory,* (**U**)*nsatisfactory,* (**NA**) *Not Applicable*
◆ *Denotes a critical element for a satisfactory score on the procedure*

Procedure Steps	1st trial	2nd trial	3rd trial
1. Wash hands.			
2. Assemble supplies and equipment.			
3. Put on gloves.			
4. Place a square of the absorbent test mat from kit on a clean paper towel.			
5. Using the dropper, place 10 drops of urine onto the center of the test mat.			
6. Remove one tablet from bottle using forceps.			
7. Do not touch tablet with fingers.			
8. Place on the test mat.			
9. Recap bottle immediately.			
10. Place one drop distilled water on tablet.			
11. Wait 5 seconds.			
12. Place a second drop of water onto tablet so water runs off tablet and onto mat.			
13. Observe color of mat around tablet after 60 seconds.			
14. Discard tablet, test mat, paper towel and used supplies in biohazard waste container.			
15. Remove and discard gloves in biohazard waste container.			
16. Wash hands.			

Procedure Steps	1st trial	2nd trial	3rd trial
17. Record date, time, and results in patient medical record.			
18. The results recorded are the same as those of the evaluator. ◆			
19. Complete the procedure within 30 minutes. ◆			

Charting

DATE	

Evaluator Comments:

Score Calculation:

For each procedural step marked U (Unsatisfactory) deduct 6 points
For each procedural step (◆) marked U (Unsatisfactory) deduct 20 points

Score calculation 100 points
− points missed

Total score

1st	2nd	3rd

Satisfactory score: 85 or above

Procedure 24-8: Preparing Urine for Microscopic Examination

Performance Objective

Task: Prepare a urine sample for microscopic examination

Conditions: Gloves, at least 15 mL of fresh, well-mixed urine, plastic urine centrifuge tubes with caps, disposable transfer pipette, test tube rack, urine centrifuge, plain glass slides and cover slips or commercially available urine plastic slides, brightfield binocular compound microscope with 10X and 40X power objectives, biohazard waste container

Standards: Complete procedure in 15 minutes, and achieve a satisfactory score on the procedure performance checklist

Scoring Key: (**S**)*atisfactory,* (**U**)*nsatisfactory,* (**NA**) *Not Applicable*
◆ *Denotes a critical element for a satisfactory score on the procedure*

Procedure Steps	1st trial	2nd trial	3rd trial
1. Wash hands.			
2. Assemble supplies and equipment.			
3. Put on gloves.			
4. Mix urine specimen with transfer pipette.			
5. Place centrifuge tube in test tube rack.			
6. Pour in 12 mL of urine.			
7. Place cap on tube.			
8. Place tube in centrifuge.			
9. Balance centrifuge by placing another centrifuge tube filled with 12 mL water and with cap directly opposite urine-filled tube in centrifuge.			
10. Centrifuge, at 1500 RPM, for 5 minutes.			
11. Remove urine tube from centrifuge.			
12. Do not shake tube.			
13. Remove cap from tube.			
14. Using plastic transfer pipette, remove clear liquid (supernatant) from top of tube, leaving 0.5 to 1.0 mL of urine on top of sediment.			
15. Discard supernatant.			
16. Resuspend sediment by gently flicking bottom of tube.			

Procedure Steps	1st trial	2nd trial	3rd trial
17. Add urine stain (if desired by physician) following manufacturer's directions.			
18. Draw up urine into pipette.			
19. Place one drop of urine mixture onto a glass slide.			
20. Add coverslip, being careful not to introduce bubbles.			
20A. Or, place one drop of urine into commercial urine slide counting chamber.			
21. Place slide onto center of microscope stage.			
22. Prepare microscope by turning on light, closing diaphragm, and keeping rheostat at a low setting.			
23. Rotate nosepiece until low power objective clicks into place.			
24. Use coarse adjustment to bring slide into coarse focus.			
25. Inform doctor or lab technician that specimen is ready for examination.			
26. After doctor has completed examination, recap centrifuge tube.			
27. Discard tube, slide, and pipette in rigid biohazard waste container.			
28. Remove and discard gloves in biohazard waste container.			
29. Wash hands.			
30. Complete the procedure within 15 minutes. ◆			

Evaluator Comments:

Score Calculation:

For each procedural step marked U (Unsatisfactory) deduct 6 points
For each procedural step (◆) marked U (Unsatisfactory) deduct 20 points

Score calculation 100 points

− points missed

Total score

1st	2nd	3rd

Satisfactory score: 85 or above

SELF-EVALUATION

Chapter 25

Phlebotomy, Hematology, and Coagulation Studies

CHAPTER FOCUS

In this chapter you learned how to obtain blood specimens by venipuncture and capillary puncture. You also learned about hematology and coagulation tests on blood specimens. Hematocrits and/or hemoglobin levels are often measured in the medical office, although blood specimens are usually sent to a hospital laboratory for complete blood counts and erythrocyte sedimentation rates. Studies related to the clotting ability of the blood are sometimes done in the office and sometimes done in a hospital laboratory.

TERMINOLOGY REVIEW

Vocabulary Matching: Match each term with its definition.

___ 1. tourniquet

___ 2. hematoma

___ 3. microhematocrit

___ 4. anemia

___ 5. hematopoiesis

___ 6. phagocytosis

___ 7. serum

___ 8. plasma

A. A decreased ability of red blood cells to carry oxygen

B. The area of the forearm inside of the elbow

C. A surface tension effect seen in narrow tubes

D. A narrow strip of rubber that is wrapped around the arm to dilate the veins for venipuncture

E. A glass or plastic tube, sealed with a rubber stopper to maintain a vacuum

F. The action that causes the fibrin clot to be removed

G. Formation of blood cells

H. A large bruised area at the puncture site, caused by blood leaking into the tissue surrounding the vein

___ 9. phlebotomy/venipuncture	I. A blood protein that contains iron molecules
___ 10. evacuated tube	J. Fainting
___ 11. antecubital	K. The liquid portion of the blood after all of the cells and clotting elements have settled and formed a clot
___ 12. hemoglobin	L. A measurement of the packed red blood cell volume
___ 13. syncope	M. The process by which white blood cells engulf bacteria and debris
___ 14. phenylketonuria	N. A metabolic condition in which an individual is unable to metabolize the amino acid phenylalanine
___ 15. sclerosed	O. Removal of a sample of blood, usually from a superficial vein
___ 16. capillary action	P. The liquid portion of blood
___ 17. fibrinolysis	Q. Hardened by repeated venipuncture

Describe the following types of blood cells:

1. agranulocyte ______________________
2. basophil ______________________
3. eosinophil ______________________
4. erythrocyte ______________________
5. granulocyte ______________________
6. leukocyte ______________________
7. neutrophil ______________________
8. polymorphonuclear leukocyte ______________________
9. platelet ______________________
10. reticulocyte ______________________
11. thrombocyte ______________________

Abbreviations: Expand each abbreviation to its complete form.

1. CBC ______________________
2. diff ______________________
3. ESR ______________________
4. Hb/Hgb ______________________

5. Hct ______________________________

6. PKU ______________________________

7. polys ______________________________

8. segs ______________________________

9. PT ______________________________

10. PTT ______________________________

11. RBC ______________________________

12. WBC ______________________________

CONTENT REVIEW QUESTIONS

1. Identify four important functions of blood.

   a. ______________________________

   b. ______________________________

   c. ______________________________

   d. ______________________________

2. Describe how blood clots, including identifying blood cells that promote clot formation.

   ____

   ____

   ____

   ____

3. Describe the location and appearance of a suitable vein for venipuncture.

   ____

   ____

   ____

   ____

4. Identify the veins of the forearm on the illustration below.

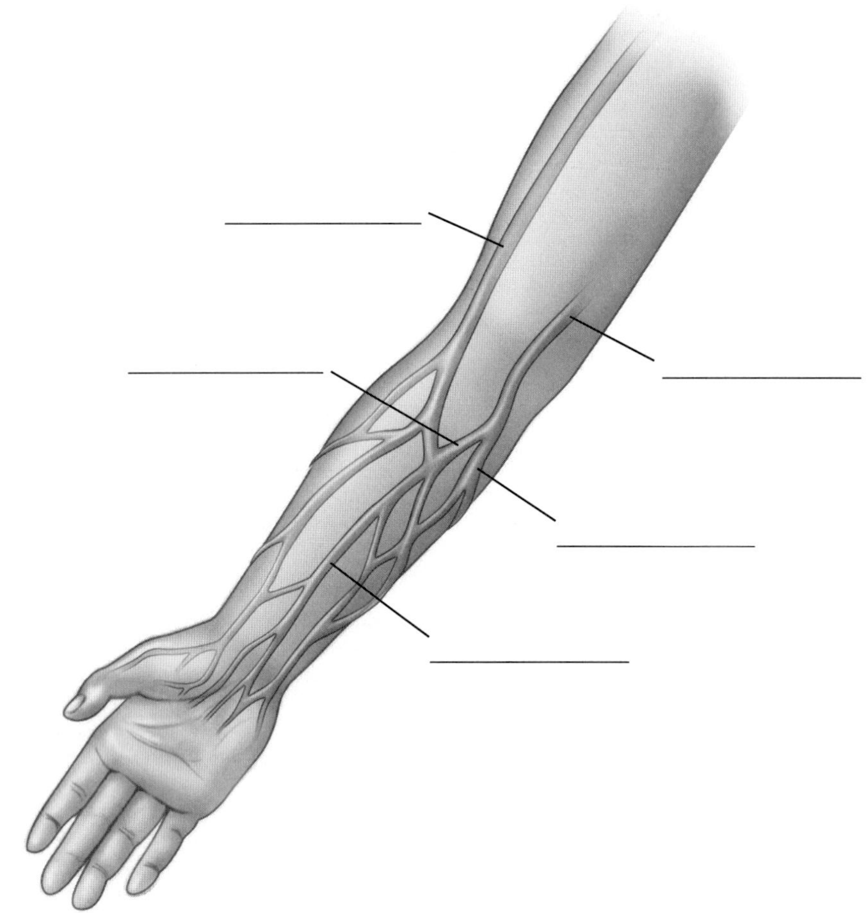

5. Identify the parts of the evacuated tube system for venipuncture on the illustration below.

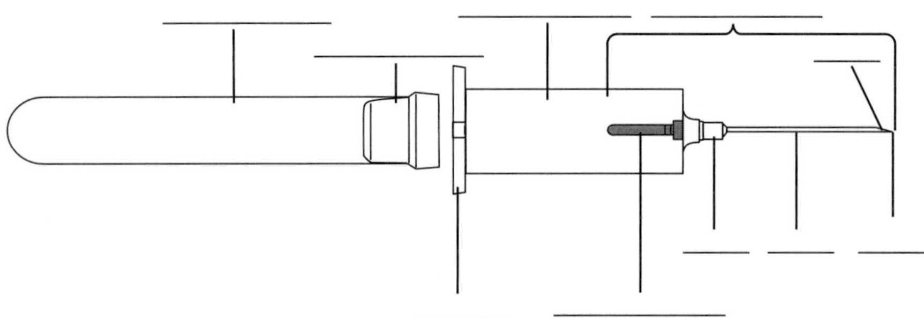

6. What happens to the blood in an evacuated tube if there is no additive? After it sits for several minutes, what is found in the tube?

____

____

____

____

7. Identify the correct order of draw for the evacuated tube method of venipuncture including the color of the rubber stopper.

____

____

____

8. What measures are used to protect the phlebotomist during venipuncture?

____

____

____

9. Identify seven reasons why blood may fail to enter the tube during venipuncture.

a. _______________

b. _______________

c. _______________

d. _______________

e. _______________

f. _______________

g. _______________

10. Why would the syringe method of venipuncture be used? What are its disadvantages compared to the vacuum tube method?

____

____

____

11. In what order are the vacuum tubes filled after drawing blood with the syringe method?

____

____

____

12. What are the advantages and disadvantages of using a butterfly needle to draw blood?

____

____

____

13. What are the five most common problems that occur during venipuncture?

a. ____

b. ____

c. ____

d. ____

e. ____

14. What are the two sites used most commonly for capillary puncture?

a. ____

b. ____

15. Identify three types of collection devices used for capillary puncture.

a. ____

b. ____

c. ____

16. Describe how a capillary puncture should be made on the finger when using a test strip.

____

____

____

17. What part of the heel can be used, and for what patients is a heel stick suitable?

____

____

____

18. What is PKU? Why do states require testing of infants?

____

____

____

19. What are the five basic elements that are identified in a CBC?

a. ____

b. ____

c. ____

d. ____

e. ____

20. What additional information is provided when a differential count is done with the CBC?

____

____

____

____

21. What is hemoglobin and what is its function?

____

____

____

____

22. Identify three ways that hemoglobin can be measured.

    a. ____

    b. ____

    c. ____

23. What is a hematocrit and what does the value indicate?

____

____

____

24. What is the ESR (erythrocyte sedimentation rate) and what do abnormal values indicate?

____

____

____

25. What do coagulation studies measure?

____

____

____

26. Describe how to collect a blood sample for a coagulation test if the blood will be sent to an outside lab.

____

____

____

27. Discuss the types of patients for whom the following coagulation tests are performed.

    a. Prothrombin time (PT) ____

    ____

    b. Partial thromboplastin time (PTT) ____

    ____

CRITICAL THINKING QUESTIONS

1. In many facilities, serum separator tubes (red and gray stopper) are drawn immediately after tubes without additives (red stopper), even though the manufacturer recommends drawing tiger top tubes after tubes containing anticoagulants. Do you think this is usually a problem? Why or why not?

2. Research the medical offices in your area to determine which offices perform venipuncture and/or capillary punctures. Determine what tests are done in the office and which tests are sent to outside laboratories. Which blood tests are most commonly performed in the office? What reasons do offices give if they do not draw blood or send blood to an outside lab for testing?

3. Look up the following blood conditions and describe them briefly. What abnormal values might be seen on the CBC or hematocrit?
   a. iron deficiency anemia
   b. sickle cell anemia
   c. polycythemia
   d. thrombocytopenia purpura

PRACTICAL APPLICATIONS

1. What should the medical assistant do or answer if the patient says any of the following things prior to venipuncture:
   a. "You are going to have trouble. They can never get my blood."

b. "I get so lightheaded when someone draws my blood." ______________________

____

____

c. "They don't like to use my left arm because I had a total mastectomy on that side ten years ago." ______________________

____

____

d. "They always use my right arm for this." ______________________

____

____

e. "Are you guys vampires or something? Why do you need so much blood?" ______________________

____

____

2. Describe what the medical assistant should do if he or she has inserted the needle for venipuncture and put the first vacuum tube on the needle, but blood is not flowing into the tube.

____

____

____

____

3. Describe what could happen if each of the following occurs while the medical assistant is performing venipuncture:

a. The medical assistant does not remember to remove the tourniquet before removing the needle from the vein. ______________________

____

b. The medical assistant forgets to label the tube of blood at the time of collection. ______________________

____

c. The blood fills half the tube of blood and then stops flowing. ______________________

____

d. The medical assistant pushes the tube onto the needle in the holder before entering the vein. ______________________

____

e. Blood for a complete blood count is collected in a tube with a red stopper. ______________________

____

f. A 26 gauge needle is used to collect a blood specimen. ______________________

____

g. The medical assistant leaves the tourniquet on for 3 minutes. ______________________

____

h. Pressure is not applied to the puncture site after the procedure.

____

____

4. Describe what could happen if each of the following occurs while the medical assistant is performing a capillary puncture:

a. The medical assistant performs the puncture while alcohol is still wet on the skin. ________

____

b. The medical assistant performs a heel stick at the back of the heel. ______________________

____

c. The medical assistant squeezes the finger to get blood or uses the first drop of blood. ______

____

d. The medical assistant warms the heel of an infant before performing a heel stick. ________

____

PROCEDURE PERFORMANCE CHECKLISTS

Procedure 25-1: Drawing Blood Using the Evacuated-Tube Method

Performance Objective

Task: Collect a venous blood specimen using the evacuated tube method

Conditions: Gloves, alcohol pad, 2 × 2 gauze squares, tourniquet, double pointed needle (20-22 gauge, 1 to 1 1/2 inch), plastic holder, evacuated tubes for tests ordered, rigid biohazard waste container, bandage

Standards: Complete the procedure in 10 minutes, and achieve a satisfactory score on the procedure performance checklist

Scoring Key: (**S**)*atisfactory,* (**U**)*nsatisfactory,* (**NA**) *Not Applicable*
◆ *Denotes a critical element for a satisfactory score on the procedure*

Procedure Steps	1st trial	2nd trial	3rd trial
1. Wash hands.			
2. Review lab slip or encounter form for tests ordered.			
3. Choose appropriate collection tubes.			
4. Gather other supplies.			
5. Screw the posterior needle into the needle holder securely.			
6. Open the alcohol pad.			
7. Place first tube in holder with stopper just making contact with the needle.			
8. Place tubes in order in easy reach of the nondominant hand.			
9. Greet patient.			
10. Explain procedure.			
11. Identify patient from lab slip.			
12. Review requisition, and ask patient about any required preparation (i.e., fasting).			
13. Visually assess patient's veins.			
14. If veins appear moderate to large, and in good condition, proceed.			
15. If veins are not visible, place a tourniquet 3–4 inches above bend in elbow.			
16. Place tourniquet behind the arm, holding an end with each hand.			

Procedure Steps	1st trial	2nd trial	3rd trial
17. Cross the ends in front, putting tension on the tourniquet.			
18. Hold the place where the tourniquet ends cross with one hand and tuck the flap of one end under, flap facing up.			
19. Locate suitable vein or try other arm.			
20. If assessment takes longer than 1 minute, release tourniquet.			
21. Put on gloves. (You may also wish to wear safety glasses or goggles.)			
22. Apply or reapply tourniquet if it has been released.			
23. Ask patient to make a fist and hold arm straight.			
24. Palpate the site to determine location and direction of vein.			
25. Clean site with alcohol wipe.			
26. Wipe area you have cleaned with gauze square or allow to dry.			
27. Pick up prepared holder with needle and tube attached.			
28. Remove needle cover.			
29. Hold equipment in dominant hand at a 15-degree angle with the bevel of the needle facing up.			
30. Stabilize vein with the thumb of nondominant hand.			
31. Penetrate the vein with a quick motion in the direction of the vein.			
32. Allow the holder to rest on your fingers against skin of patient's lower arm.			
33. Do not move holder or needle.			
34. Using nondominant hand, push the evacuated tube completely into the holder (tube should begin to fill).			
35. Allow the tube to fill by vacuum action.			
36. When tube is full, withdraw, and without moving the holder or needle, put on the next tube, following the correct order of draw.			
37. When last tube begins filling, release the tourniquet by pulling on the end that was tucked under.			
38. Remove last tube from holder.			

Procedure Steps	1st trial	2nd trial	3rd trial
39. Place gauze square over the puncture site.			
40. Be sure tourniquet has been released before removing needle. ◆			
41. Remove needle rapidly at same angle it entered.			
42. Apply pressure at puncture site after needle has been removed.			
43. Ask patient to apply pressure for 2 minutes.			
44. Do not allow patient to bend arm.			
45. Dispose of needle in rigid biohazard waste container.			
46. While patient is holding gauze square, gently rotate any tubes with additives 8–10 times to mix the blood with the additive.			
47. Label the tubes with the date, time, patient's name, doctor's name, and your initials; or apply preprinted labels.			
48. When bleeding has stopped, fold gauze square into quarters, place over puncture, and apply bandage to hold in place.			
49. After tubes have been labeled and mixed, place in the appropriate area for testing or transfer (with appropriate requisitions).			
50. If preparing for transfer, place into plastic biohazard transfer bag.			
51. Remove and discard gloves in biohazard waste container.			
52. Wash hands.			
53. Document in patient medical record the date, time, lab tests ordered, arm blood was drawn from, and any adverse reaction.			
54. Complete the procedure within 10 minutes. ◆			

Charting

DATE	

Evaluator Comments:

Score Calculation:

For each procedural step marked U (Unsatisfactory) deduct 6 points
For each procedural step (◆) marked U (Unsatisfactory) deduct 20 points

Score calculation 100 points

– points missed

Total score

1st	2nd	3rd

Satisfactory score: 85 or above

Procedure 25-2: Drawing Blood Using the Syringe Method

Performance Objective

Task: Collect a venous blood specimen using the syringe method

Conditions: Gloves, alcohol pad, 2 × 2 gauze squares, tourniquet, 20-22 gauge needle, syringe large enough to contain blood for tests ordered, evacuated tubes appropriate for tests ordered, test tube rack, rigid biohazard waste container, bandage

Standards: Complete the procedure in 10 minutes, and achieve a satisfactory score on the procedure performance checklist.

*Scoring Key: (**S**)atisfactory, (**U**)nsatisfactory, (**NA**) Not Applicable*
◆ *Denotes a critical element for a satisfactory score on the procedure*

Procedure Steps	1st trial	2nd trial	3rd trial
1. Wash hands.			
2. Review lab slip or encounter forms.			
3. Choose appropriate collection tubes.			
4. Prepare needle and syringe.			
5. Open alcohol pad.			
6. Greet patient.			
7. Explain procedure.			
8. Identify patient from lab slip.			
9. Question patient about any required preparation (i.e., fasting).			
10. Visually assess the patient's veins.			
11. If vein appears moderate to large and in good condition, proceed with collection.			
12. If veins are not visible, place a tourniquet 3–4 inches above bend in elbow.			
13. Ask patient to make a fist and palpate to find a suitable vein. If necessary, check both arms.			
14. If assessment takes longer than 1 minute, release tourniquet.			
15. Put on gloves. (You may also wish to wear safety glasses or goggles.)			
16. Apply or reapply tourniquet if it has been released.			

Procedure Steps	1st trial	2nd trial	3rd trial
17. Clean site selected.			
18. Remove needle cover.			
19. Hold syringe in dominant hand at a 15-degree angle, with thumb on top and fingers curled under the syringe.			
20. Stabilize vein with thumb of nondominant hand.			
21. Penetrate the vein with a quick motion in the direction of the vein.			
22. Pull back on plunger of syringe slowly until blood fills the syringe.			
23. Keep pulling slowly until you have obtained as much blood as necessary.			
24. Release tourniquet. ◆			
25. Place a gauze square over the puncture site.			
26. Remove needle rapidly at same angle it entered.			
27. Apply pressure to puncture site.			
28. Ask patient to apply pressure for 1 to 2 minutes.			
29. Tell patient not to bend arm.			
30. Place correct evacuated tube(s) in a test tube rack in correct order of draw.			
31. Transfer blood by inserting the needle through the rubber stopper and allowing the vacuum to pull the blood from the tubes.			
32. Do not hold tube while inserting needle.			
33. Discard needle and syringe in rigid biohazard waste container.			
34. While patient is holding gauze square, gently rotate any tubes with additives eight to 10 times to mix blood and additive.			
35. Label tubes with the date, time, patient's name, doctor's name, and your initials; or apply preprinted labels.			
36. When bleeding has stopped, fold gauze square into quarters, place over puncture, and apply bandage to hold in place.			
37. Place tubes in appropriate area for testing or for transfer (if transfer, include appropriate requisitions).			

Procedure Steps	1st trial	2nd trial	3rd trial
38. If preparing for transfer, place tubes into plastic biohazard transfer bag.			
39. Remove and discard gloves in biohazard waste container.			
40. Wash hands.			
41. Document in patient's record the date, time, lab tests requested, arm blood drawn from, and any adverse reactions.			
42. Complete the procedure within 10 minutes. ◆			

Charting

DATE	

Evaluator Comments:

Score Calculation:

For each procedural step marked U (Unsatisfactory) deduct 6 points
For each procedural step (◆) marked U (Unsatisfactory) deduct 20 points

Score calculation 100 points

– points missed

Total score

1st	2nd	3rd

Satisfactory score: 85 or above

Notes

Procedure 25-3: Drawing Blood Using the Butterfly Method

Performance Objective

Task: Collect a venous blood specimen using the butterfly method

Conditions: Gloves, alcohol pad, 2 × 2 gauze squares, tourniquet, winged-infusion set with a Luer adapter (21-23 gauge needle), plastic holder or syringe, evacuated tubes, test tube rack, rigid biohazard waste container, bandage

Standards: Complete the procedure in 10 minutes, and achieve a satisfactory score on the procedure performance checklist

Scoring Key: (**S**)*atisfactory,* (**U**)*nsatisfactory,* (**NA**) *Not Applicable*
◆ *Denotes a critical element for a satisfactory score on the procedure*

Procedure Steps	1st trial	2nd trial	3rd trial
1. Wash hands.			
2. Review lab slip or encounter form.			
3. Choose appropriate collection tubes.			
4. Gather other supplies.			
5. Prepare the winged-infusion set by attaching the end of the plastic tubing to the syringe or to the Luer adapter needle (if not already packaged together) and pulling tubing straight.			
6. If using the evacuated tube method, screw the needle into a plastic holder and place the first tube loosely into the holder with the tip of the needle just making contact with the stopper.			
7. Greet the patient.			
8. Explain the procedure.			
9. Use the lab slip to identify the patient.			
10. Question patient about any required preparation (i.e. fasting).			
11. Place tourniquet 3–4 inches above bend in elbow, 2–3 inches below elbow (for lower arm) or 1–2 inches above wrist (for back of hand).			
12. Assess the patient's veins on both arms.			
13. If assessment takes longer than one minute, release tourniquet.			
14. After you have located a suitable vein, put on gloves. (You may also wish to wear safety glasses or goggles.)			
15. Reapply tourniquet if needed and ask patient to make a fist and hold arm straight.			

Procedure Steps	1st trial	2nd trial	3rd trial
16. Palpate the site to determine location and direction of vein.			
17. Clean site with alcohol wipe.			
18. Wipe area you have cleaned with gauze square or allow to dry.			
19. Apply or reapply tourniquet if it has been released.			
20. Hold the blue wings of the butterfly needle in dominant hand, bevel up, with needle at a 15-degree angle.			
21. Enter middle of vein with one rapid motion.			
22. Stabilize vein with thumb of nondominant hand if you are afraid vein will roll.			
23. Allow the needle to rest in the vein supported by the wings.			
24. Rotate the needle if necessary until the needle rests flat.			
25. Blood will enter tubing.			
26. If using the evacuated tube method, push the first tube completely on to the needle, and allow the tube to fill by vacuum action.			
27. When full, remove tube and without moving holder or needle, put on the next tube, following, correct order of draw.			
OR, if using syringe method:			
27A. If using syringe, slowly pull back on the plunger until the syringe has filled with the desired amount of blood.			
28. When last tube begins filling, or when you have removed enough blood into the syringe, release tourniquet by pulling on the end that was tucked under. ◆			
29. Place a gauze square over the puncture site.			
30. Remove needle at the same angle it entered.			
31. Apply pressure to the puncture site after needle is out.			
32. Ask patient to apply pressure for 1 to 2 minutes.			
33. Instruct patient not to bend arm or wrist.			
34. Discard winged-infusion needle and tubing into a rigid biohazard container.			

Procedure Steps	1st trial	2nd trial	3rd trial
35. If you drew blood into a syringe, attach a new needle to the syringe to keep the tip of the syringe sterile until you transfer the blood to the evacuated tube.			
36. If you drew blood in a syringe, place the correct evacuated tube(s) in a test tube rack in the correct order of draw.			
37. Transfer blood by inserting the needle through the rubber stopper and allowing the vacuum to pull the blood into the tube.			
38. For safety, do not hold the vacuum tube while inserting the needle.			
39. While the patient is applying pressure with gauze square, gently rotate any tubes with additive 8 to 10 times to mix the blood and additive.			
40. Label the tubes with the date, time, patient's name, doctor's name, and your initials, or apply preprinted labels.			
41. When bleeding has stopped, fold gauze square into quarters, place over the puncture site, and apply a bandage to hold in place.			
42. Place tubes in appropriate area for testing, or transfer with the appropriate requisitions.			
43. Remove and discard gloves into biohazard waste container.			
44. Wash hands.			
45. Document in patient's record the date, time, tests required, arm from which blood was drawn, and any adverse reaction.			
46. Complete the procedure within 10 minutes. ◆			

Charting

DATE	

Evaluator Comments:

Score Calculation:

For each procedural step marked U (Unsatisfactory) deduct 6 points
For each procedural step (◆) marked U (Unsatisfactory) deduct 20 points

Score calculation	100 points			
	– ___ points missed	1st	2nd	3rd
	Total score			

Satisfactory score: 85 or above

Procedure 25-4: Obtaining a Capillary Blood Specimen Using a Finger Stick

Performance Objective

Task: Collect a capillary blood specimen using a finger stick

Conditions: Gloves, alcohol pads, sterile gauze, collecting device or test strip, disposable lancet, rigid biohazard waste container

Standards: Complete the procedure in 5 minutes, and achieve a satisfactory score on the procedure performance checklist

Scoring Key: **(S)***atisfactory,* **(U)***nsatisfactory,* **(NA)** *Not Applicable*
◆ *Denotes a critical element for a satisfactory score on the procedure*

Procedure Steps	1st trial	2nd trial	3rd trial
1. Wash hands.			
2. Assemble supplies and equipment.			
3. Open an alcohol pad and sterile gauze square.			
4. Identify patient.			
5. Explain procedure to patient.			
6. Clean finger with alcohol.			
7. Allow to air-dry.			
8. Put on gloves.			
9. Twist the small knob off of a manual lancet, or prepare an automatic lancet for use.			
10. Hold the finger in a downward position.			
11. Without touching the area you have cleaned, make a puncture with the sterile lancet.			
12. Dispose of lancet in a rigid biohazard waste container.			
13. Allow blood to flow freely.			
14. Wipe away first drop of blood.			
15. Collect blood in microcollection device, or apply hanging drop of blood to a test strip.			
16. When collection is complete, place sterile gauze over puncture site.			
17. Apply pressure.			

Procedure Steps	1st trial	2nd trial	3rd trial
18. When bleeding stops, apply bandage.			
19. Test specimen as appropriate.			
20. Remove and discard gloves, with soiled gauze, in biohazard waste container.			
21. Wash hands.			
22. Complete the procedure within 5 minutes. ◆			

Evaluator Comments:

Score Calculation:

For each procedural step marked U (Unsatisfactory) deduct 6 points
For each procedural step (◆) marked U (Unsatisfactory) deduct 20 points

Score calculation 100 points

– ___ points missed

Total score

1st	2nd	3rd

Satisfactory score: 85 or above

Procedure 25-5: Obtaining a Capillary Blood Specimen Using a Heel Stick

Performance Objective

Task: Collect a capillary blood specimen using a heel stick

Conditions: Warm compress, gloves, alcohol pads, sterile gauze, pediatric collection tubes or capillary tubes, sealing clay (for capillary tubes), disposable pediatric lancet, rigid biohazard waste container

Standards: Complete the procedure in 5 minutes, and achieve a satisfactory score on the procedure performance checklist

Scoring Key: (**S**)*atisfactory,* (**U**)*nsatisfactory,* (**NA**) *Not Applicable*
◆ *Denotes a critical element for a satisfactory score on the procedure*

Procedure Steps	1st trial	2nd trial	3rd trial
1. Wash hands.			
2. Assemble supplies and equipment.			
3. Open alcohol pad and sterile gauze square.			
4. Identify the infant.			
5. Explain procedure to infant's parent or caretaker.			
6. Warm infant's heel with warm compress for 5 minutes.			
7. Clean heal selected for puncture with alcohol.			
8. Allow to dry.			
9. Put on gloves.			
10. Grasp infant's heel firmly and make puncture.			
11. If using automatic lancet, press firmly against skin of heel and activate to cause puncture.			
12. Discard lancet into rigid biohazard container.			
13. Allow blood to flow freely.			
14. Wipe away first drop of blood.			
15. Collect blood specimen in desired microcollection device, and seal if necessary.			
16. When collection is complete, place sterile gauze over puncture site.			

Procedure Steps	1st trial	2nd trial	3rd trial
17. Apply pressure.			
18. When bleeding stops, apply bandage.			
19. Test specimen as appropriate.			
20. Remove and discard gloves, along with soiled gauze, in biohazard waste container.			
21. Wash hands.			
22. Complete the procedure within 5 minutes. ◆			

Evaluator Comments:

Score Calculation:

For each procedural step marked U (Unsatisfactory) deduct 6 points
For each procedural step (◆) marked U (Unsatisfactory) deduct 20 points

Score calculation 100 points

− ____ points missed

Total score

1st	2nd	3rd

Satisfactory score: 85 or above

Procedure 25-6: Obtaining a Capillary Blood Specimen for PKU Testing

Performance Objective

Task: Collect a capillary blood specimen from an infant for PKU testing

Conditions: Warm compress, disposable gloves, alcohol pads, sterile gauze, PKU test card and mailing envelope, disposable pediatric lancet, rigid biohazard container

Standards: Complete the procedure in 5 minutes, and achieve a satisfactory score on the procedure performance checklist

Scoring Key: (**S**)*atisfactory*, (**U**)*nsatisfactory*, (**NA**) *Not Applicable*
◆ *Denotes a critical element for a satisfactory score on the procedure*

Procedure Steps	1st trial	2nd trial	3rd trial
1. Wash hands.			
2. Assemble supplies and equipment.			
3. Open alcohol pad and sterile gauze square.			
4. Obtain information from parent or caregiver to complete PKU test card.			
5. Warm infant's heel with compress for about 5 minutes.			
6. Clean heel selected for puncture with alcohol.			
7. Allow to air-dry.			
8. Put on gloves.			
9. Prepare a pediatric lancet.			
10. Grasp infant's heel firmly and make puncture.			
11. If using an automatic lancet, press firmly against the skin of the heel and activate device.			
12. Discard lancet into rigid biohazard container.			
13. Allow blood to flow freely.			
14. Wipe away first drop of blood.			
15. Apply infant's heel to each circle of the PKU test card, holding heel firmly but not squeezing.			
16. Fill each circle with blood so that blood can be seen on reverse side of card.			
17. When collection is complete, place sterile gauze over puncture site.			

Procedure Steps	1st trial	2nd trial	3rd trial
18. Apply pressure.			
19. When bleeding stops, apply bandage.			
20. Remove and discard gloves, along with soiled gauze, in biohazard waste container.			
21. Wash hands.			
22. Allow test card to dry for two hours at room temperature.			
23. Place card in mailing envelope and mail within 48 hours.			
24. Record in patient's medical record that specimen was obtained and mailed to laboratory.			
25. Complete the procedure within 5 minutes. ◆			

Charting

DATE	

Evaluator Comments:

Score Calculation:

For each procedural step marked U (Unsatisfactory) deduct 6 points
For each procedural step (◆) marked U (Unsatisfactory) deduct 20 points

Score calculation 100 points

− points missed

Total score

1st	2nd	3rd

Satisfactory score: 85 or above

Procedure 25-7: Preparing a Peripheral Blood Smear

Performance Objective

Task: Prepare a blood smear for a differential count

Conditions: Gloves, alcohol pads, sterile gauze, glass slides with frosted end, disposable lancet, rigid biohazard waste container

Standards: Complete the procedure in 5 minutes, and achieve a satisfactory score on the procedure performance checklist

Scoring Key: (S)*atisfactory,* (U)*nsatisfactory,* (NA) *Not Applicable*
◆ *Denotes a critical element for a satisfactory score on the procedure*

Procedure Steps	1st trial	2nd trial	3rd trial
1. Wash hands.			
2. Assemble supplies and equipment.			
3. Label at least two slides with the patient's name and date, in pencil.			
4. Identify patient.			
5. Explain procedure to patient.			
6. Clean finger to be punctured with alcohol wipe.			
7. Allow to dry.			
8. Put on gloves.			
9. Twist the small knob off of a manual lancet, or prepare an automatic lancet for use.			
10. Hold the finger in a downward position.			
11. Without touching the area you have cleaned, make a puncture with the sterile lancet perpendicular to the fingerprint swirls.			
12. Discard lancet in a rigid biohazard container.			
13. Allow blood to flow freely.			
14. Wipe away the first drop of blood with gauze.			
15. Allow a second drop to form.			
16. With patient finger pointing down, touch drop (but not finger) to the slide about 1/4 inch from the frosted end.			
17. Hold another slide at a 30–35-degree angle.			

Procedure Steps	1st trial	2nd trial	3rd trial
18. Bring edge of spreader slide into blood drop.			
19. Spread blood over 3/4 of slide.			
20. Repeat to prepare a second slide if needed.			
21. When collection is complete, place sterile gauze over puncture site.			
22. Apply pressure.			
23. When bleeding stops, apply bandage.			
24. Allow slides to air-dry.			
25. Remove and discard gloves and soiled gauze into biohazard waste container.			
26. Wash hands.			
27. Complete the procedure within 5 minutes. ◆			

Evaluator Comments:

Score Calculation:

For each procedural step marked U (Unsatisfactory) deduct 6 points
For each procedural step (◆) marked U (Unsatisfactory) deduct 20 points

Score calculation 100 points

− points missed

Total score

1st	2nd	3rd

Satisfactory score: 85 or above

Procedure 25-8: Testing Hemoglobin Using a Hemoglobinometer

Performance Objective

Task: Test hemoglobin using a hemoglobinometer

Conditions: Gloves, alcohol pads, sterile gauze, disposable lancet, hemoglobinometer, reagent applicators, rigid biohazard waste container

Standards: Complete procedure in 10 minutes, and achieve a satisfactory score on the procedure performance checklist

Scoring Key: (**S**)*atisfactory,* (**U**)*nsatisfactory,* (**NA**) *Not Applicable*
◆ *Denotes a critical element for a satisfactory score on the procedure*

Procedure Steps	1st trial	2nd trial	3rd trial
1. Wash hands.			
2. Assemble supplies and equipment.			
3. Prepare hemoglobinometer by removing chamber and opening it so the chamber slide is visible.			
4. Identify patient.			
5. Explain procedure to patient.			
6. Clean finger selected for puncture with alcohol wipe.			
7. Allow to dry.			
8. Put on gloves.			
9. Twist small knob off of a manual lancet or prepare an automatic lancet for use.			
10. Hold finger in a downward position.			
11. Without touching area you have cleaned, make puncture with the sterile lancet.			
12. Discard lancet in rigid biohazard container.			
13. Allow blood to flow freely.			
14. Wipe away first drop of blood.			
15. Allow a second drop to form.			
16. With patient finger pointed down, touch blood (but not finger) to chamber slide.			

Procedure Steps	1st trial	2nd trial	3rd trial
17. Using a reagent stick, stir the drop of blood to hemolyze red blood cells.			
18. Holding device horizontally at eye level, turn on the light.			
19. Move slide on right side of the instrument until both sides of the split field appear to be the same shade of green.			
20. Read the scale on the side of the instrument that identifies the hemoglobin reading in grams per deciliter of blood.			
21. Dispose of biohazard waste and clean the hemoglobinometer chamber and work area.			
22. Remove and discard gloves in biohazard waste container.			
23. Wash hands.			
24. Record test results in patient medical record in gm/dL.			
25. The results recorded are the same as those of the evaluator. ◆			
26. Complete the procedure within 10 minutes. ◆			

Charting

DATE	

Evaluator Comments:

Score Calculation:

For each procedural step marked U (Unsatisfactory) deduct 6 points
For each procedural step (◆) marked U (Unsatisfactory) deduct 20 points

Score calculation 100 points

– points missed

Total score

1st	2nd	3rd

Satisfactory score: 85 or above

Procedure 25-9: Performing a Microhematocrit

Performance Objective

Task: Perform a microhematocrit test

Conditions: Gloves, alcohol pads, sterile gauze, blood sample containing EDTA (lavender stopper) or disposable lancet, capillary tubes, sealing clay, microhematocrit centrifuge and reader, rigid biohazard waste container

Standards: Complete the procedure in 10 minutes, and achieve a satisfactory score on the procedure performance checklist

Scoring Key: **(S)***atisfactory,* **(U)***nsatisfactory,* **(NA)** *Not Applicable*
◆ *Denotes a critical element for a satisfactory score on the procedure*

Procedure Steps	1st trial	2nd trial	3rd trial
1. Wash hands.			
2. Assemble supplies and equipment.			
3. Identify patient.			
4. Explain procedure to patient.			
5. Put on gloves.			
6. Remove the rubber stopper from a sample of anticoagulated blood (lavender stopper), or perform a finger puncture.			
7. Discard lancet in a rigid biohazard waste container.			
8. Hold capillary tube (heparinized tube for finger stick) at an angle to the tube of blood or second drop that has formed at the site of capillary puncture, and allow tube to fill by capillary action until 3/4 full.			
9. If using a finger or heel stick, apply gentle pressure but do not squeeze.			
10. Fill two tubes, avoiding bubbles.			
11. Seal one end of each capillary tube with sealing clay.			
12. Place capillary tubes in microhematocrit centrifuge, clay-sealed end outward.			
13. Balance centrifuge with capillary tubes opposite each other.			
14. Place cover over tubes and secure. Close centrifuge securely.			
15. Centrifuge for 5 minutes.			

Procedure Steps	1st trial	2nd trial	3rd trial
16. After centrifuge has completely stopped, open and remove cover.			
17. Remove the two tubes carefully.			
18. Align the top of sealing clay, where red cells begin, on the "O" mark of the microhematocrit reader.			
19. Move the outer disk until the reading line is aligned with the meniscus of the plasma in the tubes.			
20. Rotate the reader until the reading line lies exactly underneath the junction of the packed red cells and the buffy coat.			
21. Read the results on the scale at the outer edge of the reader.			
22. Average the two readings.			
23. Discard tubes and used supplies in biohazard waste container.			
24. Remove and discard gloves in biohazard waste container.			
25. Wash hands.			
26. Document results in the patient's medical record.			
27. The results recorded are within ±1 of the evaluator. ◆			
28. Complete the procedure within 10 minutes. ◆			

Charting

DATE	

Evaluator Comments:

Score Calculation:

For each procedural step marked U (Unsatisfactory) deduct 6 points
For each procedural step (◆) marked U (Unsatisfactory) deduct 20 points

Score calculation	100 points			
	– ____ points missed	1st	2nd	3rd
	Total score			

Satisfactory score: 85 or above

SELF-EVALUATION

Chapter 26

Microbiology, Immunology, and Chemistry

CHAPTER FOCUS

In this chapter you learned how to collect and process specimens to grow and/or test for microorganisms (microbiology), to test for antigen-antibody response (immunology or serology), and to test for chemicals in various body fluids (chemistry). The medical assistant is responsible for specimen collection, proper handling of specimens, and either the actual testing or preparing specimens and paperwork for transfer to an outside laboratory.

TERMINOLOGY REVIEW

Vocabulary Matching: Match each term with its definition.

___ 1. incubator

___ 2. high-density lipoproteins

___ 3. triglycerides

___ 4. parasite

___ 5. immunoassay

___ 6. culture medium (plural: media)

___ 7. titer

___ 8. *in vitro*

___ 9. mordant

A. A standard strength per volume of solution, used to test for the presence of antibodies

B. Antibiotic disks placed in culture medium to determine which antibiotic(s) will prevent growth of specific bacteria

C. A substance obtained from seaweed used to grow microorganisms

D. Clumping of blood cells

E. A chemical that reacts with other substances

F. An unsaturated alcohol used by the body to produce hormones

G. A test that attempts to grow microorganisms to determine the type and number of organisms present

H. A substance rich in nutrients into which a culture is placed to see if bacteria grow

I. The virus that causes infectious mononucleosis

___ 10. heterophile antibodies	J. Specific antibodies seen in infectious mononucleosis
___ 11. sensitivity	K. The substance responsible for transporting cholesterol to the liver to assist in the manufacture of bile
___ 12. culture	L. A test for the presence of a specific antibody
___ 13. agar	M. A cabinet that maintains a constant temperature
___ 14. cholesterol	N. In the laboratory or test tube
___ 15. *in vivo*	O. In the person
___ 16. low-density lipoproteins	P. Substance that transports cholesterol to blood vessels and tissues
___ 17. reagent	Q. A substance that holds stain onto a slide for microscopic examination
___ 18. agglutination	R. A combination of glycerol and fatty acids
___ 19. Epstein-Barr virus	S. Organisms that live on or in a host organism

Abbreviations: Expand each abbreviation to its complete form.

1. BUN ______________________________
2. C&S ______________________________
3. CSF ______________________________
4. EBV ______________________________
5. EIA ______________________________
6. ELISA ______________________________
7. FBS ______________________________
8. hCG ______________________________
9. HDL ______________________________
10. LDL ______________________________

CONTENT REVIEW QUESTIONS

1. Describe five items of equipment that are used specifically for microbiological testing, including what they are used for.

   a. ______________________________

   b. ______________________________

   c. ______________________________

   d. ______________________________

   e. ______________________________

2. List six safety rules for microbiological testing.

a. ______

b. ______

c. ______

d. ______

e. ______

f. ______

3. Identify four quality-control activities for the microbiology lab.

a. ______

b. ______

c. ______

d. ______

4. What is a culture?

______

______

______

5. Identify six different places or types of specimens that can be obtained for culture.

a. ______

b. ______

c. ______

d. ______

e. ______

f. ______

6. Identify three methods for collecting a urine culture.

a. ______

b. ______

c. ______

7. When are the following types of specimens observed under the microscope?

a. wet mount ______

b. hanging-drop specimen ______

c. dry smear (usually stained) ______

8. Describe the process of preparing a slide with the Gram's stain. When complete, what differentiates gram-positive from gram-negative organisms?

______

______

______

9. If a bacterial culture breaks down the agar on a blood agar plate leaving a clear area, what type of microorganism is present?

____

____

10. What is done if more than one type of bacteria grows on a culture plate?

____

____

11. How can a culture be used to estimate the number of bacteria present?

____

____

____

12. In what position are agar plates placed into an incubator? Why?

____

____

____

13. Describe sensitivity testing and identify why it is done.

____

____

____

14. What are parasites and how are they identified?

____

____

____

15. If a patient has diarrhea that doesn't respond to treatment, diarrhea with a high fever, or bloody diarrhea, what should the stool be tested for?

____

16. How is a vaginal specimen tested for trichomonas? How soon after collection must the test be done?

____

____

17. Identify two other types of parasites and describe how they are identified.

a. ____

____

b. ____

____

18. Why are serology (immunology) tests often used to diagnose viral conditions?

____

____

19. Identify four immunologic tests that may be done in the physician's office, the body fluid tested, and the disease or condition diagnosed.

    a. ____

    b. ____

    c. ____

    d. ____

20. Why is a person's blood type identified and a small sample of their blood mixed with blood from a possible donor before a transfusion? What will happen if the two blood types are incompatible? What will happen if they are compatible?

____

____

____

____

____

21. Identify three common types of immunologic tests and give an example of each.

    a. ____

    b. ____

    c. ____

22. What part of blood is used for chemistry testing?

____

____

23. Describe the following tests of blood glucose.

    a. fasting blood sugar (FBS) ____

    ____

    b. glucose tolerance test ____

    ____

    c. two-hour postprandial glucose ____

    ____

24. Describe four other chemical elements that are often tested in blood.

    a. ____

    b. ____

    c. ____

    d. ____

CRITICAL THINKING QUESTIONS

1. How did the development of staining techniques for use with the microscope by Robert Koch (1843–1910), Hans Gram (1853–1938), Franz Ziehl (1856–1926), and Fredrich Neelsen (1854–1894) help scientists with the study of bacteria?

____

____

____

____

____

____

2. Discuss how much teaching you think the medical office should do about cholesterol and the meaning of blood levels of cholesterol, LDL, HDL, and triglycerides. Does an understanding of normal levels of these substances motivate patients to watch their diet and/or take cholesterol-lowering medication? Justify your answer.

____

____

____

____

____

____

3. Do research to find information about Rh incompatibility and the problems it can cause during pregnancy. You will find some information on this topic in chapter 29, but you may need to consult other resources. Discuss this problem and describe how it is treated.

____

____

____

____

____

____

PRACTICAL APPLICATIONS

1. When collecting wound cultures, why should two cultures usually be obtained and placed in different types of transport media?

____

____

2. Why should the physician observe any wound from which the medical assistant collects a wound culture?

3. Why should the medical assistant usually collect two swabs for a routine throat culture?

4. What special steps should the medical assistant take to obtain blood cultures?

5. What special steps should the medical assistant take when handling materials for culture?

6. How should the medical assistant prepare an agar plate for a urine culture? What is the advantage of using exactly 0.001 mL of urine?

7. Identify the signs and symptoms that the patient might complain of when the physician orders each of the following types of cultures. You may need to find information about bacterial diseases of the areas involved to answer this question.

   a. wound culture

   b. urine culture

   c. throat culture

   d. blood culture

   e. vaginal culture

   f. cerebrospinal culture

8. What instructions would you give a patient who needs to collect one or more stool specimens for ova and parasites?

____

____

____

9. What can you tell a mother who is extremely upset about her child's case of head lice?

____

____

____

____

PROCEDURE PERFORMANCE CHECKLISTS

Procedure 26-1: Obtaining a Wound Specimen for Microbiological Testing

Performance Objective

Task: Obtain a wound specimen for microbiological testing

Conditions: Gloves, lab coat, sterile culture kits containing tubes, swab, and transport media (both anaerobic and aerobic culture kits may be needed), supplies to clean and redress the wound, biohazard waste container

Standards: Complete the procedure in 10 minutes, and achieve a satisfactory score on the procedure performance checklist

Scoring Key: (**S**)*atisfactory,* (**U**)*nsatisfactory,* (**NA**) *Not Applicable*
◆ *Denotes a critical element for a satisfactory score on the procedure*

Procedure Steps	1st trial	2nd trial	3rd trial
1. Wash hands.			
2. Put on personal protective equipment.			
3. Identify patient.			
4. Explain the procedure.			
5. Remove old dressing.			
6. Discard old dressing in biohazard container.			
7. Inspect wound, observing odor, color, amount of drainage, redness, and depth of wound.			
8. Remove swab from culture kit.			
9. Swab area of wound where the most exudate is seen.			
10. If collecting for both anaerobic and aerobic cultures, collect anaerobic first from deepest part of wound.			
11. Place swab in culture tube immediately.			
12. Crush transport media ampule by squeezing sides of tube firmly.			
13. Label wound culture tubes with the patient's name, date, time, and doctor's name, or apply pre-printed labels.			
14. Remove and discard gloves in biohazard waste container.			
15. Set up for sterile dressing change (see Procedure 17-9).			

Procedure Steps	1st trial	2nd trial	3rd trial
16. Put on sterile gloves.			
17. Clean wound using sterile technique.			
18. Apply sterile dressing and secure.			
19. Clean the area and discard waste in biohazard waste container.			
20. Place culture tubes in plastic biohazard transfer container.			
21. Remove and discard gloves in biohazard waste container.			
22. Wash hands.			
23. Document appearance of wound, type and amount of drainage, type and number of specimens sent to lab.			
24. Complete lab slip if needed, and place in pocket of biohazard transfer container.			
25. Transport culture tubes to lab immediately or place in incubator until lab pickup.			
26. Complete the procedure within 10 minutes. ◆			

Charting

DATE	

Evaluator Comments:

Score Calculation:

For each procedural step marked U (Unsatisfactory) deduct 6 points
For each procedural step (◆) marked U (Unsatisfactory) deduct 20 points

Score calculation 100 points
– points missed
Total score

1st	2nd	3rd

Satisfactory score: 85 or above

Procedure 26-2: Obtaining a Throat Specimen for Microbiological Testing

Performance Objective

Task: Obtain a throat specimen and prepare for processing

Conditions: Gloves, lab coat, face protection, sterile Dacron-tipped throat swabs, or Culturette (swab in container with transport media), tongue depressor

Standards: Complete procedure in 5 minutes, and achieve a satisfactory score on the procedure performance checklist

Scoring Key: (**S**)*atisfactory,* (**U**)*nsatisfactory,* (**NA**) *Not Applicable*
◆ *Denotes a critical element for a satisfactory score on the procedure*

Procedure Steps	1st trial	2nd trial	3rd trial
1. Wash hands.			
2. Put on personal protective equipment.			
3. Identify patient.			
4. Explain procedure.			
5. Instruct patient to open mouth wide.			
6. Hold tongue down with tongue depressor.			
7. Swiftly and vigorously swab tonsillar areas (use figure-of-eight motion to reach all areas).			
8. If rapid strep test is to be performed, use two swabs.			
9. If performing in-house test, perform rapid strep test or plant on agar immediately and place in incubator. **or**			
9A. If sending to lab, place in Culturette and crush transport media ampule by squeezing sides of tube firmly.			
10. If sending sample(s) out, label culture tube(s) with patient name, date, time, and doctor's name, or apply pre-printed labels.			
11. Remove and discard gloves in biohazard waste container.			
12. Wash hands.			
13. Document that specimens were obtained and tested or sent to lab.			
14. Transport culture tube(s) to lab immediately or place in incubator to wait for lab pickup.			
15. Complete the procedure within 5 minutes. ◆			

Charting

DATE	

Evaluator Comments:

Score Calculation:

For each procedural step marked U (Unsatisfactory) deduct 6 points
For each procedural step (◆) marked U (Unsatisfactory) deduct 20 points

Score calculation 100 points

− points missed

Total score

1st	2nd	3rd

Satisfactory score: 85 or above

Procedure 26-3: Preparing a Wet Mount and Hanging Drop Slide

Performance Objective

Task: Prepare a wet mount and a hanging drop slide.

Conditions: Gloves, lab coat, face protection, swab and solution containing specimen for examination, glass slide, hanging drop slide, coverslips, bacteriostatic saline and dropper, 10 percent potassium hydroxide solution, petroleum jelly, microscope, rigid biohazard waste container

Standards: Complete the procedure in 5 minutes, and achieve a satisfactory score on the procedure performance checklist.

Scoring Key: (**S**)*atisfactory,* (**U**)*nsatisfactory,* (**NA**) *Not Applicable*
◆ *Denotes a critical element for a satisfactory score on the procedure*

Procedure Steps	1st trial	2nd trial	3rd trial
1. Wash hands.			
2. Assemble supplies and equipment.			
3. Put on personal protective equipment.			
4. For wet mount, roll swab over glass slide.			
5. To prepare a saline mount, add a drop of bacteriostatic saline.			
6. Or, to prepare a potassium hydroxide mount, add a drop of potassium hydroxide.			
7. Place a coverslip over the slide.			
8. The slide is ready to be examined under the microscope.			
9. For a hanging drop slide, place a small amount of petroleum jelly around the edge of the coverslip.			
10. Place a drop of solution containing material to be examined on the coverslip.			
11. Place the hanging drop slide over the coverslip so the depression in the slide is centered over the drop of solution.			
12. Apply pressure.			
13. Turn the slide over quickly so the drop of solution hangs from the coverslip into the well of the slide.			
14. The slide is ready to be examined under the microscope.			
15. Following examination, discard slide in a rigid biohazard container.			

Procedure Steps	1st trial	2nd trial	3rd trial
16. Remove and discard gloves in biohazard waste container.			
17. Wash hands.			
18. Complete the procedure within 5 minutes. ◆			

Evaluator Comments:

Score Calculation:

For each procedural step marked U (Unsatisfactory) deduct 6 points
For each procedural step (◆) marked U (Unsatisfactory) deduct 20 points

Score calculation 100 points

− points missed

Total score

1st	2nd	3rd

Satisfactory score: 85 or above

Procedure 26-4: Preparing a Dry Smear for Staining

Performance Objective

Task: Prepare a dry smear on a microscopic slide so that it can be stained.

Conditions: Clean glass slide with frosted end, disposable gloves, lab coat, face protection, container of methanol, cotton swab or dropper, applicator sticks, thumb forceps

Standards: Complete the procedure in 10 minutes, and achieve a satisfactory score on the procedure performance checklist

Scoring Key: (**S**)*atisfactory,* (**U**)*nsatisfactory,* (**NA**) *Not Applicable*
◆ *Denotes a critical element for a satisfactory score on the procedure*

Procedure Steps	1st trial	2nd trial	3rd trial
1. Wash hands.			
2. Label slide with pencil on frosted end.			
3. Put on personal protective equipment.			
4. Place thin layer of specimen onto glass slide using dropper or swab and applicator sticks.			
5. Allow specimen to air-dry.			
6. Hold specimen with thumb forceps by frosted end.			
7. Dip slide into methanol to fix slide.			
8. Allow slide to air-dry. The slide is now ready to stain.			
9. Clean work area.			
10. Dispose of used equipment and supplies in biohazard waste container.			
11. Remove and discard gloves in biohazard container.			
12. Wash hands.			
13. Complete the procedure within 10 minutes. ◆			

Evaluator Comments:

Score Calculation:

For each procedural step marked U (Unsatisfactory) deduct 6 points
For each procedural step (◆) marked U (Unsatisfactory) deduct 20 points

Score calculation 100 points

− points missed

Total score

1st	2nd	3rd

Satisfactory score: 85 or above

Procedure 26-5: Inoculating a Culture Plate

Performance Objective

Task: Inoculate a culture plate using a throat-specimen swab

Conditions: Gloves, lab coat, face protection, specimen container containing swabs with specimen, blood agar plate, loop incinerator, platinum loop (or disposable loop), loop holder, laboratory marker, incubator, biohazard waste container

Standards: Complete the procedure in 10 minutes, and achieve a satisfactory score on the procedure performance checklist

Scoring Key: (**S**)*atisfactory,* (**U**)*nsatisfactory,* (**NA**) *Not Applicable*
◆ *Denotes a critical element for a satisfactory score on the procedure*

Procedure Steps	1st trial	2nd trial	3rd trial
1. Wash hands.			
2. Assemble equipment and supplies.			
3. Turn on loop incinerator.			
4. Prepare loop for use by placing it in a loop holder where you will be working.			
5. Put on personal protective equipment.			
6. Remove cap from container with specimen swab.			
7. Remove one of the swabs.			
8. Recap the container.			
9. Set container aside.			
10. Place a blood agar plate on the counter, agar side down.			
11. Remove the cover.			
12. Flame inoculating loop in the loop incinerator.			
13. If using disposable loops, open a package from the end away from the loops and pull out one loop by handle.			
14. Streak the top third of the plate beginning just above the middle.			
15. Reflame loop or get new loop.			
16. Go into first streak area at right angles 2–3 times and spread specimen into second quadrant of plate.			
17. Reflame loop or get new loop.			

Procedure Steps	1st trial	2nd trial	3rd trial
18. Go into second streaked area 2–3 times at right angles, and streak third quadrant of plate.			
19. Reflame loop or get new loop.			
20. Streak remainder of plate.			
21. Cover the blood agar plate.			
22. Turn it upside down.			
23. Use the laboratory marker to label the plate with the patient's name and date.			
24. Place the blood agar plate in the incubator, agar side up, or place in plastic biohazard transfer container with lab slip.			
25. If sending to outside lab, transport immediately.			
26. If placed in the incubator, record date, time, patient's name, and source of specimen in laboratory logbook.			
27. Dispose of waste in biohazard waste container.			
28. Remove and discard gloves in biohazard waste container.			
29. Wash hands.			
30. If sent to lab, document date, time, type and specimen, and lab to which it was sent in patient medical record.			
31. Complete the procedure within 10 minutes. ◆			

Charting

DATE	

Evaluator Comments:

Score Calculation:

For each procedural step marked U (Unsatisfactory) deduct 6 points
For each procedural step (◆) marked U (Unsatisfactory) deduct 20 points

Score calculation 100 points

− points missed

Total score

1st	2nd	3rd

Satisfactory score: 85 or above

Notes

Procedure 26-6: Performing a Urine Culture Using a Dip Slide Kit

Performance Objective

Task: Prepare a urine specimen for culture using a dip slide kit, and read results

Conditions: Gloves, lab coat, face protection, clean-catch midstream urine specimen (either freshly voided or refrigerated), urine dip slide kit (such as UriCheck Plus), incubator, biohazard waste container

Standards: Complete the procedure in 5 minutes, and achieve a satisfactory score on the procedure performance checklist

Scoring Key: (**S**)*atisfactory,* (**U**)*nsatisfactory,* (**NA**) *Not Applicable*
◆ *Denotes a critical element for a satisfactory score on the procedure*

Procedure Steps	1st trial	2nd trial	3rd trial
1. Wash hands.			
2. Assemble equipment and supplies.			
3. Put on personal protective equipment.			
4. Open the clean-catch midstream urine specimen without touching the inside of the container.			
5. Do not use the slide kit to collect urine.			
6. Unscrew cap of the urine dip slide kit.			
7. Remove the cap and attached slide from the vial without touching the slide or the inside of the vial.			
8. Dip slide into freshly voided urine so the agar surfaces on both sides of the slide become totally immersed.			
9. Allow excess urine to drain back into collection container.			
10. Replace agar slide back into vial.			
11. Screw cap back on, and screw on loosely.			
12. Label collection container with patient's name, date, and time, or use preprinted labels.			
13. Place slide kit in incubator at 35–37° F or place in plastic biohazard transfer container with lab slip.			
14. If sending to outside lab, transport immediately.			
15. If placed in incubator, record date, patient's name, and source of specimen in laboratory logbook.			

Procedure Steps	1st trial	2nd trial	3rd trial
16. Dispose of waste in biohazard waste container.			
17. Remove and discard gloves in biohazard waste container.			
18. Wash hands.			
19. If sent to lab, document date, time, type of specimen, and laboratory to which it was sent.			
20. Complete the procedure within 5 minutes. ◆			
21. If done in house, incubate slide for 18–24 hours.			
22. Compare growth density to chart supplied by manufacturer.			
23. Document date, time, type of test, and results in patient's medical record.			

Charting

DATE	

Evaluator Comments:

Score Calculation:

For each procedural step marked U (Unsatisfactory) deduct 6 points
For each procedural step (◆) marked U (Unsatisfactory) deduct 20 points

Score calculation 100 points
− points missed

Total score

1st	2nd	3rd

Satisfactory score: 85 or above

Procedure 26-7: Urine Pregnancy Testing

Performance Objective

Task: Perform a urine pregnancy test and determine result

Conditions: Gloves, lab coat, face protection, urine sample collected in clean container (preferably first morning specimen), minute timer, urine pregnancy test kit containing test cassettes, disposable pipettes, biohazard waste container

Standards: Complete the procedure in 5 minutes, and achieve a satisfactory score on the procedure performance checklist

Scoring Key: (**S**)*atisfactory,* (**U**)*nsatisfactory,* (**NA**) *Not Applicable*
◆ *Denotes a critical element for a satisfactory score on the procedure*

Procedure Steps	1st trial	2nd trial	3rd trial
1. Wash hands.			
2. Assemble equipment and supplies.			
3. Put on personal protective equipment.			
4. Check expiration date to be sure it has not expired.			
5. Remove test kit from pouch.			
6. Label each test kit with patient's name and date.			
7. Aspirate urine with disposable pipette.			
8. Drop three drops of urine in test well from the back of the kit.			
9. Begin timer.			
10. At exactly 3 minutes, read results.			
11. Dispose of specimen and used supplies in biohazard waste container.			
12. Remove gloves and discard in biohazard waste container.			
13. Wash hands.			
14. Record date, time, brand of test, and results in patient medical record.			
15. Complete the procedure within 5 minutes. ◆			

Charting

DATE	

Evaluator Comments:

Score Calculation:

For each procedural step marked U (Unsatisfactory) deduct 6 points
For each procedural step (◆) marked U (Unsatisfactory) deduct 20 points

Score calculation 100 points

– points missed

Total score

1st	2nd	3rd

Satisfactory score: 85 or above

Procedure 26-8: Performing a Rapid Strep Test

Performance Objective

Task: Perform and read a rapid strep test

Conditions: Gloves, lab coat, throat specimen, Strep A test kit containing test unit, extraction tube, and reagents

Standards: Complete procedure in 15 minutes, and achieve a satisfactory score on the procedure performance checklist

Scoring Key: (**S**)*atisfactory,* (**U**)*nsatisfactory,* (**NA**) *Not Applicable*
◆ *Denotes a critical element for a satisfactory score on the procedure*

Procedure Steps	1st trial	2nd trial	3rd trial
1. Wash hands.			
2. Assemble equipment and supplies.			
3. Check expiration date to be sure it has not expired.			
4. Put on personal protective equipment.			
5. Place open plastic tube in tube stand from kit box.			
6. Place the number of drops of reagent(s) as specified by the manufacturer into the testing tube.			
7. Insert specimen swab into the tube.			
8. Mix well.			
9. Allow swab to remain in tube for the length of time specified by the manufacturer.			
10. Add the number of drops of additional reagent(s) as specified by the manufacturer.			
11. Use the swab to mix the contents.			
12. Express all liquid from swab by rolling swab head against side of plastic tube and pressing slightly while withdrawing swab (or follow manufacturer's directions).			
13. Discard swab.			
14. Put cap on extraction tube.			
15. Perform test within time limit specified by manufacturer.			
16. Remove test cassette from foil pouch.			

Procedure Steps	1st trial	2nd trial	3rd trial
17. Place on level surface.			
18. Open extraction tube.			
19. Drop the number of drops specified by the manufacturer on paper in sample window of test unit.			
20. Begin timing.			
21. Read result in exactly 5 minutes (or time specified by manufacturer).			
22. If test is negative, plant culture for incubation to verify result.			
23. Discard used supplies in biohazard waste container.			
24. Remove and discard gloves in biohazard waste container.			
25. Wash hands.			
26. Record date, time, type of test, and result in patient medical record.			
27. Complete the procedure within 15 minutes. ◆			

Charting

DATE	

Evaluator Comments:

Score Calculation:

For each procedural step marked U (Unsatisfactory) deduct 6 points
For each procedural step (◆) marked U (Unsatisfactory) deduct 20 points

Score calculation 100 points

– points missed

Total score

1st	2nd	3rd

Satisfactory score: 85 or above

Procedure 26-9: Testing for Glucose Using Glucometer Elite Analyzer

Performance Objective

Task: Calibrate glucometer and measure blood glucose using a hand-held glucometer

Conditions: Gloves, Glucometer Elite blood glucose analyzer with batteries, check strip, code strip for calibration of test strips, test strips, glucose control of normal level, lancet, gauze, bandage, alcohol pad

Standards: Complete procedure in 15 minutes, and achieve a satisfactory score on the procedure performance checklist

Scoring Key: (**S**)*atisfactory,* (**U**)*nsatisfactory,* (**NA**) *Not Applicable*
◆ *Denotes a critical element for a satisfactory score on the procedure*

Procedure Steps	1st trial	2nd trial	3rd trial
1. Wash hands.			
2. Gather equipment and supplies.			
3. Check meter performance by inserting check strip into the meter with the tab toward the top of the meter.			
4. Compare result with the check strip range listed on label inside check strip box.			
5. If using a new vial of test strips, use the code strip to calibrate the instrument.			
6. Insert code strip into test slot with the function number face up and tab at the top.			
7. Beep will sound when code strip is fully in place.			
8. A second beep will sound and function number will be displayed.			
9. Remove test strip from foil packet by carefully peeling foil to the line to expose meter end of test strip.			
10. Hold end of test strip between two layers of foil.			
11. Insert test strip fully into meter.			
12. A beep will sound, followed by the function number.			
13. Pull test strip from the meter.			
14. Quickly reinsert test strip (within 2 seconds).			
15. A "C" and the function number will alternately flash on the screen.			

Procedure Steps	1st trial	2nd trial	3rd trial
16. Gently squeeze a drop of normal control fluid onto inside of the foil of test strip.			
17. Touch test end of the test strip to the drop until a beep sounds.			
18. Wait while the timer automatically times the specimen for 59 seconds.			
19. When a result appears in the meter screen, compare it to the range listed on end flap of test strip container.			
20. Remove strip and meter will automatically turn off.			
21. Record that meter was calibrated, and the results of the control, in the lab logbook.			
22. Wash hands again.			
23. Assemble supplies and equipment to test patient glucose.			
24. Identify patient.			
25. Ask patient when s/he last ate, and took insulin (if applicable).			
26. Patient should have washed and dried hands thoroughly before procedure.			
27. Explain procedure.			
28. Put on disposable gloves.			
29. Remove test strip from foil packet by carefully peeling foil to the line to expose meter end of test strip.			
30. Hold test end of strip between two layers of foil.			
31. Insert test strip fully into meter.			
32. A beep will sound, followed by the function number.			
33. Perform a finger stick with a lancet, as described in Procedure 25-4.			
34. Wipe away the first drop of blood.			
35. Touch the test end of the test strip to the blood and hold until a beep occurs.			
36. After 59 seconds the patient's glucose level will appear on the meter screen.			

Procedure Steps	1st trial	2nd trial	3rd trial
37. If you do not want to save the result, reinsert strip within 2 seconds, and remove.			
38. Discard used supplies and used test strip in biohazard waste container.			
39. Remove and discard gloves into biohazard waste container.			
40. Wash hands.			
41. Record results in patient medical record.			
42. Complete the procedure within 15 minutes. ◆			

Charting

DATE	

Evaluator Comments:

Score Calculation:

For each procedural step marked U (Unsatisfactory) deduct 6 points
For each procedural step (◆) marked U (Unsatisfactory) deduct 20 points

Score calculation 100 points

– points missed

Total score

1st	2nd	3rd

Satisfactory score: 85 or above

SELF-EVALUATION

UNIT 6 Special Populations

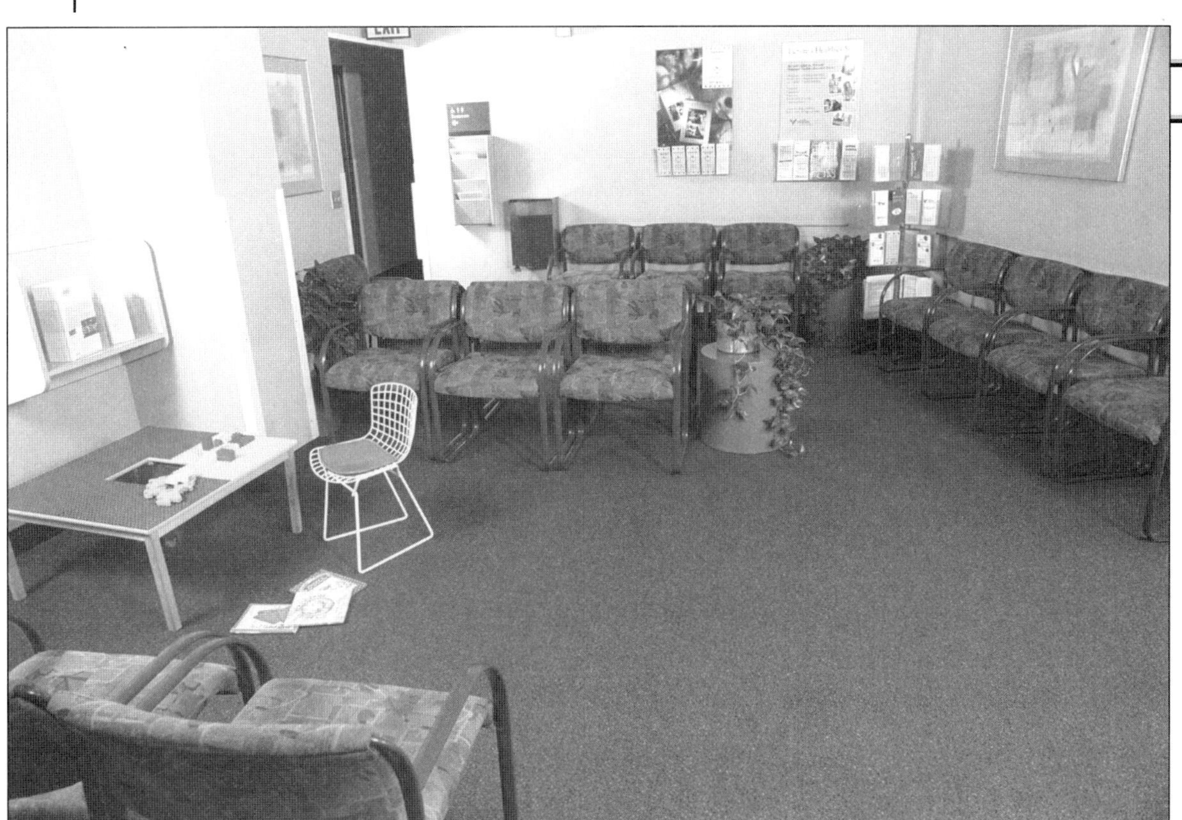

Birth to 36 months: Boys
Length-for-age and Weight-for-age percentiles

NAME ______________________

RECORD# ____________

Mother's Stature ________		Gestational		Comment
Father's Stature ________		Age: ________ Weeks		
Date	Age	Weight	Length	Head Circ.	
	Birth				

Revised November 21, 2000.
SOURCE: Developed by the National Center for Health Statistics in collaboration with the National Center for Chronic Disease Prevention and Health Promotion (2000).
http://www.cdc.gov/growthcharts

CDC

e. Two months and the mother tells you the child had a fever of 103° that morning

_______________ _______________

f. Two years and very uncooperative

_______________ _______________

4. Why would the medical assistant usually measure an apical pulse on an infant?

5. Why is blood pressure not measured routinely for infants and toddlers?

6. Why should the medical assistant wash the genitalia carefully before applying a pediatric urine collection device?

7. Identify two specific ways to immobilize an infant for safe administration of immunizations.

a. _______________

b. _______________

8. How can the medical assistant get older children to cooperate for injections?

9. Identify special precautions and/or possible side effects of each of the following immunizations:

a. DTaP _______________

b. Hib _______________

c. IPV _______________

d. Hep B _______________

e. MMR _______________

10. If a mother asks you why she cannot give her child aspirin to reduce a fever, what would you tell her?

11. Complete Case 3 (Robin Soto) on the CD-ROM.

Procedure 27-1: Measuring an Infant's Length

Performance Objective

Task: Measure an infant's length

Conditions: Examination table, table paper, marking pen/pencil, measuring tape

Standards: Complete the procedure in 5 minutes, and achieve a satisfactory score on the procedure performance checklist

Scoring Key: (**S**)*atisfactory,* (**U**)*nsatisfactory,* (**NA**) *Not Applicable*
◆ *Denotes a critical element for a satisfactory score on the procedure*

Procedure Steps	1st trial	2nd trial	3rd trial
1. Wash hands.			
2. Assemble supplies and equipment.			
3. Identify infant and parent.			
4. Explain procedure to adult.			
5. Place infant on its back on table.			
6. Using vertical board against the infant's head, place pencil mark at top of infant's head.			
7. Holding infant, stretch leg and foot down and place a mark at the bottom of the infant's heel.			
8. Ask adult to pick up infant.			
9. Measure between the two marks.			
10. If measuring tape uses centimeters, use conversion chart to covert to inches for baby's home record.			
11. Wash hands.			
12. Document length in medical record.			
13. Plot point on appropriate growth chart.			
14. The length recorded is within ±0.5 inch of the evaluator's measurement. ◆			
15. The point plotted on the growth chart is evaluated as accurate by the evaluator. ◆			
16. Complete the procedure within 5 minutes. ◆			

Charting

DATE	

Evaluator Comments:

Score Calculation:

For each procedural step marked U (Unsatisfactory) deduct 6 points
For each procedural step (◆) marked U (Unsatisfactory) deduct 20 points

Score calculation 100 points

− points missed

Total score

1st	2nd	3rd

Satisfactory score: 85 or above

Procedure 27-2: Measuring an Infant's Weight

Performance Objective

Task: Weigh an infant

Conditions: Scale with platform for infant to lie in supine position, protective underpad, clean disposable diaper, biohazard waste container

Standards: Complete the procedure in 5 minutes, and achieve a satisfactory score on the procedure performance checklist

Scoring Key: *(**S**)atisfactory, (**U**)nsatisfactory, (**NA**) Not Applicable*
◆ *Denotes a critical element for a satisfactory score on the procedure*

Procedure Steps	1st trial	2nd trial	3rd trial
1. Wash hands.			
2. Place protective underpad on scale.			
3. Balance scale at zero.			
4. Identify infant and parent.			
5. Explain procedure to adult.			
6. Ask adult to remove infant's clothes and diaper.			
7. Place infant on scale platform in supine position.			
8. Hold hand gently on infant's chest.			
9. Slowly move weights until scale bar balances.			
10. Hold hand just above infant's chest to perform final adjustment.			
11. Lift infant up and return to adult.			
12. Provide a clean disposable diaper to place on infant.			
13. If the office charts weights in kilograms and grams, use a conversion chart to convert into pounds and ounces for infant's home record.			
14. Discard underpad. If soiled, discard in biohazard waste container.			
15. Return weights to resting position.			
16. Wash hands.			
17. Document weight in medical record.			
18. Plot point on the appropriate growth chart.			

Procedure Steps	1st trial	2nd trial	3rd trial
19. The weight recorded is within ±0.5 ounce of the evaluator's measurement. ◆			
20. The point plotted on the growth chart is evaluated as accurate by the evaluator. ◆			
21. Complete the procedure within 5 minutes. ◆			

Charting

DATE	

Evaluator Comments:

Score Calculation:

For each procedural step marked U (Unsatisfactory) deduct 6 points

For each procedural step (◆) marked U (Unsatisfactory) deduct 20 points

Score calculation 100 points

− points missed

Total score

1st	2nd	3rd

Satisfactory score: 85 or above

Procedure 27-3: Measuring Head Circumference of an Infant

Performance Objective

Task: Measure an infant's head circumference

Conditions: Measuring tape

Standards: Complete the procedure in 5 minutes, and achieve a satisfactory score on the procedure performance checklist

Scoring Key: (**S**)*atisfactory*, (**U**)*nsatisfactory*, (**NA**) *Not Applicable*
◆ *Denotes a critical element for a satisfactory score on the procedure*

Procedure Steps	1st trial	2nd trial	3rd trial
1. Wash hands.			
2. Identify infant and parent.			
3. Explain procedure and cooperation that may be needed from adult.			
4. Place measuring tape snugly around infant's head at widest part (occipital to supraorbital area).			
5. Read the results in centimeters (or inches).			
6. Wash hands.			
7. Document head circumference in medical record.			
8. Plot point on the head circumference growth chart.			
9. The head circumference recorded is within ±0.5 centimeter of the evaluator's measurement. ◆			
10. The point plotted on the growth chart is evaluated as accurate by the evaluator. ◆			
11. Complete the procedure within 5 minutes. ◆			

Charting

DATE	

Evaluator Comments:

Score Calculation:

For each procedural step marked U (Unsatisfactory) deduct 6 points
For each procedural step (◆) marked U (Unsatisfactory) deduct 20 points

Score calculation	100 points			
	− points missed	1st	2nd	3rd
	Total score			

Satisfactory score: 85 or above

Procedure 27-4: Measuring Chest Circumference of an Infant

Performance Objective

Task: Measure an infant's chest circumference

Conditions: Measuring tape

Standards: Complete the procedure in 5 minutes, and achieve a satisfactory score on the procedure performance checklist

Scoring Key: (**S**)*atisfactory,* (**U**)*nsatisfactory,* (**NA**) *Not Applicable*
◆ *Denotes a critical element for a satisfactory score on the procedure*

Procedure Steps	1st trial	2nd trial	3rd trial
1. Wash hands.			
2. Identify infant and parent.			
3. Explain procedure and assistance that may be needed from adult.			
4. Place measuring tape snugly around infant's chest, just above nipple line and under axillary area.			
5. Read measurement to nearest inch or centimeter.			
6. Wash hands.			
7. Document chest circumference in medical record.			
8. The chest circumference recorded is within ±0.5 inch or 1 centimeter of the evaluator's measurement. ◆			
9. Complete the procedure within 5 minutes. ◆			

Charting

DATE	

Evaluator Comments:

Score Calculation:

For each procedural step marked U (Unsatisfactory) deduct 6 points
For each procedural step (◆) marked U (Unsatisfactory) deduct 20 points

Score calculation 100 points

− ___ points missed

Total score

1st	2nd	3rd

Satisfactory score: 85 or above

Procedure 27-5: Measuring the Apical Pulse of an Infant

Performance Objective

Task: Measure an infant's apical pulse

Conditions: Stethoscope, watch with second hand

Standards: Complete procedure in 3 minutes, and achieve a satisfactory score on the procedure performance checklist

Scoring Key: (**S**)*atisfactory,* (**U**)*nsatisfactory,* (**NA**) *Not Applicable*
◆ *Denotes a critical element for a satisfactory score on the procedure*

Procedure Steps	1st trial	2nd trial	3rd trial
1. Wash hands.			
2. Identify infant and parent.			
3. Explain procedure and assistance that may be needed from adult.			
4. Remove infant's shirt.			
5. Sit infant on exam table or place in supine position.			
6. Locate fifth intercostal space.			
7. Place stethoscope at midclavicular line to the left of sternum.			
8. Count beats for 1 minute.			
9. Note heart rate at 30 seconds in case the infant becomes too restless to continue for the full minute.			
10. If the infant becomes uncooperative, double 30-second heart rate.			
11. Wash hands.			
12. Document apical pulse in medical record.			
13. The apical pulse recorded is within ±2 beats of the evaluator's measurement.◆			
14. Note any irregular pulse.			
15. Complete the procedure within 3 minutes. ◆			

Charting

DATE	

Evaluator Comments:

Score Calculation:

For each procedural step marked U (Unsatisfactory) deduct 6 points
For each procedural step (◆) marked U (Unsatisfactory) deduct 20 points

Score calculation 100 points

− ____ points missed

Total score

1st	2nd	3rd

Satisfactory score: 85 or above

Procedure 27-6: Measuring the Respirations of an Infant

Performance Objective

Task: Measure an infant's respirations

Conditions: Watch with a second hand

Standards: Complete the procedure in 3 minutes, and achieve a satisfactory score on the procedure performance checklist

Scoring Key: **(S)***atisfactory,* **(U)***nsatisfactory,* **(NA)** *Not Applicable*
◆ *Denotes a critical element for a satisfactory score on the procedure*

Procedure Steps	1st trial	2nd trial	3rd trial
1. Wash hands.			
2. Identify infant and parent.			
3. Explain procedure and assistance that may be needed from adult.			
4. Remove infant's shirt.			
5. Place infant in supine position.			
6. Place hand over infant's chest.			
7. Count each rise and fall of the chest wall for 1 minute, using watch with second hand.			
8. Wash hands.			
9. Document respirations in medical record. Note any irregularities in sound or rhythm.			
10. The respiratory rate recorded is within ±1 of the evaluator's measurement. ◆			
11. Complete the procedure within 3 minutes. ◆			

Charting

DATE	

Evaluator Comments:

Score Calculation:

For each procedural step marked U (Unsatisfactory) deduct 6 points
For each procedural step (◆) marked U (Unsatisfactory) deduct 20 points

Score calculation	100 points			
	− points missed	1st	2nd	3rd
	Total score			

Satisfactory score: 85 or above

Procedure 27-7: Obtaining a Urine Specimen From an Infant

Performance Objective

Task: Collect a urine specimen from an infant

Conditions: Gloves, urine collection bag, cleansing cloths, biohazard waste container

Standards: Complete the procedure in 5 minutes, and achieve a satisfactory score on the procedure performance checklist

Scoring Key: (**S**)*atisfactory,* (**U**)*nsatisfactory,* (**NA**) *Not Applicable*
◆ *Denotes a critical element for a satisfactory score on the procedure*

Procedure Steps	1st trial	2nd trial	3rd trial
1. Wash hands.			
2. Identify infant and parent.			
3. Explain procedure and assistance that may be needed from adult.			
4. Remove infant's diaper.			
5. Place infant in supine position.			
6. Put on gloves.			
7. Cleanse the infant's perineal area including area beneath foreskin if infant is an uncircumcised male.			
8. Dry perineal area.			
9. Remove paper tabs from adhesive on infant urine collection bag.			
10. Apply to a male infant over penis and scrotum.			
10A. Apply to a female infant over genitalia with opening over urinary meatus.			
11. Replace diaper.			
12. Remove and discard gloves in biohazard waste bag.			
13. Wash hands.			
14. Complete placement within 5 minutes. ◆			
15. Check bag every 10 to 15 minutes.			
16. When bag is full, put on new pair of gloves.			
17. Remove diaper and remove bag carefully.			
18. Gently pull adhesive away from infant's skin, holding bag upright.			

Procedure Steps

Procedure Steps	1st trial	2nd trial	3rd trial
19. Place urine in a container.			
20. Label and test or prepare to send to a lab.			
21. Document date, time, specimen obtained, any results if testing is done in-house, or that specimen was sent to lab.			

Charting

DATE	

Evaluator Comments:

Score Calculation:

For each procedural step marked U (Unsatisfactory) deduct 6 points
For each procedural step (◆) marked U (Unsatisfactory) deduct 20 points

Score calculation 100 points

− points missed

Total score

1st	2nd	3rd

Satisfactory score: 85 or above

SELF-EVALUATION

Chapter 28

Geriatrics

CHAPTER FOCUS

In this chapter you learned about the special health needs and health problems of the geriatric population, the fastest growing group of people in the United States. Up to 50% of adult patients in a primary care practice will be over 65. Therefore, it is vital for the medical assistant to understand normal and abnormal changes of aging and to be prepared to meet the needs of the older adult.

TERMINOLOGY REVIEW

Vocabulary Matching: Match each term with its definition.

___ 1. opacity
___ 2. life expectancy
___ 3. exacerbation
___ 4. dementia
___ 5. senile
___ 6. neuropathy
___ 7. osteoporosis
___ 8. geriatric

A. A condition of memory loss, confusion, and sometimes agitation and aggression
B. The worsening of a condition or disease
C. Medical term meaning old
D. Expected length of life for a particular person at a given time
E. A lack of sensation due to reduced nerve function
F. Clouding of the lens of the eye that impairs vision
G. Loss of bone mass of over 2.5%
H. Having decreased mental functioning

CONTENT REVIEW QUESTIONS

1. Identify four developmental tasks that the older adult must complete.

   a. ______________________________

   b. ______________________________

c. ___

d. ___

2. Identify normal changes of the aging process related to each of the following:

a. height ___

b. weight ___

c. body temperature ___

d. heart rhythm ___

e. blood pressure ___

f. muscle size ___

g. gastric motility ___

h. skin ___

i. reaction time ___

j. memory ___

h. vision ___

i. hearing ___

j. taste and smell ___

k. kidneys and bladder ___

3. Identify six diseases that are common in the elderly population.

a. ___

b. ___

c. ___

d. ___

e. ___

f. ___

4. How may the elderly person react to questions if he or she has memory problems?

___

___

___

5. What is dementia, and what may cause it?

___

___

___

6. List ten ways the medical assistant can work more effectively with a patient with dementia.

a. ___

b. ___

c. ______

d. ______

e. ______

f. ______

g. ______

h. ______

i. ______

j. ______

7. What should the medical assistant keep in mind when making appointments for a patient with decreased mobility?

______

______

______

8. What safety measures should be taught to a person with decreased mobility and/or impaired balance?

______

______

______

9. How can the medical assistant assist a person with impaired vision to walk through the medical office safely?

______

______

______

10. How can the medical assistant improve verbal communication with a person whose hearing is impaired?

______

______

______

11. What additional methods can be used to communicate with a person with impaired hearing?

______

______

______

12. What is neuropathy, and how can it affect elderly patients?

______

______

______

13. What special teaching needs does a patient with neuropathy have?

____

____

____

14. What services may be available through the community to help an elderly person?

____

____

____

15. Identify at least ten indications of elder abuse.

a. ______________________________

b. ______________________________

c. ______________________________

d. ______________________________

e. ______________________________

f. ______________________________

g. ______________________________

h. ______________________________

i. ______________________________

j. ______________________________

16. What should the medical assistant do if he or she suspects that an elderly person is suffering abuse or neglect?

____

____

____

CRITICAL THINKING QUESTIONS

1. What are indications that an elderly individual or couple is no longer able to manage independent living? What are realistic ways that the medical assistant can help the elderly person and the family to respond when the person's health is at risk because of this?

____

____

____

____

____

____

2. Discuss the health of your own elderly relatives and the plans that have been made to care for them (if any). What problems arise in a family, from your own experience, when trying to balance the physical and emotional needs of the elderly with their wishes and desire for independence?

3. Do research into one of the chronic diseases that commonly affect the elderly, such as osteoporosis, Parkinson's disease, diabetes mellitus, chronic renal failure, emphysema, or chronic heart disease, and prepare a report correlating the progression of the disease to the special problems of the older adult.

SELF-EVALUATION

Chapter 29

Obstetrics

CHAPTER FOCUS

In this chapter you learned about the medical assistant's role during pregnancy and the puerperium. Medical assistants often work in OB/GYN practices and they must be ready to prepare patients for examinations and procedures during pregnancy and during follow-up visits after delivery. In addition, this chapter helps the medical assistant become familiar with much of the specialized terminology relating to pregnancy and the birth process.

TERMINOLOGY REVIEW

Vocabulary Matching: Match each term with its definition.

___ 1. stillbirth
___ 2. episiotomy
___ 3. miscarriage
___ 4. viable
___ 5. labor
___ 6. puerperium
___ 7. contraction stress test
___ 8. elective abortion
___ 9. conception
___ 10. eclampsia

A. Thick, yellowish fluid that nourishes a baby immediately after birth
B. Brownish pigmentation of the face
C. The uniting of a single sperm with an ovum, which starts pregnancy
D. Stimulation of mild contractions during fetal heart rate monitoring
E. A serious condition of pregnancy that causes convulsive seizures, coma, and death if untreated
F. Intentional termination of a pregnancy
G. The product of conception, from weeks 4 through 8 of pregnancy
H. Incision made to enlarge the vaginal opening for birth
I. The infant in utero, from the ninth week of pregnancy to birth
J. The base of the uterus, located opposite the cervix

___ 11. pica
___ 12. colostrum
___ 13. fundus
___ 14. spontaneous abortion
___ 15. gestation
___ 16. preeclampsia
___ 17. chloasma
___ 18. non-stress test
___ 19. trimester
___ 20. gravida
___ 21. fetus
___ 22. para
___ 23. obstetrics
___ 24. embryo
___ 25. supine hypotension syndrome
___ 26. prenatal
___ 27. postpartum

K. The length of time that has passed since conception
L. Total times pregnant
M. The process a woman's body goes through immediately preceding birth of a baby
N. Common term for spontaneous abortion
O. Test to correlate mother's heart rate to fetal movement and Braxton-Hicks contractions
P. The field of medicine that deals with pregnancy, childbirth, and the period immediately following childbirth
Q. Number of pregnancies that went to the age of viability
R. Craving by a pregnant woman for non-food items
S. A complication of pregnancy characterized by hypertension, albuminuria, and edema of the lower extremities
T. The time before birth
U. The weeks and months immediately following birth of a baby
V. The 6-week period immediately following childbirth
W. Natural expulsion of a fetus for unknown reasons
X. Birth of a dead fetus of the age of viability
Y. Low blood pressure while an expectant mother lies on her back
Z. Three-month period; there are three during pregnancy
AA. Able to survive

Abbreviations: Expand each abbreviation to its complete form.

1. Ab ______________________________
2. CST ______________________________
3. EDC ______________________________
4. EDD ______________________________
5. LMP ______________________________

CONTENT REVIEW QUESTIONS

1. Describe how the ovum is fertilized and implants in the uterus.

2. Why is extensive prenatal care recommended for the health of the mother and fetus?

3. What type of care is usually received by a woman during the actual birth of her baby?

4. What are presumptive signs of pregnancy? Identify five.
   a.
   b.
   c.
   d.
   e.

5. What are probable signs of pregnancy? Who usually identifies the probable signs?

6. Identify four positive signs of pregnancy.
   a.
   b.
   c.
   d.

7. Discuss changes that occur in each of the following body systems during pregnancy:
   a. weight gain
   b. uterus and cervix

c. breasts ______________________________

____

____

d. endocrine system ______________________________

____

____

f. circulatory system ______________________________

____

____

g. respiratory system ______________________________

____

____

h. gastrointestinal system ______________________________

____

____

i. urinary system ______________________________

____

____

j. musculoskeletal system ______________________________

____

____

8. What are psychological changes that may occur

a. during the first trimester? ______________________________

____

____

b. during the second trimester? ______________________________

____

____

c. during the third trimester? ______________________________

____

____

9. What happens during the first prenatal visit?

____

____

____

____

10. When taking a patient's obstetric history, what is included in the following terms?

a. Gravida ________________________________

____

b. Para ________________________________

____

c. Abortions ________________________________

____

11. Identify ten diagnostic tests that are usually done on the first prenatal visit.

a. ____________________ f. ____________________

b. ____________________ g. ____________________

c. ____________________ h. ____________________

d. ____________________ i. ____________________

e. ____________________ j. ____________________

12. What will be monitored on each follow-up prenatal visit?

____

____

____

13. Describe how the following are measured:

a. fetal heart rate ________________________________

____

b. height of the uterine fundus ________________________________

____

14. Describe the following special diagnostic tests and identify their use during pregnancy.

a. Ultrasonography ________________________________

____

b. Chorionic villus sampling ________________________________

____

c. Amniocentesis ______________________________

____

d. Maternal alpha-fetoprotein analysis ______________________________

____

15. What is a non-stress test and when is it used? A contraction stress test?

____

____

____

16. Identify seven signs of impending labor.

a. ______________ e. ______________

b. ______________ f. ______________

c. ______________ g. ______________

d. ______________

17. What are the four stages of labor?

a. ______________________________

b. ______________________________

c. ______________________________

d. ______________________________

18. Identify five signs of true labor and five signs of false labor.

True labor	False labor

19. Identify signs and symptoms of problems during the first few days after delivery.

____

____

____

____

20. What is the normal sequence of lochia (discharge) following delivery?

____

____

____

____

21. Describe the six-week postpartum visit.

____

____

____

____

CRITICAL THINKING QUESTIONS

1. Discuss trends in infant mortality rates, maternal mortality rates, and numbers of maternal hospitalizations for severe complications. In what parts of society are these rates the highest? What interventions might reduce them?

____

____

____

____

____

____

2. Do research to find more information on one of the following complications of pregnancy: preeclampsia and eclampsia, gestational diabetes, placenta previa, abruptio placenta, inadequate cervix. Prepare a report and share it with your classmates.

3. Many OB/GYN practices hire registered nurses to work with pregnant patients. Do you think that a medical assistant is qualified to assume this role, or is it better to have a nurse? Give reasons for your answer.

____

____

____

____

____

____

PRACTICAL APPLICATIONS

1. Calculate the EDC (due date) for the following women using Nagele's rule:

   a. Sarah Graham LMP 2/16/01 ______________________

   b. Michelle Parsons LMP 3/28/01 ______________________

   c. Denise Worthing LMP 6/22/01 ______________________

2. Determine the numbers for Para, Gravida, and Abortion (using Roman numerals) for each of the following pregnant patients:

   a. Sarah Graham tells you that she has one child following an uneventful pregnancy, her only other pregnancy.

      P: _______ Gr: _______ Ab: _______

   b. Michelle Parsons already has three children, including one set of twins. She had a spontaneous abortion last year.

      P: _______ Gr: _______ Ab: _______

   c. Denise Worthing has never had a pregnancy that went to term although she has been pregnant three times before, each time ending in a spontaneous abortion.

      P: _______ Gr: _______ Ab: _______

3. Identify five areas of teaching needs, giving specific information about what a pregnant patient needs to be taught.

   a. ______________________________

   b. ______________________________

   c. ______________________________

   d. ______________________________

   e. ______________________________

4. As Sarah Graham nears the end of her pregnancy, she calls the office to report that she is having painful contractions that have increased from every 5 minutes to every 4 minutes, and that they are becoming longer and more intense. In addition, she reports a small amount of bloody discharge shortly before the contractions began. What should the medical assistant tell her?

   ____

   ____

   ____

   ____

5. As Joanne Caitlin, a primigravida, nears the end of her pregnancy, she calls the office to report that she is having contractions that are painful. The contractions are 7 minutes apart and have not changed in interval or intensity. The pain is abdominal and not increasing in intensity. What should the medical assistant tell her?

   ____

   ____

   ____

   ____

Procedure 29-1: Assisting with the First Prenatal Visit

Performance Objective

Task: Assist a pregnant patient during her first prenatal visit

Conditions: Gloves, patient gown, drape, water-based lubricant, sphygmomanometer, stethoscope, watch with second hand, measuring tape, Doppler or Fetoscope, supplies and equipment for Pap smear (Procedure 16-2), supplies and equipment for pregnancy test (Procedure 26-7), supplies and equipment for venipuncture (Procedure 25-1), supplies and equipment for dipstick urinalysis (Procedure 24-4), biohazard waste container

Standards: Complete procedure in 20 minutes, and achieve a satisfactory score on the procedure performance checklist

Scoring Key: (**S**)*atisfactory,* (**U**)*nsatisfactory,* (**NA**) *Not Applicable*
◆ *Denotes a critical element for a satisfactory score on the procedure*

Procedure Steps	1st trial	2nd trial	3rd trial
1. Identify patient.			
2. If patient has not brought a first voided urine specimen, ask her to empty bladder and collect a random specimen.			
3. Wash hands.			
4. Put on non-sterile gloves.			
5. Perform urine pregnancy test and dipstick urinalysis.			
6. Discard waste in biohazard waste container.			
7. Remove and discard gloves in biohazard waste container.			
8. Wash hands.			
9. Ask patient to remove shoes.			
10. Weigh patient.			
11. Measure pulse, respirations, and blood pressure.			
12. Depending on office policy, prenatal blood work may be drawn at this time, or the patient may be instructed to visit an outpatient lab.			
13. Chart all results in patient record.			
14. Accompany patient to exam room.			

Procedure Steps	1st trial	2nd trial	3rd trial
15. Set up all equipment and supplies for physical exam, Pap smear, and bimanual pelvic exam.			
16. Ask patient to undress fully, put on gown, and sit on exam table.			
17. Give patient gown and drape, and leave room to provide privacy.			
18. Assist patient and doctor as needed during exam, Pap smear, and bimanual pelvic exam, wearing gloves to handle specimens.			
19. Assist patient to get into various positions for exam.			
20. At end of bimanual pelvic exam, assist patient back to supine position and store stirrups.			
21. After doctor has measured height of fundus, instruct patient to dress.			
22. Provide tissues to remove water-based lubricant.			
23. Label and place slide for Pap test and specimens for culture (if any) into mailer and/or plastic laboratory transport bags.			
24. Dispose of used supplies in biohazard waste container.			
25. Remove gloves and discard in biohazard waste container.			
26. Wash hands.			
27. Complete all lab slips and include with specimens.			
28. Chart all procedures and patient concerns in patient record.			
29. Complete the procedure within 20 minutes. ◆			
30. Schedule follow-up prenatal visit.			

Charting

DATE	

Evaluator Comments:

Score Calculation:

For each procedural step marked U (Unsatisfactory) deduct 6 points
For each procedural step (◆) marked U (Unsatisfactory) deduct 20 points

Score calculation 100 points

− ______ points missed

Total score

1st	2nd	3rd

Satisfactory score: 85 or above

Notes

Procedure 29-2: Assisting with Follow-up Prenatal Visits

Performance Objective

Task: Assist a patient during follow-up prenatal visits

Conditions: Gloves, patient gown and drape, water-based lubricant, sphygmomanometer, stethoscope, watch with second hand, measuring tape, Doppler or Fetoscope, gel, supplies and equipment for hemoglobin testing (Procedure 23-9) or micro-hematocrit (Procedure 23-10), supplies and equipment for dipstick urinalysis (Procedure 24-4), biohazard waste container

Standards: Complete the procedure in 20 minutes, and achieve a satisfactory score on the procedure performance checklist

Scoring Key: (**S**)*atisfactory,* (**U**)*nsatisfactory,* (**NA**) *Not Applicable*
◆ *Denotes a critical element for a satisfactory score on the procedure*

Procedure Steps	1st trial	2nd trial	3rd trial
1. Identify patient.			
2. Ask patient to empty bladder and collect random urine specimen.			
3. Wash hands.			
4. Put on gloves.			
5. Test urine for protein, ketones, and glucose using dipstick.			
6. Discard waste in biohazard waste container.			
7. Remove and discard gloves in biohazard waste container.			
8. Wash hands.			
9. Ask patient to remove shoes.			
10. Weigh patient.			
11. Measure pulse, respirations, and blood pressure.			
12. Document weight and vital signs in patient record.			
13. If office policy, question patient about symptoms such as nausea, vomiting, bleeding, etc., and document in pregnancy flow sheet.			
14. If done in the office, measure hemoglobin or hematocrit levels at regular intervals (or send patient to lab).			
15. Chart all results in patient record.			
16. Accompany patient to exam room.			

Procedure Steps	1st trial	2nd trial	3rd trial
17. Instruct patient to undress from the waist down and provide gown and drape.			
18. Provide Doppler or Fetoscope, gel, and tape measure to doctor to routinely check fetal heart tones and fundal growth measurements.			
19. Assist doctor and patient as necessary in positioning patient in either supine or lithotomy positions.			
20. Record information such as fetal heart rate and height of fundus, as directed by doctor.			
21. Wash hands.			
22. Complete the procedure within 20 minutes. ◆			
23. Schedule follow-up prenatal visit.			

Charting

DATE	

Evaluator Comments:

Score Calculation:

For each procedural step marked U (Unsatisfactory) deduct 6 points
For each procedural step (◆) marked U (Unsatisfactory) deduct 20 points

Score calculation 100 points
− points missed

Total score

1st	2nd	3rd

Satisfactory score: 85 or above

Procedure 29-3: Assisting with Postpartum Visits

Performance Objective

Task: Assist a patient during her postpartum visit(s)

Conditions: Gloves, sphygmomanometer and stethoscope, supplies and equipment for hemoglobin testing or hematocrit testing, supplies and equipment for Pap smear, biohazard waste container

Standards: Complete procedure in 20 minutes, and achieve a satisfactory score on the procedure performance checklist

Scoring Key: (**S**)*atisfactory,* (**U**)*nsatisfactory,* (**NA**) *Not Applicable*
◆ *Denotes a critical element for a satisfactory score on the procedure*

Procedure Steps	1st trial	2nd trial	3rd trial
1. Identify and greet patient.			
2. Wash hands.			
3. Ask patient to remove shoes.			
4. Weigh patient.			
5. Measure pulse, respiration, and blood pressure.			
6. Document weight and vital signs in patient record.			
7. If office policy includes assessment, ask patient about lochia, cramping or other discomfort, and general concerns.			
8. Document results of assessment.			
9. If done in office, measure hemoglobin or hematocrit level.			
10. Accompany patient to exam room.			
11. Set up all equipment and supplies for physical exam, Pap smear, and bimanual pelvic exam.			
12. Instruct patient to undress from waist down and provide gown and drape.			
13. Assist patient and doctor as needed during exam, Pap smear, and bimanual pelvic exam wearing gloves to handle specimens.			
14. Assist patient to get into various positions for exam.			
15. At end of bimanual pelvic exam, assist patient back to supine position and store stirrups.			
16. Instruct patient to dress.			
17. Provide patient with tissues to remove lubricant.			

Procedure Steps	1st trial	2nd trial	3rd trial
18. Label and place slide for Pap test and specimens for culture (if any) into mailer and/or plastic laboratory transport bags.			
19. Dispose of used supplies in biohazard waste container.			
20. Remove gloves and discard in biohazard waste container.			
21. Wash hands.			
22. Complete all lab slips and include with specimens.			
23. Complete the procedure within 20 minutes. ◆			
24. Schedule follow-up appointment if ordered by doctor.			

Charting

DATE	

Evaluator Comments:

Score Calculation:

For each procedural step marked U (Unsatisfactory) deduct 6 points
For each procedural step (◆) marked U (Unsatisfactory) deduct 20 points

Score calculation 100 points
– points missed

Total score

1st	2nd	3rd

Satisfactory score: 85 or above

SELF-EVALUATION

Chapter 30

Patients with Chronic and Terminal Diseases

CHAPTER FOCUS

Chronic diseases have become an expected part of life as life expectancy has increased during the 20th century. Often patients with chronic disease are elderly, but many younger people also experience chronic conditions. In this chapter you have learned about chronic diseases and actions that the medical assistant can take to assist patients during treatment for such conditions. Death may be the eventual outcome of a chronic condition, and this needs to be confronted as a natural process. At the same time the medical assistant is supporting the dying patient, he or she must remain conscious of personal feelings about death and dying.

TERMINOLOGY REVIEW

Vocabulary Matching: Match each term with its definition.

___	1. chemotherapy	A.	A tumor with harmless cells
___	2. remission	B.	Outlook for future health
___	3. terminal	C.	A state of wasting and/or malnutrition due to illness
___	4. Kaposi's sarcoma	D.	Treatment using anticancer drugs
___	5. neoplasm	E.	Measurable loss of function
___	6. prognosis	F.	A document that gives the designated person the ability to make all legal decisions for an individual, including medical decisions
___	7. cachexia	G.	Cancer treatment using various types of radiation
___	8. benign	H.	When a patient is not expected to live more than six months
___	9. impairment	I.	The extent to which a person cannot perform normal activities
___	10. radiation therapy	J.	An organization that provides end-of-life comfort and care

___ 11. opportunistic infection

___ 12. mortality rate

___ 13. palliative

___ 14. living will

___ 15. handicap

___ 16. disability

___ 17. durable power of attorney

___ 18. necrosis

___ 19. immunotherapy

___ 20. syndrome

___ 21. hospice

K. Disturbance of functioning that may be physical or psychological

L. Cancer treatment using measures to stimulate the immune system

M. A document executed by an individual that gives medical professionals instructions about how that person wishes to be treated in the event he or she becomes incompetent

N. A rare type of skin cancer, often seen in patients who are HIV-positive

O. A time when symptoms disappear or improve

P. A group of related signs and symptoms

Q. The rate of deaths due to a particular disease or condition

R. Destruction of tissue from ulceration and infection

S. Tumors

T. Infections that occur because of a patient's decreased immunity

U. Care that relieves symptoms without providing a cure

CONTENT REVIEW QUESTIONS

1. Identify four major areas in which the medical assistant may play a role to coordinate the care of a patient with a chronic disease or condition.

   a. ___

   b. ___

   c. ___

   d. ___

2. What may make it difficult for the medical assistant and family members to maintain a positive attitude when working with a patient whose chronic disease is progressing?

   ___

   ___

   ___

3. How do a hospital and a hospice differ?

   ___

   ___

   ___

4. Identify five factors that influence attitudes about death of patients among health care providers.

   a. ___

   b. ___

c. ___

d. ___

e. ___

5. Describe each of the five stages of the grieving process identified by Elizabeth Kübler-Ross.

   a. Denial ___

   b. Anger ___

   c. Bargaining ___

   d. Depression ___

   e. Acceptance ___

6. Discuss how the stages of grieving usually occur.

___

7. Identify seven manifestations of grief.

   a. ___

   b. ___

   c. ___

   d. ___

   e. ___

   f. ___

   g. ___

8. Identify two historical documents that provide basic principles to determine how medical research should be conducted.

   a. ___

   b. ___

9. What role do financial issues play for dying patients?

____

____

____

____

10. Describe each of the following measures to formalize decisions about dying:

a. DNR order _______________

____

b. Living will or health care proxy _______________

____

c. Durable power of attorney _______________

____

11. What are three methods of classifying cancers?

a. _______________

b. _______________

c. _______________

12. What are the four general groups of risk factors for cancer?

a. _______________

b. _______________

c. _______________

d. _______________

13. What are important measures to improve survival rates of several types of cancer?

____

____

____

14. How do malignant tumors grow and spread?

____

____

____

15. Describe three local effects that a tumor may have.

a. _______________

b. _______________

c. _______________

16. Describe four systemic effects of cancer.

a. ____________________

b. ____________________

c. ____________________

d. ____________________

17. How do cancerous tumors spread to distant parts of the body?

____

____

____

____

18. Give two examples of each of the following diagnostic methods that can be used to identify benign or malignant tumors.

a. tissue examination ____________________

b. imaging studies ____________________

c. endoscopic tests ____________________

d. laboratory tests ____________________

19. Describe the three general types of treatments for cancer.

a. ____________________

____

b. ____________________

____

c. ____________________

____

20. How is AIDS transmitted from one person to another?

____

____

____

21. Describe the four stages of HIV infection.

a. ____________________

____

b. ____________________

____

c. ____________________

____

d. ____________________

____

22. Discuss the legal implications of HIV testing.

23. What is the treatment for AIDS and HIV infection?

24. What should a health care worker do if he or she experiences an accidental needlestick or is directly exposed to body fluids?

CRITICAL THINKING QUESTIONS

1. Mandatory testing for syphilis before marriage has been required for decades, yet there is no mandatory testing for HIV. Discuss the medical and historical factors that result in this difference.

2. Do you have a living will or health care proxy? Why or why not? Discuss the emotional response when a person thinks about formulating such a document.

3. Should a patient whose blood was drawn by a needle that later sticks an employee be allowed to refuse to be tested for HIV? Defend your position.

4. Describe a personal experience that you have had with loss and grieving. What stages did you go through? How did you work with your own feelings? How were health care personnel helpful to you (or how could they have been helpful)?

PRACTICAL APPLICATIONS

1. A patient with metastatic cancer tells you, "I saw a person on a respirator on a TV show last night. I hope no one ever puts me on one of those things. I want to die without all those tubes in me." How could the medical assistant answer to determine if the patient has put an appropriate advance directive in place?

2. A patient who has been told to schedule a mammogram says, "If I have cancer, I really don't want to know. So many of my relatives have died from it. I would really rather just forget about it." How could you answer this patient?

3. A patient with advanced chronic disease says, "If I can just hold on until June so that I can go to my daughter's graduation, I won't ask for anything else." What stage of the grieving process do you think the person is in? How would you respond?

____

____

____

____

____

____

4. A patient fears that he or she might have been exposed to HIV. The patient asks you, "Why do I have to wait three months to be tested? I want to know if I have it now." What would you answer?

____

____

____

____

____

____

SELF-EVALUATION

c. poisoning

d. drowning

If possible, identify or create pamphlets to instruct parents in ways to prevent injuries.

2. Identify emergency medical supplies and/or first-aid kits in at least two buildings at your school. Question staff and students to determine if they are aware of the locations and supplies available. Who is responsible for maintaining these supplies?

PRACTICAL APPLICATIONS

1. Identify eight types of equipment and/or supplies that might be found on a crash cart but would not be found in a first-aid kit.

a.

e.

b.

f.

c.

g.

d.

h.

2. If the physician orders oxygen by nasal cannula at 4 L/minute for a patient, what must the medical assistant do to carry out the order?

3. Identify how a medical assistant might differentiate between a severe asthma attack and anaphylactic shock.

4. A patient calls the medical office, reporting that she has burned her hand by grabbing a hot curling iron that was falling from a shelf, without realizing that the iron was turned on. She reports that the palm of her hand is red and that blisters have started to form. What additional information would you ask her? What classification of burns do you believe she has? What would you advise her to do?

5. Under what circumstances would the medical assistant apply pressure to an artery to try to control bleeding?

6. If a patient who is known to experience angina pectoris has an episode of chest pain in the medical office, what should the medical assistant do? What additional measures might the physician instruct the medical assistant to take? Under what circumstances might the physician instruct the medical assistant to call an ambulance?

7. How would the medical assistant instruct a patient to induce vomiting after ingesting a poison if recommended by the Poison Control Center or a physician? How should the patient follow up?

8. What should the medical assistant do if a patient suddenly experiences a nosebleed in the waiting room?

PROCEDURE PERFORMANCE CHECKLISTS

Procedure 31-1: Checking Contents of Emergency Box/Crash Cart

Performance Objective

Task: Check the contents of an emergency box or crash cart for completeness

Conditions: Crash cart or emergency box, inventory-control sheet, disposable sealing or locking mechanism

Standards: Complete procedure in 10 minutes, and achieve a satisfactory score on the procedure performance checklist.

Scoring Key: (**S**)*atisfactory,* (**U**)*nsatisfactory,* (**NA**) *Not Applicable*
◆ *Denotes a critical element for a satisfactory score on the procedure*

Procedure Steps	**1st trial**	**2nd trial**	**3rd trial**
1. Open crash cart or emergency box.			
2. Check contents of each drawer, or contents of emergency box.			
3. Identify each item on inventory control sheet.			
4. Check expiration of each item.			
5. Record findings.			
6. Replace any expired or missing items.			
7. Secure crash cart using easily opened disposable locking device.			
8. Complete the procedure within 10 minutes. ◆			

Evaluator Comments:

Score Calculation:

For each procedural step marked U (Unsatisfactory) deduct 6 points
For each procedural step (◆) marked U (Unsatisfactory) deduct 20 points

Score calculation 100 points

− points missed

	1st	2nd	3rd
Total score			

Satisfactory score: 85 or above

Notes

Procedure 31-2: Assisting the Choking Victim

Performance Objective

Task: Assist a patient who is choking

Conditions: None

Standards: Complete the procedure in 5 minutes, and achieve a satisfactory score on the procedure performance checklist

*Scoring Key: (**S**)atisfactory, (**U**)nsatisfactory, (**NA**) Not Applicable*
◆ *Denotes a critical element for a satisfactory score on the procedure*

Procedure Steps

Procedure Steps	1st trial	2nd trial	3rd trial
1. Identify that patient is choking.			
2. Place thumb side of your fist against patient's middle abdomen.			
3. Grasp your fist with opposed hand.			
4. Make quick upward thrusts on patient's abdomen.			
5. Continue thrusts until object is dislodged or patient becomes unconscious.			
6. Assist patient to a sitting position once object is dislodged and patient is breathing freely.			
7. Wash hands.			
8. If choking occurred in the medical office, record description of event in patient's medical record.			
9. Complete the procedure within 5 minutes. ◆			

Charting

DATE	

Evaluator Comments:

Score Calculation:

For each procedural step marked U (Unsatisfactory) deduct 6 points
For each procedural step (◆) marked U (Unsatisfactory) deduct 20 points

Score calculation 100 points

− ___ points missed

Total score

1st	2nd	3rd

Satisfactory score: 85 or above

Procedure 31-3: Administering Oxygen by Nasal Cannula or Face Mask

Performance Objective

Task: Administer oxygen by nasal cannula or face mask

Conditions: Oxygen in portable tank or wall unit, oxygen mask or nasal cannula, flow meter and tubing

Standards: Complete the procedure in 10 minutes, and achieve a satisfactory score on the procedure performance checklist

Scoring Key: (**S**)*atisfactory,* (**U**)*nsatisfactory,* (**NA**) *Not Applicable*
◆ *Denotes a critical element for a satisfactory score on the procedure*

Procedure Steps	1st trial	2nd trial	3rd trial
1. Identify patient.			
2. Read doctor's order.			
3. Explain procedure to patient.			
4. Assemble equipment.			
5. Wash hands.			
6. Measure patient's pulse, respiration rate, quality of respiration, and note the patient's color.			
7. Record observations.			
8. Place mask comfortably on patient's face, covering mouth and nose, or			
8A. Place prongs of nasal cannula into patient's nose and loop tubing behind patient's ears and adjust to fit snugly under patient's chin.			
9. Connect tubing to oxygen tank.			
10. Open valve so that oxygen is flowing and adjust flow rate to that ordered by the physician.			
11. Assess patient after 5 minutes.			
12. Notify doctor if patient still has respiratory difficulty after 5 minutes.			
13. Document actions and patient response in the medical record.			
14. The oxygen was adjusted to the exact flow rate ordered by the physician. ◆			
15. Complete the procedure within 10 minutes. ◆			

Charting

DATE	

Evaluator Comments:

Score Calculation:

For each procedural step marked U (Unsatisfactory) deduct 6 points
For each procedural step (◆) marked U (Unsatisfactory) deduct 20 points

Score calculation 100 points

− points missed

Total score

1st	2nd	3rd

Satisfactory score: 85 or above

Procedure 31-4: Caring for Burns

Performance Objective

Task: Perform burn care for a patient

Conditions: Cotton cloth, water

Standards: Complete the procedure in 5 minutes, and achieve a satisfactory score on the procedure performance checklist

*Scoring Key: (**S**)atisfactory, (**U**)nsatisfactory, (**NA**) Not Applicable*
◆ *Denotes a critical element for a satisfactory score on the procedure*

Procedure Steps

Procedure Steps	1st trial	2nd trial	3rd trial
1. Remove source of burn to stop burning process.			
2. Assess severity of burn.			
3. Assess patient's respiration.			
4. Call 911 or emergency number for moderate or severe burns.			
5. Flush chemical burns or thermal burns that have not penetrated the dermis with cool water, sterile if possible.			
6. If burns have penetrated dermis, cover burn with non-adhering cotton cloth.			
7. Continue to monitor respiration status.			
8. If burns occurred in the medical office, record description of event and actions taken in patient's medical record.			
9. Complete the procedure within 5 minutes. ◆			

Charting

DATE	

Evaluator Comments:

Score Calculation:

For each procedural step marked U (Unsatisfactory) deduct 6 points
For each procedural step (◆) marked U (Unsatisfactory) deduct 20 points

Score calculation	100 points			
	− ____ points missed	1st	2nd	3rd
	Total score			

Satisfactory score: 85 or above

Procedure 31-5: Controlling Bleeding

Performance Objective

Task: Control moderate to severe bleeding

Conditions: Gloves, sterile dressing, gown and eye protection, mask, biohazard waste container

Standards: Complete the procedure in 10 minutes, and achieve a satisfactory score on the procedure performance checklist

Scoring Key: (**S**)*atisfactory,* (**U**)*nsatisfactory,* (**NA**) *Not Applicable*
◆ *Denotes a critical element for a satisfactory score on the procedure*

Procedure Steps	1st trial	2nd trial	3rd trial
1. Identify patient.			
2. If bleeding is severe, call 911 or emergency number.			
3. Wash hands (if possible).			
4. Put on PPE (if possible and if available).			
5. Assemble equipment.			
6. Explain procedure to patient if patient is conscious.			
7. Apply dressing over open wound and press firmly. (Use sterile dressing if available.)			
8. If the wound is on an arm or hand, elevate above heart level.			
9. Continue pressure for several minutes to assure clotting.			
10. If bleeding persists and seeps through dressing, continue pressure.			
11. When bleeding has subsided, cover with fresh dressing.			
12. Wash hands.			
13. Discard soiled dressings, gloves, and other supplies in a biohazard waste container.			
14. If bleeding occurred in the medical office, record description of event and actions taken in patient's medical record.			
15. Complete the procedure within 10 minutes. ◆			

Charting

DATE	

Evaluator Comments:

Score Calculation:

For each procedural step marked U (Unsatisfactory) deduct 6 points
For each procedural step (◆) marked U (Unsatisfactory) deduct 20 points

Score calculation	100 points			
	− points missed	1st	2nd	3rd
	Total score			

Satisfactory score: 85 or above

Procedure 31-6: Applying a Splint

Performance Objective

Task: Apply a splint to an extremity

Conditions: Straps for securing splint, flat surface to immobilize extremity, padding

Standards: Complete the procedure in 10 minutes, and achieve a satisfactory score on the procedure performance checklist

Scoring Key: (**S**)*atisfactory,* (**U**)*nsatisfactory,* (**NA**) *Not Applicable*
◆ *Denotes a critical element for a satisfactory score on the procedure*

Procedure Steps	1st trial	2nd trial	3rd trial
1. Assess patient for fracture or dislocation.			
2. If available, call 911 or emergency number.			
3. Assemble equipment.			
4. Explain what you are attempting to do to immobilize extremity.			
5. Place padded rigid surface along injured extremity.			
6. Wrap several layers of strapping around extremity and rigid surface.			
7. Assure that extremity is not mobile.			
8. If fracture or dislocation occurred in the medical office, record description of event and actions taken in patient's medical record.			
9. Complete the procedure within 10 minutes. ◆			

Charting

DATE	

Evaluator Comments:

Score Calculation:

For each procedural step marked U (Unsatisfactory) deduct 6 points
For each procedural step (◆) marked U (Unsatisfactory) deduct 20 points

Score calculation	100 points			
	− ___ points missed	1st	2nd	3rd
	Total score			

Satisfactory score: 85 or above

Procedure 31-7: Cleaning Minor Wounds

Performance Objective

Task: Clean minor wound using aseptic technique

Conditions: Sterile dressing(s), sterile gauze squares, sterile gloves, sterile water or other sterile solution, sterile basin, sterile drapes, adhesive tape, biohazard waste container

Standards: Complete the procedure in 10 minutes, and achieve a satisfactory score on the procedure performance checklist

Scoring Key: (**S**)*atisfactory,* (**U**)*nsatisfactory,* (**NA**) *Not Applicable*
◆ *Denotes a critical element for a satisfactory score on the procedure*

Procedure Steps	1st trial	2nd trial	3rd trial
1. Identify patient.			
2. Visually assess wound.			
3. Assemble supplies.			
4. Wash hands.			
5. Prepare a sterile field containing a sterile basin.			
6. Pour sterile water or other solution ordered by the physician into sterile basin.			
7. Add sterile gauze squares and sterile forceps to the sterile field. (A sterile syringe may also be used to irrigate the wound.)			
8. Open packaged dressings.			
9. Place absorbent underpad below the wound area.			
10. Drape wound if needed.			
11. Position biohazard bag close by.			
12. Put on sterile gloves.			
13. Clean wound site using one swipe per gauze pad or swab in a downward motion, or irrigate from cleaner area to less clean area.			
14. Dry wound using gentle patting motion with new gauze squares.			
15. Cover wound with sterile dressing.			
16. Anchor dressing with adhesive tape or conforming gauze bandage.			
17. Discard soiled supplies in biohazard bag.			

Procedure Steps	**1st trial**	**2nd trial**	**3rd trial**
18. Remove and discard gloves in biohazard bag.			
19. Wash hands.			
20. Document in patient medical record.			
21. Complete the procedure within 10 minutes. ◆			

Charting

DATE	

Evaluator Comments:

Score Calculation:

For each procedural step marked U (Unsatisfactory) deduct 6 points
For each procedural step (◆) marked U (Unsatisfactory) deduct 20 points

Score calculation	100 points			
	− points missed	1st	2nd	3rd
	Total score			

Satisfactory score: 85 or above

SELF-EVALUATION

UNIT 7

Patient Teaching and Follow-up

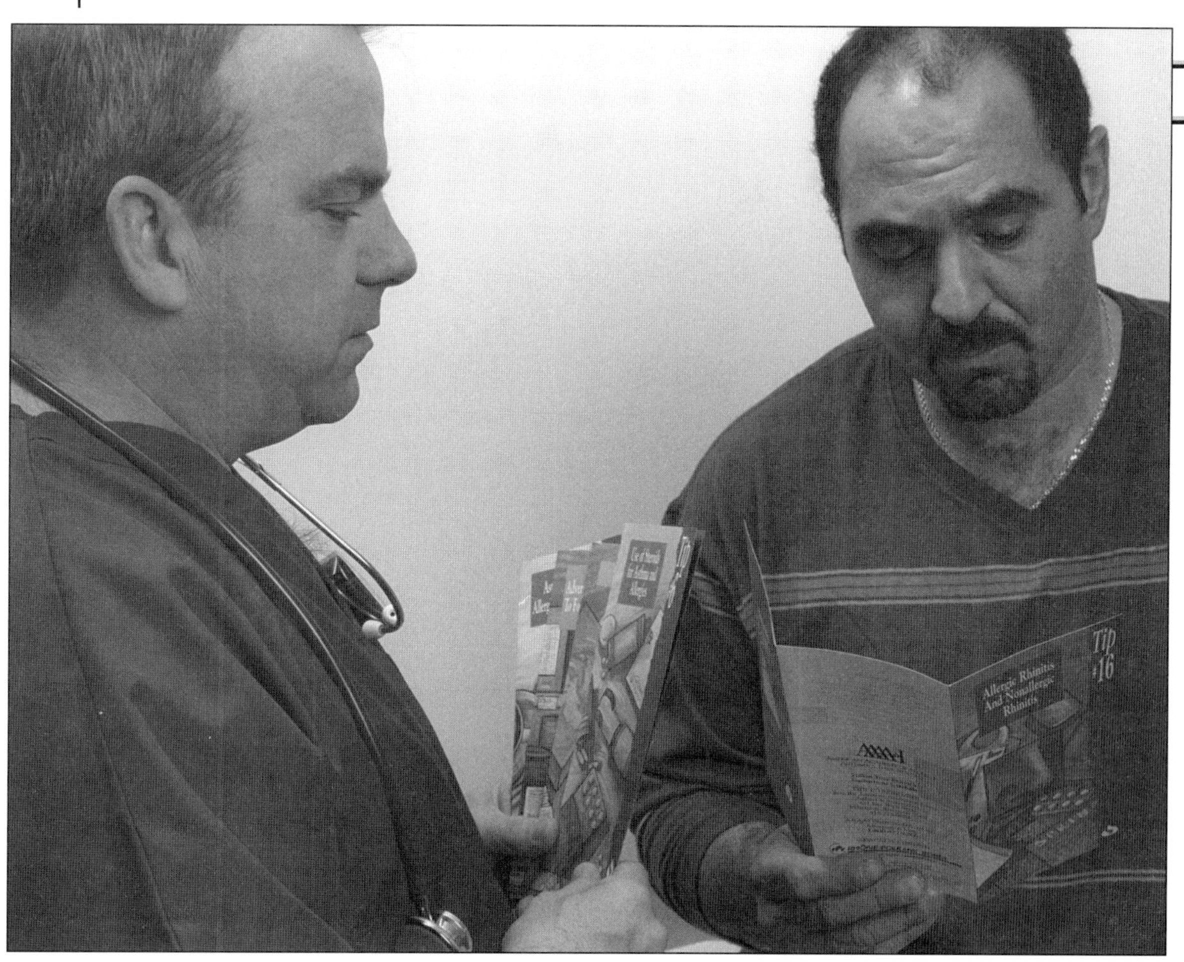

Chapter 32

Teaching Patients in the Medical Office

CHAPTER FOCUS

Patient teaching is a vital part of caring for patients in the medical office, and the medical assistant must be able to teach patients and adapt teaching to the needs of special populations. This chapter described various learning styles and discusses various teaching strategies and their appropriate uses. It also presented specific information about teaching patients with casts and ambulatory aids such as a cane, walker, or crutches.

TERMINOLOGY REVIEW

Vocabulary Matching: Match each term with its definition.

___ 1. Swing-through gait

___ 2. Forearm crutches

___ 3. Three-point gait

___ 4. Swing-to gait

___ 5. Axillary crutches

___ 6. Two-point gait

___ 7. Four-point gait

___ 8. Platform crutches

A. Crutches with a shelflike device to support the lower arms

B. Moving each leg with the opposite crutch

C. Moving the crutches forward, then swinging both legs up to the crutches

D. Aluminum crutches with hand grips and cuffs that fit around the lower arms

E. The most common type of crutches, with extensions above the hand grips that end a little below the armpits

F. Moving both crutches with the affected leg

G. Moving each crutch and each leg as a separate operation

H. Moving the crutches forward, then swinging both legs beyond the crutches

Definitions: Define the following domains for learning.

1. Cognitive ____

2. Affective ____

3. Psychomotor ______________________________________

CONTENT REVIEW QUESTIONS

1. Identify four factors that can interfere with learning.
   a. ________________________________
   b. ________________________________
   c. ________________________________
   d. ________________________________
2. Identify four ways that retention of newly learned material can be improved.
   a. ________________________________
   b. ________________________________
   c. ________________________________
   d. ________________________________
3. What are two intellectual processes of the cognitive domain?
   a. ________________________________
   b. ________________________________
4. What are four areas of the affective domain of learning?
   a. ________________________________
   b. ________________________________
   c. ________________________________
   d. ________________________________
5. How does a person learn in the psychomotor domain of learning?

6. Identify eight barriers to learning and the domains in which they occur.

   a. ______________________________
   b. ______________________________
   c. ______________________________
   d. ______________________________
   e. ______________________________
   f. ______________________________
   g. ______________________________
   h. ______________________________

7. What are the five steps of the teaching process?

   a. ______________________________
   b. ______________________________
   c. ______________________________
   d. ______________________________
   e. ______________________________

8. Why are specific learning objectives helpful for the teaching and learning process?

   ____
   ____
   ____
   ____

9. Describe four factors that must be considered when adapting teaching to the individual learner.

   a. ______________________________
   b. ______________________________
   c. ______________________________
   d. ______________________________

10. Describe seven teaching strategies that can be used in the medical office.

   a. ______________________________
   b. ______________________________
   c. ______________________________
   d. ______________________________
   e. ______________________________
   f. ______________________________
   g. ______________________________

11. What are the five parts of a written teaching plan?

 a. ______________________________

 b. ______________________________

 c. ______________________________

 d. ______________________________

 e. ______________________________

12. What should be included in the documentation after patient teaching?

____

____

____

____

13. How can the medical assistant validate patient learning?

____

____

____

____

14. Which areas of patient teaching are necessary for a patient and/or family member when a cast is applied?

____

____

____

____

15. In which hand should a person hold a cane if he or she has weakness of one leg? If he or she is generally weak?

____

____

____

____

16. Why should the top of an axillary crutch end at least two finger-widths below the axilla?

____

____

____

____

17. Which crutch gaits can be used by a person who has poor balance or weakness in both lower extremities?

18. Which crutch gait can be used by a person with one extremity that is non-weight-bearing?

19. What are the advantages and disadvantages of using a walker instead of a cane?

20. In which areas does a patient often need instruction before having a gastrointestinal procedure?

21. Describe the medical assistant's role in teaching patients about medication.

CRITICAL THINKING QUESTIONS

1. After you have completed the teaching plan in the section below, describe if it is helpful to you to expend the energy to create a written teaching plan. Give reasons for your answer.

2. Have you as a student been using the instructional objectives at the beginning of each chapter and procedure as tools for your own learning? If so, how are they helpful? If not, do you think they could help you to focus on important material?

3. Based on your own experience, do the medical assistants in your area play a large or small role in patient teaching? What do you think makes the difference in the medical assistant's willingness and ability to teach patients effectively?

PRACTICAL APPLICATIONS

1. How would the medical assistant vary his or her approach if he or she had to teach each of the following patients to take a vision exam for the first time?

   a. 4-year-old child

   b. 8-year-old child

   c. 14-year-old adolescent

   d. 34-year-old man

   e. 80-year-old woman

2. Identify three specific things you would ask a person to do in order to evaluate that your teaching of the three-point crutch gait with non-weight-bearing of the right leg had been effective. Describe exactly what you would look for in each.

   a. ______________________________

   ____

   b. ______________________________

   ____

   c. ______________________________

   ____

3. If written instructions for a barium enema included taking a bottle of magnesium citrate the night before the test, eating a fat-free supper, and taking two Fleet enemas the morning of the test, identify four specific things that the patient could tell you to demonstrate that he or she understood the instructions.

   a. ______________________________

   b. ______________________________

   c. ______________________________

   d. ______________________________

4. How might the radiologist in the x-ray department evaluate that the patient had or had not completely understood the instructions for the bowel prep for a barium enema?

   ____

   ____

   ____

   ____

5. What adaptations to teaching about a restricted diet would you need to make for the following patients:

   a. A patient who speaks only Spanish ______________________________

   ____

   b. A patient with poor vision ______________________________

   ____

   c. A patient who is mentally retarded ______________________________

   ____

   d. A patient who is hard of hearing ______________________________

   ____

6. Create a written teaching plan for the patient presented in your textbook, Warren Blake, a 23-year-old newly diagnosed insulin-dependent diabetic, to measure his blood sugar using a glucometer using the teaching plan forms on the following pages. Use information from Chapter 25 and Chapter 26.

TEACHING PLAN

TOPIC: ____________________

Patient Information:

Teaching Goal:

Material to Be Taught:

Learning Objectives	Teaching Method/ Audio-Visual Aids	When Teaching Planned	Evaluation Methods/Indications that Teaching Was Effective

TEACHING PLAN

Learning Objectives	Teaching Method/ Audio-Visual Aids	When Teaching Planned	Evaluation Methods/Indications that Teaching Was Effective

TEACHING PLAN

Learning Objectives	Teaching Method/ Audio-Visual Aids	When Teaching Planned	Evaluation Methods/Indications that Teaching Was Effective

TEACHING PLAN

Learning Objectives	Teaching Method/ Audio-Visual Aids	When Teaching Planned	Evaluation Methods/Indications that Teaching Was Effective

Procedure 32-1: Teaching a Patient to Use a Cane

Performance Objective

Task: Teach a patient to use a cane

Conditions: Cane

Standards: Complete the procedure in 15 minutes, and achieve a satisfactory score on the procedure performance checklist

Scoring Key: (**S**)*atisfactory,* (**U**)*nsatisfactory,* (**NA**) *Not Applicable*
◆ *Denotes a critical element for a satisfactory score on the procedure*

Procedure Steps	1st trial	2nd trial	3rd trial
1. Identify patient.			
2. Explain procedure.			
3. Measure cane to make sure top reaches to patient's hip, so the patient's elbow is slightly flexed.			
4. Adjust cane height if necessary.			
5. Instruct patient to move cane forward about 6 inches.			
6. Instruct patient to move affected leg forward to be parallel to cane.			
7. Instruct patient to move unaffected leg forward and about 6 inches ahead of the cane.			
8. Demonstrate use of cane for the patient if needed.			
9. Ask patient to demonstrate walking with the cane.			
10. Document instruction and patient achievement in patient medical record.			
11. Complete the procedure within 15 minutes. ◆			

Charting

DATE	

Evaluator Comments:

Score Calculation:

For each procedural step marked U (Unsatisfactory) deduct 6 points
For each procedural step (◆) marked U (Unsatisfactory) deduct 20 points

Score calculation	100 points			
	− points missed	1st	2nd	3rd
	Total score			

Satisfactory score: 85 or above

Procedure 32-2: Teaching a Patient to Use Crutches

Performance Objective

Task: Teach a patient to use crutches

Conditions: Crutches with crutch tips, axillary padding, and padding on hand grips

Standards: Complete procedure in 20 minutes, and achieve a satisfactory score on the procedure performance checklist

*Scoring Key: (**S**)atisfactory, (**U**)nsatisfactory, (**NA**) Not Applicable*
◆ *Denotes a critical element for a satisfactory score on the procedure*

Procedure Steps	1st trial	2nd trial	3rd trial
1. Identify patient.			
2. Explain procedure.			
3. Adjust crutches and hand grips to fit patient.			
4. Check height of crutches after they have been adjusted to be sure they end at least two finger-widths below the axilla.			
5. Check height of hand grips to be sure that arms are slightly bent.			
6. Instruct patient to stand with crutches about 4 inches to the side of the legs and 4 to 6 inches ahead of the foot.			
7. Verify that patient is placing correct amount of weight on affected leg.			
8. Instruct patient to move crutches and legs to achieve crutch gait with appropriate weight-bearing status.			
9. Demonstrate appropriate gait for patient.			
10. Guide patient to use appropriate gait.			
11. Coach patient as he or she uses appropriate gait.			
12. Allow patient to practice until comfortable with gait.			
13. Instruct patient on correct method to ascend and descend stairs.			
14. Demonstrate ascending and descending stairs for patient.			
15. Allow patient to practice until comfortable on stairs.			
16. Document instruction and patient performance in patient medical record.			
17. Complete the procedure within 20 minutes. ◆			

Charting

DATE	

Evaluator Comments:

Score Calculation:

For each procedural step marked U (Unsatisfactory) deduct 6 points
For each procedural step (◆) marked U (Unsatisfactory) deduct 20 points

Score calculation 100 points

− points missed

	1st	2nd	3rd
Total score			

Satisfactory score: 85 or above

Procedure 32-3: Teaching a Patient to Use a Walker

Performance Objective

Task: Teach a patient to use a walker

Conditions: Walker

Standards: Complete the procedure in 15 minutes, and achieve a satisfactory score on the procedure performance checklist

Scoring Key: (**S**)*atisfactory,* (**U**)*nsatisfactory,* (**NA**) *Not Applicable*
◆ *Denotes a critical element for a satisfactory score on the procedure*

Procedure Steps	1st trial	2nd trial	3rd trial
1. Identify patient.			
2. Explain procedure.			
3. Adjust walker height so patient can hold it comfortably when standing, with the walker slightly ahead of his or her body.			
4. Instruct patient to pick up or push walker using hand grips and move it forward about 6 inches.			
5. Instruct patient to set walker down securely and walk forward into the walker's "cage," holding the hand grips for support.			
6. Allow patient to practice, and observe.			
7. Demonstrate how to fold walker for storage.			
8. Document instruction and patient performance in patient medical record.			
9. Complete the procedure within 15 minutes. ◆			

Charting

DATE	

Evaluator Comments:

Score Calculation:

For each procedural step marked U (Unsatisfactory) deduct 6 points
For each procedural step (◆) marked U (Unsatisfactory) deduct 20 points

Score calculation	100 points			
	− points missed	1st	2nd	3rd
	Total score			

Satisfactory score: 85 or above

SELF-EVALUATION

Chapter 33

Maintaining Health: Nutrition, Exercise, and Self-Examination

CHAPTER FOCUS

In this chapter you learned basic information about nutrition, modified diets, exercise, and principles of breast and testicular self-examination. In addition, you learned how to apply principles of modified diet, exercise, and medication to assist the patient with diabetes mellitus to maintain optimum health.

TERMINOLOGY REVIEW

Vocabulary Matching: Match each term with its definition.

___ 1. polydipsia
___ 2. flexion
___ 3. polyuria
___ 4. hyperextension
___ 5. insulin reaction
___ 6. rotation
___ 7. extension
___ 8. pronation
___ 9. hyperglycemia
___ 10. abduction
___ 11. hypoglycemia
___ 12. supination
___ 13. inversion
___ 14. oral hypoglycemic

A. Increase in the angle between the bones of a joint
B. High blood sugar
C. Drop in blood sugar as a result of too much insulin
D. Medication that stimulates the insulin-producing cells to produce more insulin
E. Lateral movement away from the body's midline
F. Extreme hunger
G. Passage of large amounts of urine
H. Extreme thirst
I. Lateral movement toward the body's midline
J. Turning soles of the feet outward
K. Low blood sugar
L. Decrease in the angle between the bones of a joint
M. Turning the soles of the feet inward
N. Turning the wrist so that the hand faces down

___ 15. adduction

___ 16. polyphagia

___ 17. eversion

O. Turning the wrist so that the hand faces up

P. Turning a bone on its axis

Q. Extension of the bones of a joint beyond 180°

Definitions: Insert the correct word to complete the sentence.

1. ______________________ exercise is performed without assistance.
2. ______________________ exercise involves muscle contraction without movement.
3. During ______________________ exercise, a helper moves a person's joints for him or her to maintain mobility of the joints and muscles.
4. ______________________ exercise includes walking, jogging, bicycle riding, and swimming.
5. ______________________ exercise involves applying tension against muscle groups during movement.

Abbreviations: Expand each abbreviation to its complete form.

1. ADL ______________________
2. IDDM ______________________
3. LDL ______________________
4. NIDDM ______________________
5. ROM ______________________
6. HDL ______________________

CONTENT REVIEW QUESTIONS

1. What is the organizing principle of the food-guide pyramid?

____

____

____

2. Identify the two forms in which carbohydrate is found.

   a. ______________________

   b. ______________________

3. Identify health dietary sources of carbohydrates.

____

____

____

4. If all fats are eliminated from the diet, which essential fatty-acid deficiency occurs?

____

____

5. Differentiate between high-density lipoproteins and low-density lipoproteins.

____

____

____

6. What type of fat should be avoided in the diet?

____

____

____

7. Why are foods such as eggs, meat, fish, and poultry called high-quality or complete proteins?

____

____

8. What is the function of protein in the body?

____

____

9. Differentiate between fat-soluble and water-soluble vitamins and give examples of each type.

____

____

____

10. Identify two good dietary sources for each of the following vitamins and minerals:

a. Vitamin A ______________________________

b. Vitamin C ______________________________

c. Vitamin D ______________________________

d. Thiamine ______________________________

e. Riboflavin ______________________________

f. Niacin ______________________________

g. Calcium ______________________________

h. Iron ______________________________

i. Iodine ______________________________

11. How is calcium used by the body?

12. Why is water an important part of a healthy diet?

13. What is a liquid diet, and when is it used?

14. What are three strategies that have been used to promote weight loss?

a.

b.

c.

15. Identify when a moderate sodium-restricted diet is recommended.

16. When patients have elevated cholesterol, what type of management may the physician initiate?

17. What are four important things to tell a patient about exercise?

a.

b.

c.

d.

18. Why should a patient examine his or her skin regularly?

19. Who should perform regular breast examination? Testicular examination? How often?

____

____

____

20. What are five goals of dietary management for patients with diabetes mellitus?

a. ____

b. ____

c. ____

d. ____

e. ____

21. How does adjustment of each of the following help a diabetic to maintain health?

a. Diet ____

____

b. Exercise ____

____

c. Medication ____

____

22. When insulin is prescribed for a patient with diabetes, what are six specific areas of teaching for the patient to take his or her insulin properly and respond to adverse effects?

a. ____

b. ____

c. ____

d. ____

e. ____

f. ____

23. Describe three aspects of foot care for diabetic patients.

a. ____

b. ____

c. ____

CRITICAL THINKING QUESTIONS

1. Based on your study of this chapter, identify six specific recommendations you would make for yourself to adopt a healthier lifestyle. Analyze your recommendations and determine how likely you are to adopt them. What factors would motivate you? What factors would make change unlikely?

____

____

____

____

____

____

____

____

____

2. Prepare a detailed teaching plan for one of the following patients using the forms that follow this section of the chapter.

   a. James Robb is a 72-year-old man who had a stroke (CVA) 4 months ago. His left leg is a little weak and he has been advised to use a cane when walking. His left arm is almost totally paralyzed and he has been advised to wear a sling when walking to support his arm and shoulder. Mr. Robb and his wife need to learn how to perform range-of-motion exercises for his left arm. Mr. Robb thinks he will be able to do the exercises himself with his right arm if he is shown how to do it.

   b. Warren Blake, the newly diagnosed diabetic presented in "On the Job" in Chapter 32, has been prescribed a 1500-2000 calorie ADA diet, which almost exactly mirrors the recommendations of the dietary food pyramid. He is supposed to have two snacks, one in the afternoon and one before bedtime. He is also supposed to limit fat to less than 30% of daily calories and cholesterol to under 300 mg per day. In addition, he needs to learn to recognize the signs and symptoms of diabetic ketoacidosis and insulin reaction.

   c. Diane Calorie, a 58-year-old woman, has been a Type I diabetic for 10 years, but she has recently been switched from a single type of insulin to a mixture of regular and NPH insulin. She needs to learn how to draw up two types of insulin in a single syringe. In addition, the physician has asked you to review foot care with her, since her feet are dry and cracked.

PRACTICAL APPLICATIONS

1. Analyze the following food eaten during one day by a 175-pound man. For each food, identify the type of food according to the food-guide pyramid. Compare the total number of servings of each type of food with those recommended. How would you instruct this man to modify his diet?

Breakfast:	**# Servings**	**Food Group**
1 cup of corn flakes	____________	____________
with sugar	____________	____________
and 1/2 cup milk	____________	____________
3/4 cup orange juice	____________	____________
coffee with cream	____________	____________
and sugar	____________	____________
1 donut	____________	____________
Lunch		
Tuna fish sandwich	____________	____________
with 2 oz tuna	____________	____________
lettuce, tomato,	____________	____________
and mayonnaise	____________	____________
Snack		
Small package of potato chips	____________	____________
Chocolate bar	____________	____________
Dinner		
1 cup pasta with tomato sauce	____________	____________
and 6 ounces chicken	____________	____________
green salad (1 cup)	____________	____________
with 2 ounces of cheese	____________	____________
2 Tbsp salad dressing	____________	____________
3/4 cup ice cream	____________;	____________

Total servings: Grain ____________ Fruit/Veg ____________ Milk ____________

Meat ____________ Eat sparingly ____________

Recommendations:

____

____

____

2. Identify specific recommendations you would make to a patient for whom the physician recommended a moderate sodium-restricted diet.

____

____

____

____

3. Identify specific foods to avoid and recommendations for a patient who is supposed to avoid saturated fat and reduce cholesterol.

____

____

____

____

____

4. How would you explain the onset, peak action, and duration of each of the following types of insulin to a patient?

   a. Regular insulin ____

   ____

   b. Lente or NPH insulin ____

   ____

   c. Mixtures with NPH/regular insulin _______________________________

   ____

TEACHING PLAN

TOPIC: ______________________

Patient Information:

Teaching Goal:

Material to Be Taught:

Learning Objectives	Teaching Method/ Audio-Visual Aids	When Teaching Planned	Evaluation Methods/Indications that Teaching Was Effective

TEACHING PLAN

Learning Objectives	Teaching Method/ Audio-Visual Aids	When Teaching Planned	Evaluation Methods/Indications that Teaching Was Effective

TEACHING PLAN

Learning Objectives	Teaching Method/ Audio-Visual Aids	When Teaching Planned	Evaluation Methods/Indications that Teaching Was Effective

TEACHING PLAN

Learning Objectives	Teaching Method/ Audio-Visual Aids	When Teaching Planned	Evaluation Methods/Indications that Teaching Was Effective

PROCEDURE PERFORMANCE CHECKLISTS

Procedure 33-1: Teaching Range-of-Motion Exercises

Performance Objective

Task: Teach a patient and/or family member to perform range-of-motion exercises

Conditions: Treatment table, pillows

Standards: Complete the procedure in 30 minutes, and achieve a satisfactory score on the procedure performance checklist

Scoring Key: (**S**)*atisfactory,* (**U**)*nsatisfactory,* (**NA**) *Not Applicable*
◆ *Denotes a critical element for a satisfactory score on the procedure*

Procedure Steps	1st trial	2nd trial	3rd trial
1. Wash hands.			
2. Identify patient and any others to be included in teaching.			
3. Explain that range-of-motion exercises are usually done in sequence from the head down.			
4. Explain that every joint should be moved through its full range of motion to the extent that this can be done without excessive pain or force.			
5. Ask patient to move each muscle group through normal range of motion to best ability, in order to gauge active range of motion.			
6. Demonstrate each motion.			
7. Ask the patient to return the demonstration.			
8. Explain how a patient can use a strong extremity to assist a weak extremity if needed.			
9. Demonstrate active assistive exercises if needed for the patient.			
10. Explain how an assistant may assist the patient and/or perform the exercises if one or more extremities are paralyzed.			
11. Demonstrate passive exercises if needed for the patient.			
12. Include full range of motion for each of the following: head and neck; right shoulder, elbow, wrist, fingers; left shoulder, elbow, wrist, fingers; right hip, knee, ankle, toes; left hip, knee, ankle, toes; torso; and spine.			
13. Ask if the patient or assistant has any questions.			

Procedure Steps	1st trial	2nd trial	3rd trial
14. Wash hands.			
15. Document teaching and patient/assistant performance in patient medical record.			
16. Complete the procedure within 30 minutes. ◆			

Charting

DATE	

Evaluator Comments:

Score Calculation:

For each procedural step marked U (Unsatisfactory) deduct 6 points
For each procedural step (◆) marked U (Unsatisfactory) deduct 20 points

Score calculation 100 points

− points missed

Total score

1st	2nd	3rd

Satisfactory score: 85 or above

Procedure 33-2: Teaching Breast Self-examination

Performance Objective

Task: Teach a woman to perform breast self-examination

Conditions: Treatment table, pillows, model of breast containing an abnormal lump

Standards: Complete the procedure in 20 minutes, and achieve a satisfactory score on the procedure performance checklist

Scoring Key: (**S**)*atisfactory*, (**U**)*nsatisfactory*, (**NA**) *Not Applicable*
◆ *Denotes a critical element for a satisfactory score on the procedure*

Procedure Steps	1st trial	2nd trial	3rd trial
1. Wash hands.			
2. Identify patient.			
3. Explain importance of monthly breast self-examination.			
4. Instruct patient to perform exam about one week after the beginning of her menstrual period.			
5. Instruct patient in proper technique to palpate breasts using model.			
6. Instruct patient on procedure to examine right breast while lying down.			
7. Instruct patient on procedure to examine left breast while lying down.			
8. Instruct patient on procedure to examine right breast while standing up.			
9. Instruct patient on procedure to examine left breast while standing up.			
10. Instruct patient on procedure to examine breasts visually using a mirror.			
11. Ask if the patient has any questions.			
12. Wash hands.			
13. Document instruction in patient medical record.			
14. Complete the procedure within 20 minutes. ◆			

Charting

DATE	

Evaluator Comments:

Score Calculation:

For each procedural step marked U (Unsatisfactory) deduct 6 points
For each procedural step (◆) marked U (Unsatisfactory) deduct 20 points

Score calculation 100 points

− points missed

	1st	2nd	3rd
Total score			

Satisfactory score: 85 or above

Procedure 33-3: Teaching Testicular Self-examination

Performance Objective

Task: Teach a man to perform testicular self-examination

Conditions: Model of testes containing abnormal lump

Standards: Complete the procedure in 20 minutes, and achieve a satisfactory score on the procedure performance checklist

Scoring Key: (**S**)*atisfactory*, (**U**)*nsatisfactory*, (**NA**) *Not Applicable*
◆ *Denotes a critical element for a satisfactory score on the procedure*

Procedure Steps	1st trial	2nd trial	3rd trial
1. Wash hands.			
2. Identify patient.			
3. Explain the importance of monthly testicular examination.			
4. Instruct patient to perform exam on same day each month.			
5. Instruct patient of symptoms of testicular cancer.			
6. Instruct patient on proper technique for self-examination using testicular model.			
7. Ask patient to demonstrate technique using model.			
8. Instruct the patient to examine each testicle gently.			
9. Instruct the patient to palpate up along each spermatic cord.			
10. Ask if the patient has any questions.			
11. Wash hands.			
12. Document teaching in patient medical record.			
13. Complete the procedure within 20 minutes. ◆			

Charting

DATE	

Evaluator Comments:

Score Calculation:

For each procedural step marked U (Unsatisfactory) deduct 6 points
For each procedural step (◆) marked U (Unsatisfactory) deduct 20 points

Score calculation	100 points			
	– points missed	1st	2nd	3rd
	Total score			

Satisfactory score: 85 or above

SELF-EVALUATION

Chapter 34

Oral Follow-up

CHAPTER FOCUS

In this chapter you learned basic information about how the medical assistant schedules follow-up for a patient, such as diagnostic tests, therapy, a consultation by another physician, or surgery. Often the patient requires a referral form or preauthorization in order for his or her insurance company to pay. In addition, the medical assistant may refer a patient to a community agency, and this may also require a physician's authorization and/or referral form.

TERMINOLOGY REVIEW

Vocabulary Matching: Match each term with its definition.

__ 1. preauthorization

__ 2. ORIF

__ 3. recall file

__ 4. authorization number

__ 5. referral

__ 6. PAT

A. The number issued by the insurance company to verify permission for a test or procedure

B. A file of reminders to call patients

C. Pre-Authorization for tests

D. Prior approval by an insurance company for treatment or test

E. On referral information form

F. An authorization from a primary care provider for treatment by or visits to a specialist or other health care practitioner

G. Open reduction, internal fixation

H. Preadmission testing

CONTENT REVIEW QUESTIONS

1. Give an example when a follow-up appointment might need to be scheduled:

   a. On a specific day ____

b. At a particular time of day ______________________________

c. After a certain day ______________________________

2. What instructions might the medical assistant need to give a patient about a follow-up appointment?

____

____

3. Give an example of treatment that the medical assistant might give a patient between appointments.

____

____

4. What system might the office use if the patient's follow-up visit cannot be scheduled because it is several months in the future?

____

____

5. How can the office remind patients about appointments?

____

____

6. What information is necessary for a medical assistant to schedule a diagnostic test at a facility such as the hospital radiology department?

____

____

____

7. What should the medical assistant document in the patient's medical record after scheduling a diagnostic test for the patient?

____

____

____

8. How might the office handle informing patients of diagnostic test results?

____

____

____

9. Why is it usually necessary to obtain preauthorization before surgery, certain diagnostic tests, and some kinds of therapy?

____

____

____

10. Where will preadmission testing be performed before surgery?

____

____

____

11. If a patient will have inpatient surgery, how should the medical assistant schedule it?

____

____

____

12. What is the difference between a referral and a preauthorization?

____

____

____

13. What are three common reasons for a referral?

a. _______________

b. _______________

c. _______________

CRITICAL THINKING QUESTIONS

1. Do research to find out what types of surgery are done as day surgery and what types of surgery are done as inpatient surgery in your geographic area. Identify trends that have increased the number of day surgeries over the past ten years.

____

____

____

____

____

____

PRACTICAL APPLICATIONS

1. For each of the following patients, indicate if there is any special date or time of day that lab tests and/or follow-up appointments should be scheduled and any instructions you should give to the patient.

   a. Schedule Michelle Jaynes, R/O diabetes mellitus, for FBS and 2-hour postprandial blood sugar at the hospital lab, then follow up with U/A in the office.

   ____

   ____

b. Schedule Hyland Morris for a complete physical examination. His insurance pays for one physical exam per year. His last exam was on October 6th of the previous year.

c. Schedule Mary Ann Jenkins for a follow-up appointment in one month. She has been complaining that her eyelids start to droop as the day wears on.

2. Obtain preoperative instructions for at least one surgical procedure that is done in your area. You can often find such instructions on the hospital website. Compare instructions with those found by your classmates. Role-play what you would tell a patient.

3. Complete a referral form (found at the end of this section) for Dr. Hughes to sign. The patient's name is Agnes Mitchell. She is being referred by Dr. Joann Hughes at Blackburn Primary Care Associates, PC, 1990 Turquoise Drive, Blackburn, WI 54937, to see Dr. Winston Gray, a cardiologist whose address is 662 Area Form Drive, Blackburn, WI 54937. Her insurance number is 2452687 and the suffix # is -02. Her date of birth is 6/13/25. She is being referred for consultative opinion and necessary diagnostic studies (not to exceed three visits). Her diagnosis is cardiac arrythmia and dyspnea on exertion.

4. Complete a referral form (found at the end of this section) for Dr. Lawler to sign. The patient's name is Melissa Taylor, birth date 2/01/87. She is being referred by Dr. Howard Lawler at Blackburn Primary Care Associates, PC 1990 Turquoise Drive, Blackburn, WI 54937, to see Dr. Eileen Brauer, an dermatologist, for a consultative opinion only. Dr. Brauer's address is 9 Main Street, Blackburn, WI 54937. Melissa's diagnosis is acne vulgaris.

Health Plan Referral Form

REFERRAL NUMBER: A06

WRITTEN REFERRALS ARE REQUIRED FOR ALL SERVICES, EXCEPT FOR ROUTINE YEARLY EYE EXAMS, ORAL SURGERY, LAB, DIAGNOSTIC & RADIOLOGICAL SERVICES.

(1) Patient Name: ______________________ (2) Date of Referral: ____ / /

(3) Patient Identification Number: ______________ (4) SUFFIX # REQUIRED [|] (5) Date of Birth: ____ / /

(6) Referred From: ______________________ [ ] Provider ID # (7) I.P.A. No. [|]
NAME OF PERSONAL CARE PHYSICIAN

(8) ______________________
ADDRESS OF PERSONAL CARE PHYSICIAN

Referred To: ______________________ [ ] Provider ID #
NAME OFSPECIALTY CARE PHYSICIAN/PROVIDER/EMERGENCY

(10) ______________________
ADDRESS OF SPECIALTY CARE PHYSICIAN/PROVIDER/EMERGENCY

REFERRAL STATUS: (CHECK ONE)
In I.P.A. ☐ ☐ ☐ ☐

REASON FOR REFERRAL (STATE DIAGNOSIS): ______________________

SERVICES REQUESTED (CHECK ONE)

REFERRAL VALID FOR TWELVE MONTHS FROM DATE OF REFERRAL.

☐ Consultative OPINION. (One (1) visit only) CONTACT PCP PRIOR TO INITIATING TREATMENT.

☐ SECOND SURGICAL OPINION ONLY (Surgery is not to be performed by this provider)

☐ Consultative OPINION and NECESSARY DIAGNOSTIC STUDIES. (Not to exceed three (3) visits)

☐ Consultative OPINION and NECESSARY DIAGNOSTIC STUDY AND TREATMENT. **Indicate number of visits** [ ]

☐ Mental Health EVALUATION: Circle one (1) or two (2) visits only. (FOR PCP USE ONLY)

☐ Substance Abuse Outpatient EVALUATION: Circle one (1) or two (2) visits only. (FOR PCP USE ONLY)

☐ Mental Health/Substance Abuse Treatment (PSYCHIATRIC REVIEWER USE ONLY) subsequent visits, indicate number [ ]

AUTHORIZATION FOR MENTAL HEALTH OR SUBSTANCE ABUSE OUTPATIENT SERVICES DOES NOT OVERRIDE BENEFIT MAXIMUMS.

☐ Therapies (type of therapy: __________). **Indicate number of visits** [ ] (PT not to exceed six (6) visits per referral)

☐ Obstetrical Treatment. Designate duration of care: ______________________

☐ Emergency Room Treatment. Date of service: ______ / ______ / ______

SEPARATE REFERRAL FORM REQUIRED FOR EACH EMERGENCY ROOM DATE OF SERVICE

Note: Only those services included in the Health Plan Description of Benefits will be covered. If you have any questions contact your Professional Relations Coordinator.

I have enclosed a clinical document summary, have performed the following diagnostic studies, and am supplying the information to assist you.

DIAGNOSTIC PROCEDURES	DATE OF SERVICE	RESULTS

INSTRUCTIONS

PCP:
- Complete Form
- Send Health Plan Copy and Specialist Copy to Specialist
- Retain PCP Copy for your file

SPECIALIST:
- For Referrals to another Specialist Consult W/ PCP
- Send Health Plan Copy to Appropriate Address (see above)

ER AUTHORIZATION
- Send Health Plan Copy to Appropriate Address (see above)
- Retain Copy for your file
- Be sure to notify

X ______________________ / /
SIGNATURE OF PERSONAL CARE PHYSICIUAN — AUTHORIZATION DATE

X ______________________ / /
SIGNATURE OF PHYSICIAN REVIEWER* — AUTHORIZATION DATE

*ALL OUT OF PLAN REFERRALS REQUIRE PHYSICIAN REVIEWER SIGNATURE

Health Plan Referral Form

REFERRAL NUMBER: A06

WRITTEN REFERRALS ARE REQUIRED FOR ALL SERVICES, EXCEPT FOR ROUTINE YEARLY EYE EXAMS, ORAL SURGERY, LAB, DIAGNOSTIC & RADIOLOGICAL SERVICES.

(1) Patient Name: ______________________ (2) Date of Referral: ____ / ____ / ____

(3) Patient Identification Number: ______________ (4) SUFFIX # REQUIRED ☐☐ (5) Date of Birth: ____ / ____ / ____

(6) Referred From: ______________________ NAME OF PERSONAL CARE PHYSICIAN ☐ Provider ID # (7) I.P.A. No. ☐☐

(8) ______________________ ADDRESS OF PERSONAL CARE PHYSICIAN

Referred To: ______________________ NAME OFSPECIALTY CARE PHYSICIAN/PROVIDER/EMERGENCY ☐ Provider ID #

(10) ______________________ ADDRESS OF SPECIALTY CARE PHYSICIAN/PROVIDER/EMERGENCY

REFERRAL STATUS: (CHECK ONE) In I.P.A. ☐ ☐ ☐ ☐

REASON FOR REFERRAL (STATE DIAGNOSIS): ______________________

SERVICES REQUESTED (CHECK ONE)

REFERRAL VALID FOR TWELVE MONTHS FROM DATE OF REFERRAL.

☐ Consultative OPINION. (One (1) visit only) CONTACT PCP PRIOR TO INITIATING TREATMENT.

☐ SECOND SURGICAL OPINION ONLY (Surgery is not to be performed by this provider)

☐ Consultative OPINION and NECESSARY DIAGNOSTIC STUDIES. (Not to exceed three (3) visits)

☐ Consultative OPINION and NECESSARY DIAGNOSTIC STUDY AND TREATMENT. **Indicate number of visits** ☐

☐ Mental Health EVALUATION: Circle one (1) or two (2) visits only. (FOR PCP USE ONLY)

☐ Substance Abuse Outpatient EVALUATION: Circle one (1) or two (2) visits only. (FOR PCP USE ONLY)

☐ Mental Health/Substance Abuse Treatment (PSYCHIATRIC REVIEWER USE ONLY) subsequent visits, indicate number ☐

AUTHORIZATION FOR MENTAL HEALTH OR SUBSTANCE ABUSE OUTPATIENT SERVICES DOES NOT OVERRIDE BENEFIT MAXIMUMS.

☐ Therapies (type of therapy: ____________). **Indicate number of visits** ☐ (PT not to exceed six (6) visits per referral)

☐ Obstetrical Treatment. Designate duration of care: ______________________

☐ Emergency Room Treatment. Date of service: ____ / ____ / ____

SEPARATE REFERRAL FORM REQUIRED FOR EACH EMERGENCY ROOM DATE OF SERVICE

Note: Only those services included in the Health Plan Description of Benefits will be covered. If you have any questions contact your Professional Relations Coordinator.

I have enclosed a clinical document summary, have performed the following diagnostic studies, and am supplying the information to assist you.

DIAGNOSTIC PROCEDURES	DATE OF SERVICE	RESULTS

INSTRUCTIONS

PCP:
- Complete Form
- Send Health Plan Copy and Specialist Copy to Specialist
- Retain PCP Copy for your file

SPECIALIST:
- For Referrals to another Specialist Consult W/ PCP
- Send Health Plan Copy to Appropriate Address (see above)

ER AUTHORIZATION
- Send Health Plan Copy to Appropriate Address (see above)
- Retain Copy for your file
- Be sure to notify

X ______________________ ____ / ____ / ____
SIGNATURE OF PERSONAL CARE PHYSICIUAN — AUTHORIZATION DATE

X ______________________ ____ / ____ / ____
SIGNATURE OF PHYSICIAN REVIEWER* — AUTHORIZATION DATE

*ALL OUT OF PLAN REFERRALS REQUIRE PHYSICIAN REVIEWER SIGNATURE

PROCEDURE PERFORMANCE CHECKLISTS

Procedure 34-1: Scheduling Diagnostic Tests

Performance Objective

Task: Schedule a diagnostic test for a patient

Conditions: Patient medical record, insurance information, name of test or procedure to be scheduled, telephone, telephone number and department of facility that will perform test

Standards: Complete the procedure in 15 minutes, and achieve a satisfactory score on the procedure performance checklist

Scoring Key: (**S**)*atisfactory,* (**U**)*nsatisfactory,* (**NA**) *Not Applicable*
◆ *Denotes a critical element for a satisfactory score on the procedure*

Procedure Steps	1st trial	2nd trial	3rd trial
1. Assemble necessary information.			
2. From patient medical record or requisition filled out by doctor, determine test or procedure to be scheduled.			
3. Determine time frame for performing the test.			
4. Ask patient about preferred times and/or days.			
5. Determine facility where test will be performed.			
6. Locate facility telephone number.			
7. If necessary, obtain preauthorization from patient's insurance carrier.			
8. Call facility to schedule test.			
9. Confirm date and time with patient.			
10. Provide any verbal instructions to patient about test preparations.			
11. Provide any written instructions to patient about test preparations.			
12. Document scheduled procedures and instructions given in the patient medical record.			
13. If required, send test requisition paperwork to the facility.			
14. Complete the procedure within 15 minutes. ◆			

Charting

DATE	

Evaluator Comments:

Score Calculation:

For each procedural step marked U (Unsatisfactory) deduct 6 points
For each procedural step (◆) marked U (Unsatisfactory) deduct 20 points

Score calculation 100 points

− points missed

Total score

1st	2nd	3rd

Satisfactory score: 85 or above

Procedure 34-2: Scheduling a Surgical Procedure

Performance Objective

Task: Schedule a surgical procedure for a patient

Conditions: Patient medical record, insurance information, name of surgical procedure to be scheduled, telephone, telephone number and department of facility that will perform the surgery

Standards: Complete the procedure in 30 minutes, and achieve a satisfactory score on the procedure performance checklist

Scoring Key: (**S**)*atisfactory,* (**U**)*nsatisfactory,* (**NA**) *Not Applicable*
◆ *Denotes a critical element for a satisfactory score on the procedure*

Procedure Steps	1st trial	2nd trial	3rd trial
1. Assemble necessary information.			
2. From the patient's medical record, determine the surgical procedure to be performed and the patient's diagnosis.			
3. Determine the time frame for performing the surgery.			
4. Ask the patient about preferred days and/or times.			
5. Determine where the surgery will be performed.			
6. Locate the telephone number of facility where surgery will be performed.			
7. Obtain preauthorization from patient's medical insurance carrier.			
8. Call facility and schedule the surgery.			
9. Confirm the date and time with the patient.			
10. Arrange for preadmission testing (PAT) with either the hospital, primary-care doctor, or a laboratory acceptable to the patient's insurance carrier.			
11. Provide the patient with any necessary verbal instructions.			
12. Provide the patient with any necessary written instructions.			
13. Document the scheduled surgery and instructions in the patient's medical record.			
14. Complete the procedure within 30 minutes. ◆			

Charting

DATE	

Evaluator Comments:

Score Calculation:

For each procedural step marked U (Unsatisfactory) deduct 6 points
For each procedural step (◆) marked U (Unsatisfactory) deduct 20 points

Score calculation 100 points

– ___ points missed

Total score

1st	2nd	3rd

Satisfactory score: 85 or above

Procedure 34-3: Completing a Referral Form for Managed Care

Performance Objective

Task: Complete a referral form for a managed-care provider

Conditions: Patient medical record, insurance information, information about the service to be provided, referral form or computer terminal, telephone, telephone number of patient's insurance company

Standards: Complete the procedure in 15 minutes, and achieve a satisfactory score on the procedure performance checklist

Scoring Key: (**S**)*atisfactory,* (**U**)*nsatisfactory,* (**NA**) *Not Applicable*
◆ *Denotes a critical element for a satisfactory score on the procedure*

Procedure Steps	**1st trial**	**2nd trial**	**3rd trial**
1. Assemble necessary information.			
2. From patient medical record or the doctor, determine services for which the patient is being referred.			
3. If necessary, obtain preauthorization from insurance carrier.			
4. Complete the referral form.			
5. If preauthorization is required, submit form to the patient's insurance company for approval.			
6. Retain copy of referral for patient medical record.			
7. Give remaining copies to the patient to submit when service is received, or send referral to provider's office ahead of patient.			
8. Instruct patient on how to make appointment, or assist patient to make the appointment.			
9. File referral form in patient medical record.			
10. Complete the procedure within 15 minutes. ◆			

Charting

DATE	

Evaluator Comments:

Score Calculation:

For each procedural step marked U (Unsatisfactory) deduct 6 points
For each procedural step (◆) marked U (Unsatisfactory) deduct 20 points

Score calculation	100 points			
	− points missed	1st	2nd	3rd
	Total score			

Satisfactory score: 85 or above

SELF-EVALUATION

Chapter 35

Written Follow-up

CHAPTER FOCUS

It is important for a medical assistant to be able to prepare letters and envelopes and to transcribe reports in order to assist the medical office with follow-up after patient visits. Written follow-up may be mailed or transmitted electronically (via fax or e-mail), and the medical assistant must also know how to provide these services. The medical assistant must remember to obtain the patient's permission before releasing any information.

TERMINOLOGY REVIEW

Vocabulary Matching: Match each term with its definition.

__ 1. e-mail

__ 2. modified block letter style

__ 3. collate

__ 4. postage meter

__ 5. left-justified

__ 6. simplified letter style

__ 7. transcription

__ 8. block letter style

A. Business letter style in which all lines are left-justified

B. To correct all errors in a document, if possible before printing it

C. To arrange pages of a document in the proper sequence

D. A system for transmitting written messages from computer to computer

E. All lines starting at the left margin

F. A machine that sends and receives information over the phone lines and prints the information on paper

G. A business letter style in which body text is left-justified, but the date line, complementary close, and signature line are centered or right-justified

H. A business-letter style in which the first line on each paragraph of the body text is indented and the rest of the lines are left-justified

___ 9. right-justified — I. All lines ending at the right margin

___ 10. semi-block letter style — J. A business letter that resembles a memorandum, with a subject line in capitals and no complementary close

___ 11. template — K. A machine that weighs and automatically stamps outgoing mail with the proper amount of postage

___ 12. fax (facsimile) — L. An incomplete document that serves as a pattern

___ 13. proofread — M. Transferring information dictated by the doctor into written documents using a typewriter or computer

Definitions: Define each of the following classifications of mail and special services.

1. Express mail ______________________________
2. Priority mail ______________________________
3. First-class mail ______________________________
4. Bound printed matter ______________________________
5. Media mail ______________________________
6. Fourth-class mail (parcel post) ______________________________
7. Return receipt ______________________________
8. Registered mail ______________________________
9. Certified mail ______________________________
10. Insured mail ______________________________

CONTENT REVIEW QUESTIONS

1. When is it necessary for a patient to sign a form allowing the physician to request medical records from another physician or a hospital?

____

____

2. When must the patient sign a form allowing information regarding treatment to be sent to an attorney or liability insurance company?

____

____

3. Where is the return address placed on a number 10 envelope?

____

____

The recipient's address?

____

4. Why does the postal service recommend that all instructions such as "Personal" be placed on the left side below the inside address and above the recipient's address?

____

____

5. Where should mailing instructions be placed on the envelope (e.g., "Via Air Mail")?

____

____

6. What types of reports do doctors dictate in the medical office?

____

____

____

____

7. How is the history and physical examination formatted?

____

____

____

____

8. Describe the medical assistant's role in proofreading a transcribed report.

____

____

____

____

9. Identify three ways to send written follow-up reports.

a. ____

b. ____

c. ____

10. How does the medical assistant prepare mail using a postage meter?

____

____

____

____

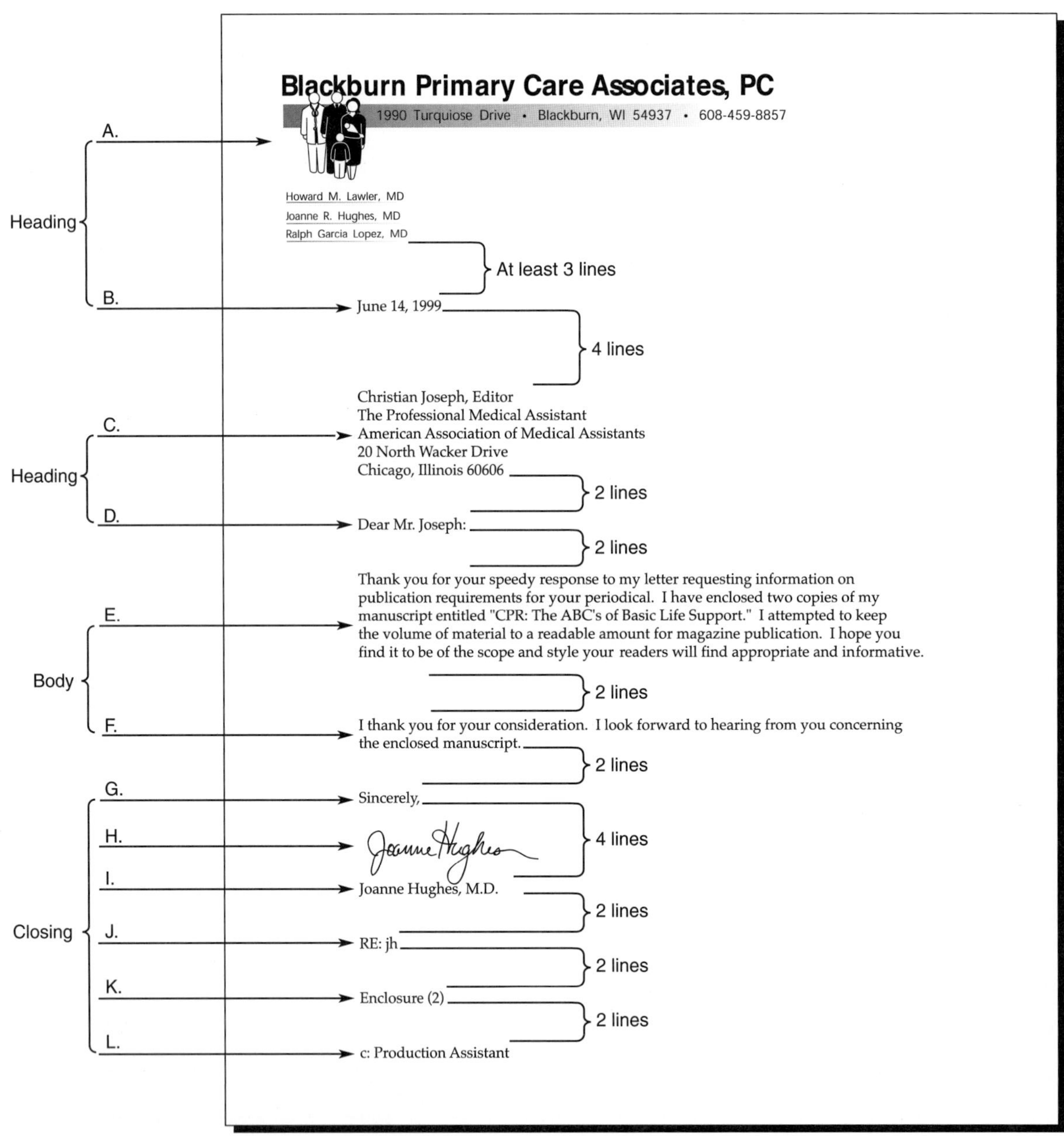
Blackburn Primary Care Associates, PC
1990 Turquiose Drive • Blackburn, WI 54937 • 608-459-8857
Howard M. Lawler, MD
Joanne R. Hughes, MD
Ralph Garcia Lopez, MD
June 14, 1999
Christian Joseph, Editor
The Professional Medical Assistant
American Association of Medical Assistants
20 North Wacker Drive
Chicago, Illinois 60606
Dear Mr. Joseph:
Thank you for your speedy response to my letter requesting information on publication requirements for your periodical. I have enclosed two copies of my manuscript entitled "CPR: The ABC's of Basic Life Support." I attempted to keep the volume of material to a readable amount for magazine publication. I hope you find it to be of the scope and style your readers will find appropriate and informative.
I thank you for your consideration. I look forward to hearing from you concerning the enclosed manuscript.
Sincerely,
Joanne Hughes
Joanne Hughes, M.D.
RE: jh
Enclosure (2)
c: Production Assistant
Heading
A.
B.
At least 3 lines
4 lines
Heading
C.
D.
2 lines
2 lines
Body
E.
F.
2 lines
2 lines
Closing
G.
H.
I.
J.
K.
L.
4 lines
2 lines
2 lines
2 lines

11. Identify each of the parts of a business letter shown on the previous page.

a. ______________________

b. ______________________

c. ______________________

d. ______________________

e. ______________________

f. ______________________

g. ______________________

h. ______________________

i. ______________________

j. ______________________

k. ______________________

l. ______________________

12. Describe how a fax (facsimile) is sent.

____

____

____

____

13. Why should information that could be compromising to a patient never be sent by fax?

____

____

____

____

14. What mail should the medical assistant open?

____

____

____

____

15. If the medical assistant opens mail for a physician, how should each piece of mail be treated?

____

____

____

____

16. What special features are often found on copy machines to facilitate making copies of lengthy documents?

CRITICAL THINKING QUESTIONS

1. Discuss the advantages and disadvantages of the following systems of preparing progress notes for the medical record: handwritten notes, dictated and transcribed notes, or use of a computer system in which progress note information is dictated or keyed directly into a computerized record.

2. Some physicians take patient questions using e-mail and answer questions at a specified time during the day. What are the advantages and disadvantages of this method for the physician? For the patient?

PRACTICAL APPLICATIONS

1. Using written guidelines obtained from the post office or from the website of the United States Postal Service (www.usps.gov), prepare an up-to-date chart of postage for postcards and first class mail per unit of weight.

2. Prepare, key, and print a letter from Dr. Joann Hughes at Blackburn Primary Care Associates, PC, 1990 Turquoise Drive, Blackburn, WI 54937 to Robert Ricigliano, 224 Lakeview Drive, Blackburn, WI 54937, informing him that the results of his recent blood work indicate that his blood sugar may be elevated and that he should make an appointment to see Dr. Hughes to discuss this finding. Use full block format for the letter. Include a reference line using Dr. Hughes' and your own initials. Prepare a mailing envelope for the letter.

3. Prepare, key, and print a letter requesting information about color copiers to ABC Business Machines, 128 Curve Street, Blackburn, WI 54937. Use your own name and the address of Blackburn Primary Care Associates, PC, as given in Question 2. You are interested in the size of available machines, the number of copies per minute, whether they can enlarge and reduce copy size, and if they can feed multiple originals. Use modified block format for the letter. Indicate that you have sent a copy to Sharon Dillard, the office manager of the practice. Prepare a mailing envelope for the letter.

4. Prepare a history and physical report using the following information and the figure showing the Format for History and Physical Examination Report. Proofread the report carefully before handing it in. Use today's date for this report about Natalie Simpson, ID number 01012, a patient of Dr. Ralph Garcia Lopez. Natalie Simpson comes to the office today with complaints of difficulty swallowing for the past three weeks. She states that it feels like her throat is closed and she can't get food to go down. Her past history is noncontributory. Her mother is alive and well. Her father has ASHD with a quadruple bypass three years ago. Siblings are alive and well. She is a secretary who smokes one package of cigarettes per day, and does not drink alcohol or use drugs. The review of systems is noncontributory.

   Physical examination reveals a thin woman of lower than normal weight. Normocephalic, pupils equal, round, and react to light. No masses palpated in the neck. Mouth, nose, and throat clear to inspection. Lungs clear. Heart rate normal sinus rhythm. Abdomen soft. Genital examination deferred. Reflexes normal. Gait normal.

   Impression: Dysphagia, R/O space occupying lesion
   Plan: CBC and SMA-12, barium swallow and CT scan of the head, trial of antispasmodic medication and recheck in 2 weeks.

5. Proofread the following note. Circle all corrections including words that are incorrectly spelled, missing words, and errors of punctuation and capitalization. Place the correct form in the space to the right of the line with the error.

This 72 yearold pateint was seen in	______72-year-old____patient
the office today with complaints of ecsessive	a. ________________
soreness and stifness in the right hip for the	b. ________________
past three months	c. ________________
SUBJECTIVE: the patint states that she no longer	d. ________________
is ability to walk up staires even three or 4.	e. ________________
OBJECTIVE: Vital signs normal, a exray done	f. ________________
this morning reveels a naraowed joint space	g. ________________
but the bone margins are normal.	h. ________________
ASSESSMENT: Joint pain and stifness probably	i. ________________
due to ostioarthritis but r/o reumatoid arthrtis.	j. ________________
PLAN: cbc and reumatoid factor, start pateint	k. ________________
on NSAIDs. RTO in 2 weeks.	l. ________________

Format for History and Physical Examination Report

Patient Name:	**Date:**
Patient ID Number:	**Physician:**

MEDICAL HISTORY:

CHIEF COMPLAINT:	Description of chief complaint
PRESENT ILLNESS:	Description of history of chief complaint
PAST HISTORY:	Past medical history
FAMILY HISTORY:	Health status of immediate family
SOCIAL HISTORY:	Social, occupational and personal factors
REVIEW OF SYSTEMS:	Response to systematic questions
EENT:	about eyes, ears, nose, throat
GI:	about gastrointestinal tract
GU:	about genitourinary tract
CR:	about cardiac and respiratory systems

PHYSICAL EXAMINATION:

GENERAL:	General appearance, weight
HEENT:	Findings from examination of the head, eyes, nose, and throat
LUNGS:	Findings from examination of the lungs
HEART:	Findings from examination of the heart
ABDOMEN:	Findings from examination of the abdomen
GENITALIA:	Findings from examination of the genitalia
EXTREMITIES:	Findings from examination of the extremities

IMPRESSION:

1. First problem or possible diagnosis
2. Second problem or possible diagnosis
3. Each additional problem or possible diagnosis follows

PLAN:

1. First planned test or treatment
2. Each additional planned test or treatment follows
3. The final entry may give a date for follow-up

6. Prepare a memorandum using today's date from Sharon Dillard, Office Manager, to all employees about a new policy regarding personal telephone calls. Use the Memorandum Form found on the following page. The memorandum reminds staff that personal telephone calls should not be made or accepted using office telephones except in the case of emergencies. There is a pay telephone in the lobby of the building for staff to use during scheduled breaks.

7. Identify the mail classification you would use and any special services needed to send the following items by mail:

   a. The patient's monthly bill

   b. A package weighing 2 pounds containing an incorrect order of medical supplies that must be returned to the supplier

   c. A copy of a medical report for a patient who became severely ill on vacation and will be following up this week with her own doctor 500 miles away

   d. A letter informing a patient that he or she should seek a new physician within 3 weeks due to failure to keep appointments

   e. A package that weighs 15 ounces, containing a present for the doctor's daughter who is at college in another state

   f. A letter containing a check to pay for medical supplies

MEMORANDUM

Date:

To:

From:

Subject:

PROCEDURE PERFORMANCE CHECKLISTS

Procedure 35-1: Composing a Business Letter

Performance Objective

Task: Compose and key a business letter

Conditions: Letterhead stationary, blank stationery, typewriter or computer and printer

Standards: Complete the procedure in 20 minutes, and achieve a satisfactory score on the procedure performance checklist

Scoring Key: (**S**)*atisfactory,* (**U**)*nsatisfactory,* (**NA**) *Not Applicable*
◆ *Denotes a critical element for a satisfactory score on the procedure*

Procedure Steps	1st trial	2nd trial	3rd trial
1. Assemble materials.			
2. Determine recipient's address.			
3. Decide on letter format.			
4. Formulate content of letter.			
5. Write rough draft.			
6. Set appropriate margins and tabs.			
7. Insert date on third line below letterhead.			
8. Place inside address four to 10 lines below date.			
9. Place salutation two lines below inside address.			
10. Begin body of letter two lines below salutation.			
11. Summarize contents in final paragraph.			
12. Place complimentary close two lines below final paragraph.			
13. Place name of person who is sending letter four lines below complimentary close, allowing space for signature.			
14. If necessary, add reference line or lines.			
15. If letter is longer than one page, make sure second page and all later pages are printed on non-letterhead stationery.			
16. Spell-check letter if using computer.			
17. Proofread letter after it is printed out or typed.			

Procedure Steps	1st trial	2nd trial	3rd trial
18. Have individual sending letter sign it.			
19. Make a copy of the signed letter.			
20. The letter is formatted correctly and has no spelling or typographical errors. ◆			
21. Complete the procedure within 20 minutes. ◆			

Evaluator Comments:

Score Calculation:

For each procedural step marked U (Unsatisfactory) deduct 6 points
For each procedural step (◆) marked U (Unsatisfactory) deduct 20 points

Score calculation 100 points

– points missed

	1st	2nd	3rd
Total score			

Satisfactory score: 85 or above

Procedure 35-2: Addressing an Envelope

Performance Objective

Task: Address an envelope for mailing

Conditions: Envelope, typewriter, or computer and printer

Standards: Complete the procedure in 10 minutes, and achieve a satisfactory score on the procedure performance checklist

Scoring Key: (**S**)*atisfactory,* (**U**)*nsatisfactory,* (**NA**) *Not Applicable*
◆ *Denotes a critical element for a satisfactory score on the procedure*

Procedure Steps	1st trial	2nd trial	3rd trial
1. Determine exact address to be used.			
2. Select an envelope of appropriate size.			
3. Key the address in capital letters without punctuation near the center of the envelope using a typewriter or computer or key the address on a mailing label.			
4. If using an envelope without letterhead, key the return address in the upper left-hand corner using the same guidelines or key the return address on a mailing label.			
5. Add any special notations, if necessary, below the return address and above the address.			
6. Add any mailing instructions, if necessary, below the return address and above the address.			
7. Place folded letter or other item(s) to be mailed in envelope.			
8. Seal envelope.			
9. Weigh if necessary.			
10. Place necessary postage on the envelope.			
11. The envelope is formatted correctly and there are no spelling or typographical errors. ◆			
12. Complete the procedure within 10 minutes. ◆			

Evaluator Comments:

Score Calculation:

For each procedural step marked U (Unsatisfactory) deduct 6 points
For each procedural step (◆) marked U (Unsatisfactory) deduct 20 points

Score calculation 100 points

− points missed

Total score

1st	2nd	3rd

Satisfactory score: 85 or above

Procedure 35-3: Transcribing a Dictated Letter or Report

Performance Objective

Task: Transcribe dictation

Conditions: Letterhead stationery, blank stationery, or printer paper; transcription machine, headphones, tape containing dictation, computer and printer or typewriter

Standards: Complete the procedure in 20 minutes, and achieve a satisfactory score on the procedure performance checklist

Scoring Key: (**S**)*atisfactory,* (**U**)*nsatisfactory,* (**NA**) *Not Applicable*
◆ *Denotes a critical element for a satisfactory score on the procedure*

Procedure Steps	1st trial	2nd trial	3rd trial
1. Assemble materials.			
2. Decide on format for letter or report.			
3. While listening to dictation, key the material on the typewriter or computer keyboard.			
4. For a letter, be sure to include a reference line using initials of the person who dictated in capital letters, followed by your initials in lowercase letters.			
5. Spell-check if using computer.			
6. Proofread carefully and print if using a computer.			
7. Have letter signed or report initialed.			
8. If letter, make copy of signed letter.			
9. The letter or report is formatted correctly and contains no more than two typographical or spelling errors. ◆			
10. Complete the procedure within 20 minutes. ◆			

Evaluator Comments:

Score Calculation:

For each procedural step marked U (Unsatisfactory) deduct 6 points
For each procedural step (◆) marked U (Unsatisfactory) deduct 20 points

Score calculation 100 points

− points missed

Total score

1st	2nd	3rd

Satisfactory score: 85 or above

Procedure 35-4: Preparing Outgoing Mail

Performance Objective

Task: Prepare outgoing mail

Conditions: Letters, other items to be mailed, postage scale stamps or postage meter

Standards: Complete the procedure in 20 minutes, and achieve a satisfactory score on the procedure performance checklist

Scoring Key: (**S**)*atisfactory,* (**U**)*nsatisfactory,* (**NA**) *Not Applicable*
◆ *Denotes a critical element for a satisfactory score on the procedure*

Procedure Steps	1st trial	2nd trial	3rd trial
1. Assemble all letters and other items to be mailed.			
2. Be sure each item has been inserted in properly addressed envelope.			
3. Make sure every envelope has been sealed.			
4. Sort envelopes according to size.			
5. Make sure every envelope has a return address.			
6. Place appropriate postage on each envelope, using stamps or a postage meter. Weigh letters if necessary.			
7. Set aside any letters that must be taken to the post office for special treatment (i.e., priority mail over 1 lb., letters to be sent return receipt, certified mail, or registered mail)			
8. Complete the procedure within 20 minutes. ◆			

Evaluator Comments:

Score Calculation:

For each procedural step marked U (Unsatisfactory) deduct 6 points
For each procedural step (◆) marked U (Unsatisfactory) deduct 20 points

Score calculation 100 points

– points missed

	1st	2nd	3rd
Total score			

Satisfactory score: 85 or above

Notes

Procedure 35-5: Sending a Fax

Performance Objective

Task: Send a fax

Conditions: Fax machine, cover sheet, document to be faxed

Standards: Complete the procedure in 30 minutes, and achieve a satisfactory score on the procedure performance checklist

Scoring Key: (**S**)*atisfactory,* (**U**)*nsatisfactory,* (**NA**) *Not Applicable*
◆ *Denotes a critical element for a satisfactory score on the procedure*

Procedure Steps	1st trial	2nd trial	3rd trial
1. Prepare the cover sheet with name and fax number of recipient, and number of pages in the fax (including the cover sheet).			
2. Organize all pages to be faxed, with cover sheet first.			
3. Place pages in fax machine, as instructed in machine's user manual.			
4. Enter the fax number, including 1 and area code for long distance, and/or any number to get outside the office's internal system to an outside line (i.e., "9").			
5. Verify fax number as it appears on display screen.			
6. Press correct button to send fax.			
7. Check to make sure fax has been sent.			
8. If error report is printed, resend the fax.			
9. If machine prints confirmation message, place on top of the fax before filing.			
10. File the original document appropriately.			
11. Complete the procedure within 30 minutes. ◆			

Evaluator Comments:

Score Calculation:

For each procedural step marked U (Unsatisfactory) deduct 6 points
For each procedural step (◆) marked U (Unsatisfactory) deduct 20 points

Score calculation 100 points

− ___ points missed

Total score

1st	2nd	3rd

Satisfactory score: 85 or above

Procedure 35-6: Preparing Copies of Multiple-Page Documents

Performance Objective

Task: Prepare copies of a document with multiple pages

Conditions: Photocopy machine, paper, document to be copied, stapler, staples, staple remover

Standards: Complete the procedure in 30 minutes, and achieve a satisfactory score on the procedure performance checklist

Scoring Key: (**S**)*atisfactory,* (**U**)*nsatisfactory,* (**NA**) *Not Applicable*
◆ *Denotes a critical element for a satisfactory score on the procedure*

Procedure Steps	1st trial	2nd trial	3rd trial
1. Assemble all pages of document(s) to be copied.			
2. If all or part of document(s) to be copied are stapled, remove staples.			
3. If the material to be copied includes all or part of a patient's medical record, verify that there is a signed release of information waiver.			
4. Set the size, number of copies, and proper switch for machine to collate and staple (if the machine does so).			
5. Press start.			
6. After copies have been made, if they are not collated, do so.			
7. If the machine does not staple, staple if necessary.			
8. If the patient will be charged for copying, verify number of pages.			
9. Submit number of pages the patient will be charged for to the person responsible for billing.			
10. Complete the procedure within 30 minutes. ◆			

Evaluator Comments:

Score Calculation:

For each procedural step marked U (Unsatisfactory) deduct 6 points
For each procedural step (◆) marked U (Unsatisfactory) deduct 20 points

Score calculation	100 points			
	− ____ points missed	1st	2nd	3rd
	Total score			

Satisfactory score: 85 or above

SELF-EVALUATION

UNIT 8 Financial Management and Health Insurance

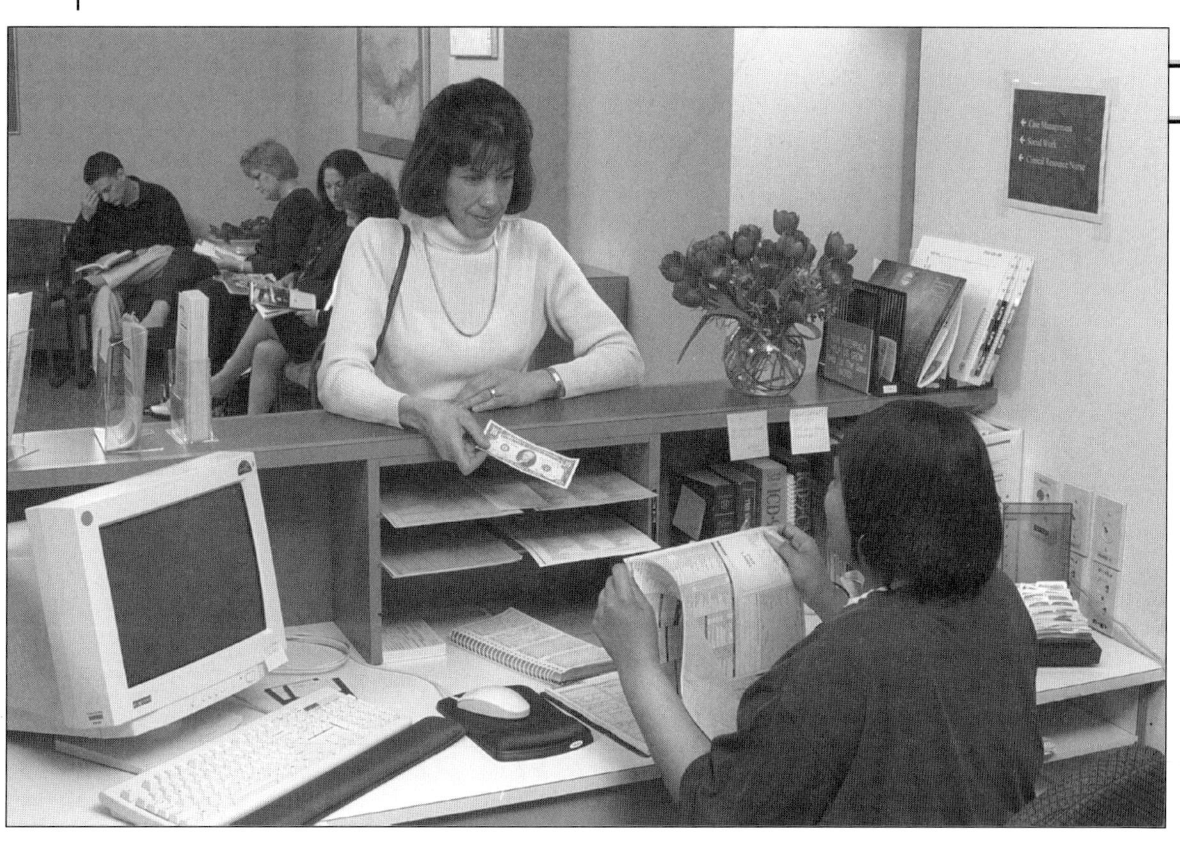

Samatha Hill

Chapter 36

Managing Practice Finances

CHAPTER FOCUS

In this chapter you learned how to manage the financial aspects of a medical practice. Depending on the size of the practice, medical assistants may perform only some of these procedures, but the medical assistant must have a clear understanding of office finances in order to function effectively. In this chapter, you learned how to prepare charge slips (encounter forms), post charges and payments, fill out a day sheet, balance a day sheet, prepare a bank deposit, prepare a check, and reconcile a bank statement.

TERMINOLOGY REVIEW

Vocabulary Matching: Match each term with its definition.

___ 1. credit

___ 2. disbursement

___ 3. fee schedule

A 4. accounts payable

___ 5. reconcile (an account)

___ 6. adjustment

___ 7. restrictive endorsement

___ 8. charge

___ 9. accounts receivable

___ 10. debit

___ 11. payee

___ 12. ABA number

A. The total amount of money owed to the practice for services performed

B. Person or company to whom a check is written

C. An alteration in the amount owed by the patient after the charge has been entered

D. The unique number assigned to an individual bank

E. An amount added to an account (e.g., for payment received)

F. Money paid out for bills owed

G. A list of charges for the various procedures a doctor performs

H. To make sure that an account balances

I. An endorsement on a check that limits the bank's powers

J. The set fee the doctor seeks for performing a service

K. An amount subtracted from an account (e.g., for money disbursed)

L. Money owed by the practice to creditors

Definitions: Insert the correct word to complete the sentence.

1. A means of keeping track of charges for services and payments made at the time of the patient visit is called a ______________________.
2. A written record of each transaction and the practice's total income for a single day is called the ______________________.
3. A card or sheet of paper on which are recorded charges to a patient for services and payment by the patient is called a ______________________ ______________________.
4. The form on which the services provided to the patient, as well as the proper diagnostic and procedure codes, is reported is called a/an ______________________ or ______________________.

CONTENT REVIEW QUESTIONS

1. If patient charges are recorded manually using a pegboard system, in what three places are these charges usually recorded?

   a. ______________________

   b. ______________________

   c. ______________________

2. If patient charges are recorded using a computer billing program, where must the data about the charge be entered? Why is it sufficient to enter the data once?

   ____

3. How is a patient charge posted to a patient account using the pegboard system?

   ____

4. Why is a more complex type of charge slip (called an encounter form or superbill) usually used in a medical office?

   ____

5. If the office typically charges $30.00 to perform an EKG, is this the amount paid by all patients? Why or why not?

   ____

6. How does the medical assistant know what to charge a patient for a specific procedure?

____

____

____

7. Identify four demographic and four financial pieces of information found on a patient's ledger card (or in a computer ledger account).

a. ______________________ e. ______________________

b. ______________________ f. ______________________

c. ______________________ g. ______________________

d. ______________________ h. ______________________

8. Differentiate between the cash and the accrual methods of accounting.

____

____

____

9. When an insurance company pays an amount that is lower than the usual charge, how is the patient's balance due returned to zero?

____

____

____

10. Describe the services and function of a checking account.

____

____

____

11. What is the advantage of maintaining a savings account or money market savings account compared to a checking account?

____

____

____

12. Describe what a check is and its advantage over currency.

____

____

____

13. Identify four ways that checks can be generated to pay bills and information recorded about the check.

a. ____

b. ____

c. ______________________________

d. ______________________________

14. What should the medical assistant do if he or she writes a check incorrectly?

____

____

____

15. Who signs the checks to pay bills for a medical practice?

____

____

____

16. What is necessary before a check can be cashed or deposited? How is this handled in a medical office?

____

____

____

17. Identify five reasons why the monthly bank statement may not agree with the medical office's calculation of the bank balance in a checking account.

a. ______________________________

b. ______________________________

c. ______________________________

d. ______________________________

e. ______________________________

18. What financial accounts does a medical office usually have, and what do those accounts include?

____

____

____

19. Why are expenses posted to a particular column when bills are paid?

____

____

____

20. How is a petty cash fund (account) managed?

____

____

____

CRITICAL THINKING QUESTIONS

1. Identify and discuss measures to prevent misuse of funds and/or embezzlement in a medical practice. Why are these necessary?

____

____

____

____

____

2. Working with your classmates, obtain charge slips from at least three family practice medical groups. Compare the type of slips to each other and the form included in the exercises for this chapter. Are they all encounter forms? How is information arranged? What codes are included? Which form do you prefer? Why?

____

____

____

____

____

PRACTICAL APPLICATIONS

1. Prepare encounter forms for the following patients for 10/12/XX. Enter the following information on the forms (found at the end of this section): the name and address of the person responsible for the bill (guarantor), the patient's name, the patient number, the doctor number (found beside the doctor's name on the upper right-hand corner of the form), date of birth, telephone number, name of insurance company, and the certificate number (insurance policy number) of the insured.

June St. Cyr	Patient number: 1010
16 Winston Terrace	Established patient of Dr. Lawler
Blackburn, WI 54937	Name of insured: self
(555) 459-1000	Insurance plan: Standard Health HMO
DOB: 2/23/1962	Policy #000-AD9876
Robert Ricigliano	Patient number: 5010
224 Lakeview Drive	New patient of Dr. Hughes
Blackburn, WI 54937	Name of insured: self
(555) 459-1111	Insurance plan: Standard Health Care Indemnity
DOB: 1/31/1947	Policy #000-4518
Mary Ann St. Cyr	Patient number: 3010
16 Winston Terrace	Established patient of Dr. Lawler
Blackburn, WI 54937	Name of insured: June St. Cyr (see above)
(555) 459-1000	Insurance plan: Standard Health HMO
DOB: 6/4/1982	Policy #000-AD9876

James Winston	Patient number: 1020
25 Magnolia Lane	Established patient of Dr. Lopez
Blackburn, WI 54937	Name of insured: self
(555) 459-1222	Insurance plan: Medicare
DOB: 12/14/1932	Policy #000-70-7000A

Marie Richards	Patient number: 5020
19 Maple Street	New patient of Dr. Lopez
Blackburn, WI 54937	Name of insured: John Richards
(555) 459-1333	Insurance plan: Standard Health HMO
DOB: 11/9/1967	Policy #000-JT4268

2. Create a ledger card for each of the patients listed in Question 1 using the forms found at the end of this section. For the purposes of this exercise, include the patient's name, last name first, in the top left corner, the name and address of the person responsible for the bill in the box marked "statement to," and the previous balance (as noted in Question 3). Place the name of the insured, the insurance plan, and the policy number in the upper right-hand corner.

3. Enter information from previous visits on the ledger cards for these established patients. Usually all charges from one day are placed on the same line of the ledger card using procedure codes. Calculate each patient's balance.

June St. Cyr			
7/22/XX	99212, 90703	Charge $53.00	Payment $10.00
Mary Ann St. Cyr			
7/14/XX	99212, 94010	Charge $98.00	Payment $10.00
James Winston			
9/1/XX	99213, 81002, 93000	Charge $122.00	Payment $50.00

4. Using the fee schedule for Blackburn Medical Associates found following this section, complete the encounter forms by adding the charges for each of the following patients for 10/12/XX. Check the correct box for the procedure (or add a procedure with its code under "Other" if there is no preprinted box). For the established patients, enter the previous balance from the patient's ledger card and total the new balance.

Robert Ricigliano	99205 Comprehensive Office Visit 93000 EKG, 12 lead Payment $15.00 (Check #602; Bank number 48-72)
Marie Richards	99202 Expanded Office visit 93000 EKG, 12 lead 81002 Urinalysis Payment $10.00 (Check #2881; Bank number 52-31)
June St. Cyr	99211 Nurse/minimal visit 35415 Venipuncture Payment: $10.00 (Check #817; Bank number 288-11)
Mary Ann St. Cyr	99212 Focused Office Visit Payment: $10.00 (Check #818; Bank number 288-11)
James Winston	93015 Stress EKG, Treadmill

5. Record the information for the five patients listed in Question 4 on the first five lines of the day sheet that follows this section. In addition, record the following payments received in the mail on both the patient ledger cards and lines six through ten of the day sheet.

   Insurance payment for June St. Cyr
      Payment in full for charges of 7/22/XX, $ 43.00
      (Check #288; Bank number 24-82)
      Enter adjustment so that all charges for 7/22/XX are paid.

   Insurance payment for Mary Ann St. Cyr
      Payment in full for charges of 7/14/XX, $ 79.00
      (Check #289; Bank number 24-82)
      Enter adjustment so that all charges for 7/14/XX are paid.

   Insurance payment for James Winston
      Payment for charges of 9/1/XX, $30.40
      (Check #622; Bank number 862-11)
      Allowable charge $88.00, patient portion $57.60 (includes annual deductible plus 20% of allowable charge); Mr. Winston has already paid the deductible. Enter adjustment so that all charges for 9/1/XX will be paid after Mr. Winston pays $7.60 (patient responsibility as identified by Medicare).

6. Prepare a deposit slip entering each check received in the order listed on the day sheet.

7. Total the day sheet (Columns A through E) and complete the daily arithmetic proof of posting. Be sure the day sheet balances.

8. Write checks to pay the following bills beginning with check number 1837 found at the end of this section. Use 10/12/XX as the date. The balance brought forward is $4482.21. Calculate the balance earned forward after each check is written.

   a. Write a check for $822.00 to Mitchell Associates for rent.

   b. Write a check for $329.62 to ABC Pharmacy for medical supplies.

   c. Write a check for $219.64 to Holt Office Supply for office supplies.

9. Enter the three checks you have written on the disbursement record found at the end of this section. In addition, enter a deposit of $254.00 (made on 10/11/XX) and a deposit of $48.91 (made on 10/10/XX).

10. Reconcile a bank statement using the form at the end of this section based on the following information:
    The new balance identified by the bank is $4,328.92. Two deposits are shown in your register but not on this statement, namely $254.00 and $48.91. There are three outstanding checks for $822.00, $329.62, and $219.64. Identify the amount that should be shown as the balance in your check register.

    ____

11. You need to buy dishwashing soap, a sponge, and napkins for the office kitchen, and the office manager instructs you to take $10.00 from the petty cash fund and purchase these items at the local drug store. When you go to the petty cash box it contains $2.00, receipts, and a slip identifying that $25.00 was added to a previous balance of $1.25 two weeks ago. The office manager writes a check for $25.00, and instructs you to cash it as part of your errand. When you return, she asks you to total the receipts for medical or office supplies and other (miscellaneous) items, enter the totals on the disbursement record you began in Question 8, and move the receipts for the items you are entering to the folder with the disbursement record. Also, you must determine

if the account balances. The following receipts are in the drawer: Postage – $4.75; Tissues and thermometer covers – $4.00; Lunch for physician – $8.00; Coffee and creamer – $7.50. Does the account balance? Should you place the receipt from your purchases today in the petty cash box or add it to the disbursement record? Why?

____

____

____

12. Using the Lytec medical billing program on the CD-ROM, follow the tutorial instructions at the end of this book to perform the activities from the first four questions above on the computer (i.e., prepare encounter forms, enter the new patients, post charges, post payments, post adjustments, and print a completed day sheet).

FEE SCHEDULE

BLACKBURN PRIMARY CARE ASSOCIATES, PC
1990 Turquiose Drive
Blackburn, WI 54937
608-459-8857

Federal Tax ID Number: **00-0000000**

BCBS Group Number: 14982
Medicare Group Number: 14982

OFFICE VISIT, NEW PATIENT

Focused, 99201	$45.00
Expanded, 99202	$55.00
Intermediate, 99203	$60.00
Extended, 99204	$95.00
Comprehensive, 99205	$195.00
Consultation, 99245	$250.00

OFFICE VISIT, ESTABLISHED PATIENT

Minimal, 99211	$40.00
Focused, 99212	$48.00
Intermediate, 99213	$55.00
Extended, 99214	$65.00
Comprehensive, 99215	$195.00

OFFICE PROCEDURES

EKG, 12 lead, 93000	$55.00
Stress EKG, Treadmill, 93015	$295.00
Sigmoidoscopy, Flex; 45330	$145.00
Spirometry, 94010	$50.00
Cerumen Removal, 69210	$40.00
Collection & Handling	
Lab Specimen, 99000	$9.00
Venipuncture, 35415	$9.00
Urinalysis, 81000	$20.00
Urinalysis, 81002 (Dip Only)	$12.00
Influenza Injection, 90724	$20.00
Pneumococcal Injection, 90732	$20.00
Oral Polio, 90712	$15.00
DTaP, 90700	$20.00
Tetanus Toxoid, 90703	$15.00
MMR, 90707	$25.00
HIB, 90737	$20.00
Hepatitis B, newborn to age 11 years, 90744	$60.00
Hepatitis B, 11-19 years, 90745	$60.00
Hepatitis B, 20 years and above 90746	$60.00
Intramuscular Injection, 90788	
Penicillin	$30.00
Cephtriaxone	$25.00
Solu-Medrol	$23.00
Vitamin B-12	$13.00
Subcutaneous Injection, 90782	
Epinephrine	$18.00
Susphrine	$25.00
Insulin, U-100	$15.00

COMMON DIAGNOSTIC CODES

Ischemic Heart Disease	414.9
w/o myocardial infarction	411.89
w/coronary occlusion	411.81
Hypertension, Malignant	401.0
Benign	401.1
Unspecified	401.9
w/congest. heart failure	402.91
Asthma, Bronchial	493.9
w/ COPD	493.2
allergic, w/ S.A.	493.91
allergic, w/o S.A.	493.90
Kyphosis	737.10
w/osteoporosis	733.0
Osteoporosis	733.00
Otitis Media, Acute	382.9
Chronic	382.9

Blackburn Primary Care Associates, PC
1990 Turquoise Drive
Blackburn, WI 54937
(608) 459-8857

Howard M. Lawler, MD 11
Joanne R. Hughes, MD 21
Ralph Garcia Lopez, MD 31
TAX ID NO. 00-00000000

GUARANTOR NAME AND ADDRESS	PATIENT NO.	PATIENT NAME	DOCTOR NO.	DATE

DATE OF BIRTH	TELEPHONE NO.	INSURANCE CODE	INSURANCE DESCRIPTION	CERTIFICATE NO.

OFFICE - NEW				OFFICE - ESTABLISHED				OFFICE - CONSULT				PREVENTIVE CARE - ADULT			
X	CPT	SERVICE	FEE	X	CPT	SERVICE	FEE	X	CPT	SERVICE	FEE	X	CPT	SERVICE	FEE
	99201	Prob Foc/Straight			99211	Nurse/Minimal			99241	Prob/Foc/Straight			99385	18-39 Initial	
	99202	Exp Prob/Straight			99212	Prob Foc/Straight			99242	Exp Prob/Straight			99386	40-64 Initial	
	99203	Detailed/Low			99213	Exp Prob/Low			99243	Detailed/Low			99387	65+ Initial	
	99204	Compre/Moderate			99214	Detailed/Moderate			99244	Compre/Moderate			99395	18-39 Periodic	
	99205	Compre/High			99215	Compre/High			99245	Compre/High			99396	40-64 Periodic	
													99397	65+ Periodic	
GASTROENEROLOGY				**CARDIOLOGY & HEARING**				**INJECTIONS & IMMUNIZATION**				**REPAIR & DERMATOLOGY**			
X	CPT	SERVICE	FEE	X	CPT	SERVICE	FEE	X	CPT	SERVICE	FEE	X	CPT	SERVICE	FEE
	45300	Sigmoidoscopy Rig			93000	EKG (Global)			86585	TB Skin Test			17110	Warts: #	
	45305	Sigmoid Rig w/bx			93015	Stress Test (Global)			90716	Varicella Vaccine				Tags: #	
	45330	Sigmoidoscopy Flex			93224	Holter (Global)			90724	Flu Vaccine				Lesion Excis	
	45331	Sigmoid Flex w/bx			93225	Holter Hook Up			90732	Pneumovax				Lesion Destruct	
	45378	Colonoscopy Diag			93227	Holter Interpretation			90718	TD Immunization			SIZE CM:	SITE:	
	45380	Colonoscopy w/bx			94010	Pulm Function Test							MALIG:	PREMAL/BEN:	
	46600	Anoscopy			92551	Audiometry Screen			90782	Injection IM*				(Check One Above)	
									90788	Injection IM Antibiot*				Simple Closure	
OTHER				**SUPPLIES/DRUGS***						Injection joint*				Intermed Closure	
				DRUG NAME:				SM	MED	MAJOR			SIZE CM:	SITE:	
				UNIT/MEASURE:						(circle one)					
				QUANTITY				FOR ALL INJECTIONS, SUPPLY DRUG					10060	I&D Abscess	
								INFORMATION					10080	I&D Cyst	

DIAGNOSTIC CODES: ICD-9-CM

☐ 789.0 Abdominal Pain
☐ 795.0 Abnormal Pap Smear
☐ 706.1 Acne Vulgaris
☐ 477.0 Allergic Rhinitis
☐ 285.9 Anemia, NOS
☐ 281.0 Pernicious
☐ 411.1 Angina, Unstable
☐ 427.9 Arythmia, NOS
☐ 440.9 Arteriosclerosis
☐ 714.0 Arthritis, Rheumatoid
☐ 414.0 ASHD
☐ 493.90 Asthma, Bronchial W/O Status Ast.
☐ 493.91 Asthma, Bronchial W/Status Ast.
☐ 466.1 Bronchiolitis, Acute
☐ 466.0 Bronchitis, Acute
☐ 727.3 Bursitis
☐ 786.50 Chest Pain
☐ 574.20 Cholelithiasis
☐ 372.30 Conjunctivitis, Unspecified
☐ 564.0 Constipation
☐ 496 COPD
☐ 692.9 Dermatitis, Allergic
☐ 250.01 Diabetes Mellitus, ID
☐ 250.00 Diabetes Mellitus, NID
☐ 558.9 Diarrhea
☐ 562.11 Diverticulitis
☐ 562.10 Diverticulosis

☐ 782.3 Edema
☐ 492.8 Emphysema
☐ V16.0 Family History Of Diabetes
☐ 780.6 Fever of Undetermined Origin
☐ 578.9 G.I. Bleeding, Unspecified
☐ 727.41 Ganglion of Joint
☐ 535.0 Gastritis, Acute
☐ V72.3 Arythmia, NOS
☐ 748.0 Headache
☐ 550.90 Hernia, Inguinal, NOS
☐ 054.9 Herpes Simplex
☐ 053.9 Herpes Zoster
☐ 708.9 Hives/Urticaria
☐ 401.1 Hypertension, Benign
☐ 401.0 Hypertension, Malignant
☐ 402.90 Hypertension, W/O CHF
☐ 244.9 Hypothyroidism, Primary
☐ 380.4 Impacted Cerumen
☐ 487.1 Influenza
☐ 564.1 Irritable Bowel Syndrome
☐ 464.0 Laryngitis, Acute
☐ 454.9 Leg Varicose Veins
☐ 424.0 Mitral Valve Prolapse
☐ 412 Myocardial Infarction, Old
☐ 715.90 Osteoarthritis, Unspec. Site
☐ 620.2 Ovarian Cyst

☐ 614.9 Pelvic Inflammatory Disease
☐ 685.1 Pilonidal Cyst
☐ 462 Pharyngitis, Acute
☐ 627.1 Postmenopausal Bleeding
☐ 625.4 Premenstrual Tension
☐ 782.1 Rash
☐ 569.3 Rectal Bleeding
☐ 398.90 Rheumatic Heart Disease, NOS
☐ 431.9 Sinusitis, Acute, NOS
☐ 782.1 Skin Eruption, Rash
☐ 845.00 Sprain, Ankle
☐ 848.9 Sprain, Muscle, Unspec. Site
☐ 785.6 Swollen Glands
☐ 246.9 Thyroid Disease, Unspecified
☐ 463 Tonsillitis, Acute

☐ 474.0 Tonsillitis, Chronic
☐ 465.9 Upper Respiratory Infection, Acute
☐ 599.0 Urinary Tract Infection
☐ V03.9 Vaccination/Bacterial Dis.
☐ V06.8 Vaccination/Combination
☐ V04.8 Vaccination, Influenza
☐ 616.10 Vaginitis, Vulvitis, NOS
☐ 780.4 Vertigo
☐ 787.0 Vomiting, Nausea
☐ ____ ____________
☐ ____ ____________
☐ ____ ____________
☐ ____ ____________

RETURN APPOINTMENT

_______ Days
_______ Weeks
_______ Months

Authorization Number:

▶ ____________________

BALANCE DUE

DATE OF SERVICE	CPT CODE	DIAGNOSIS CODE(S)	CHARGE

Place of Service:
( ) Office
( ) Emergency Room
( ) Inpatient Hospital
( ) Outpatient Hospital
( ) Nursing Home

TOTAL CHARGE	$
AMOUNT PAID	$
PREVIOUS BAL	$
BALANCE DUE	$

Check #: ____________

(Circle Method of Payment)
CASH CHECK MC VISA

Physician's Signature

▶ ____________________________

Blackburn Primary Care Associates, PC
1990 Turquoise Drive
Blackburn, WI 54937
(608) 459-8857

Howard M. Lawler, MD	11
Joanne R. Hughes, MD	21
Ralph Garcia Lopez, MD	31
TAX ID NO. 00-00000000	

GUARANTOR NAME AND ADDRESS	PATIENT NO.	PATIENT NAME	DOCTOR NO.	DATE

DATE OF BIRTH	TELEPHONE NO.	INSURANCE CODE	INSURANCE DESCRIPTION	INSURANCE CERTIFICATE NO.

OFFICE - NEW

X	CPT	SERVICE	FEE
	99201	Prob Foc/Straight	
	99202	Exp Prob/Straight	
	99203	Detailed/Low	
	99204	Compre/Moderate	
	99205	Compre/High	

OFFICE - ESTABLISHED

X	CPT	SERVICE	FEE
	99211	Nurse/Minimal	
	99212	Prob Foc/Straight	
	99213	Exp Prob/Low	
	99214	Detailed/Moderate	
	99215	Compre/High	

OFFICE - CONSULT

X	CPT	SERVICE	FEE
	99241	Prob/Foc/Straight	
	99242	Exp Prob/Straight	
	99243	Detailed/Low	
	99244	Compre/Moderate	
	99245	Compre/High	

PREVENTIVE CARE - ADULT

X	CPT	SERVICE	FEE
	99385	18-39 Initial	
	99386	40-64 Initial	
	99387	65+ Initial	
	99395	18-39 Periodic	
	99396	40-64 Periodic	
	99397	65+ Periodic	

GASTROENEROLOGY

X	CPT	SERVICE	FEE
	45300	Sigmoidoscopy Rig	
	45305	Sigmoid Rig w/bx	
	45330	Sigmoidoscopy Flex	
	45331	Sigmoid Flex w/bx	
	45378	Colonoscopy Diag	
	45380	Colonoscopy w/bx	
	46600	Anoscopy	

CARDIOLOGY & HEARING

X	CPT	SERVICE	FEE
	93000	EKG (Global)	
	93015	Stress Test (Global)	
	93224	Holter (Global)	
	93225	Holter Hook Up	
	93227	Holter Interpretation	
	94010	Pulm Function Test	
	92551	Audiometry Screen	

INJECTIONS & IMMUNIZATION

X	CPT	SERVICE	FEE
	86585	TB Skin Test	
	90716	Varicella Vaccine	
	90724	Flu Vaccine	
	90732	Pneumovax	
	90718	TD Immunization	
	90782	Injection IM*	
	90788	Injection IM Antibiot*	
		Injection joint*	
	SM	MED MAJOR	
		(circle one)	

FOR ALL INJECTIONS, SUPPLY DRUG INFORMATION

REPAIR & DERMATOLOGY

X	CPT	SERVICE	FEE
	17110	Warts: #	
		Tags: #	
		Lesion Excis	
		Lesion Destruct	
	SIZE CM:	SITE:	
	MALIG:	PREMAL/BEN:	
		(Check One Above)	
		Simple Closure	
		Intermed Closure	
	SIZE CM:	SITE:	
	10060	I&D Abscess	
	10080	I&D Cyst	

OTHER

SUPPLIES/DRUGS*

DRUG NAME:	
UNIT/MEASURE:	
QUANTITY	

DIAGNOSTIC CODES: ICD-9-CM

- ☐ 789.0 Abdominal Pain
- ☐ 795.0 Abnormal Pap Smear
- ☐ 706.1 Acne Vulgaris
- ☐ 477.0 Allergic Rhinitis
- ☐ 285.9 Anemia, NOS
- ☐ 281.0 Pernicious
- ☐ 411.1 Angina, Unstable
- ☐ 427.9 Arythmia, NOS
- ☐ 440.9 Arteriosclerosis
- ☐ 714.0 Arthritis, Rheumatoid
- ☐ 414.0 ASHD
- ☐ 493.90 Asthma, Bronchial W/O Status Ast.
- ☐ 493.91 Asthma, Bronchial W/Status Ast.
- ☐ 466.1 Bronchiolitis, Acute
- ☐ 466.0 Bronchitis, Acute
- ☐ 727.3 Bursitis
- ☐ 786.50 Chest Pain
- ☐ 574.20 Cholelithiasis
- ☐ 372.30 Conjunctivitis, Unspecified
- ☐ 564.0 Constipation
- ☐ 496 COPD
- ☐ 692.9 Dermatitis, Allergic
- ☐ 250.01 Diabetes Mellitus, ID
- ☐ 250.00 Diabetes Mellitus, NID
- ☐ 558.9 Diarrhea
- ☐ 562.11 Diverticulitis
- ☐ 562.10 Diverticulosis
- ☐ 782.3 Edema
- ☐ 492.8 Emphysema
- ☐ V16.0 Family History Of Diabetes
- ☐ 780.6 Fever of Undetermined Origin
- ☐ 578.9 G.I. Bleeding, Unspecified
- ☐ 727.41 Ganglion of Joint
- ☐ 535.0 Gastritis, Acute
- ☐ V72.3 Arythmia, NOS
- ☐ 748.0 Headache
- ☐ 550.90 Hernia, Inguinal, NOS
- ☐ 054.9 Herpes Simplex
- ☐ 053.9 Herpes Zoster
- ☐ 708.9 Hives/Urticaria
- ☐ 401.1 Hypertension, Benign
- ☐ 401.0 Hypertension, Malignant
- ☐ 402.90 Hypertension, W/O CHF
- ☐ 244.9 Hypothyroidism, Primary
- ☐ 380.4 Impacted Cerumen
- ☐ 487.1 Influenza
- ☐ 564.1 Irritable Bowel Syndrome
- ☐ 464.0 Laryngitis, Acute
- ☐ 454.9 Leg Varicose Veins
- ☐ 424.0 Mitral Valve Prolapse
- ☐ 412 Myocardial Infarction, Old
- ☐ 715.90 Osteoarthritis, Unspec. Site
- ☐ 620.2 Ovarian Cyst
- ☐ 614.9 Pelvic Inflammatory Disease
- ☐ 685.1 Pilonidal Cyst
- ☐ 462 Pharyngitis, Acute
- ☐ 627.1 Postmenopausal Bleeding
- ☐ 625.4 Premenstrual Tension
- ☐ 782.1 Rash
- ☐ 569.3 Rectal Bleeding
- ☐ 398.90 Rheumatic Heart Disease, NOS
- ☐ 431.9 Sinusitis, Acute, NOS
- ☐ 782.1 Skin Eruption, Rash
- ☐ 845.00 Sprain, Ankle
- ☐ 848.9 Sprain, Muscle, Unspec. Site
- ☐ 785.6 Swollen Glands
- ☐ 246.9 Thyroid Disease, Unspecified
- ☐ 463 Tonsillitis, Acute
- ☐ 474.0 Tonsillitis, Chronic
- ☐ 465.9 Upper Respiratory Infection, Acute
- ☐ 599.0 Urinary Tract Infection
- ☐ V03.9 Vaccination/Bacterial Dis.
- ☐ V06.8 Vaccination/Combination
- ☐ V04.8 Vaccination, Influenza
- ☐ 616.10 Vaginitis, Vulvitis, NOS
- ☐ 780.4 Vertigo
- ☐ 787.0 Vomiting, Nausea
- ☐ ____ ____________
- ☐ ____ ____________
- ☐ ____ ____________
- ☐ ____ ____________

RETURN APPOINTMENT

______ Days
______ Weeks
______ Months

Authorization Number:

▶ ____________________

BALANCE DUE

DATE OF SERVICE	CPT CODE	DIAGNOSIS CODE(S)	CHARGE

Place of Service:
( ) Office
( ) Emergency Room
( ) Inpatient Hospital
( ) Outpatient Hospital
( ) Nursing Home

TOTAL CHARGE	$
AMOUNT PAID	$
PREVIOUS BAL	$
BALANCE DUE	$

Check #: ____________

(Circle Method of Payment)
CASH CHECK MC VISA

Physician's Signature

▶ ______________________________

Blackburn Primary Care Associates, PC
1990 Turquoise Drive
Blackburn, WI 54937
(608) 459-8857

Howard M. Lawler, MD 11
Joanne R. Hughes, MD 21
Ralph Garcia Lopez, MD 31
TAX ID NO. 00-00000000

GUARANTOR NAME AND ADDRESS	PATIENT NO.	PATIENT NAME			DOCTOR NO.	DATE
	DATE OF BIRTH	TELEPHONE NO.	INSURANCE CODE	DESCRIPTION	CERTIFICATE NO.	

X	CPT	OFFICE - NEW SERVICE	FEE	X	CPT	OFFICE - ESTABLISHED SERVICE	FEE	X	CPT	OFFICE - CONSULT SERVICE	FEE	X	CPT	PREVENTIVE CARE - ADULT SERVICE	FEE
	99201	Prob Foc/Straight			99211	Nurse/Minimal			99241	Prob/Foc/Straight			99385	18-39 Initial	
	99202	Exp Prob/Straight			99212	Prob Foc/Straight			99242	Exp Prob/Straight			99386	40-64 Initial	
	99203	Detailed/Low			99213	Exp Prob/Low			99243	Detailed/Low			99387	65+ Initial	
	99204	Compre/Moderate			99214	Detailed/Moderate			99244	Compre/Moderate			99395	18-39 Periodic	
	99205	Compre/High			99215	Compre/High			99245	Compre/High			99396	40-64 Periodic	
													99397	65+ Periodic	

X	CPT	GASTROENEROLOGY SERVICE	FEE	X	CPT	CARDIOLOGY & HEARING SERVICE	FEE	X	CPT	INJECTIONS & IMMUNIZATION SERVICE	FEE	X	CPT	REPAIR & DERMATOLOGY SERVICE	FEE
	45300	Sigmoidoscopy Rig			93000	EKG (Global)			86585	TB Skin Test			17110	Warts: #	
	45305	Sigmoid Rig w/bx			93015	Stress Test (Global)			90716	Varicella Vaccine				Tags: #	
	45330	Sigmoidoscopy Flex			93224	Holter (Global)			90724	Flu Vaccine				Lesion Excis	
	45331	Sigmoid Flex w/bx			93225	Holter Hook Up			90732	Pneumovax				Lesion Destruct	
	45378	Colonoscopy Diag			93227	Holter Interpretation			90718	TD Immunization			SIZE CM:	SITE:	
	45380	Colonoscopy w/bx			94010	Pulm Function Test							MALIG:	PREMAL/BEN:	
	46600	Anoscopy			92551	Audiometry Screen			90782	Injection IM*				(Check One Above)	
									90788	Injection IM Antibiot*				Simple Closure	
		OTHER				SUPPLIES/DRUGS*				Injection joint*				Intermed Closure	
						DRUG NAME:			SM	MED MAJOR			SIZE CM:	SITE:	
						UNIT/MEASURE:				(circle one)					
						QUANTITY			FOR ALL INJECTIONS, SUPPLY DRUG				10060	I&D Abscess	
									INFORMATION				10080	I&D Cyst	

DIAGNOSTIC CODES: ICD-9-CM

- ☐ 789.0 Abdominal Pain
- ☐ 795.0 Abnormal Pap Smear
- ☐ 706.1 Acne Vulgaris
- ☐ 477.0 Allergic Rhinitis
- ☐ 285.9 Anemia, NOS
- ☐ 281.0 Pernicious
- ☐ 411.1 Angina, Unstable
- ☐ 427.9 Arythmia, NOS
- ☐ 440.9 Arteriosclerosis
- ☐ 714.0 Arthritis, Rheumatoid
- ☐ 414.0 ASHD
- ☐ 493.90 Asthma, Bronchial W/O Status Ast.
- ☐ 493.91 Asthma, Bronchial W/Status Ast.
- ☐ 466.1 Bronchiolitis, Acute
- ☐ 466.0 Bronchitis, Acute
- ☐ 727.3 Bursitis
- ☐ 786.50 Chest Pain
- ☐ 574.20 Cholelithiasis
- ☐ 372.30 Conjunctivitis, Unspecified
- ☐ 564.0 Constipation
- ☐ 496 COPD
- ☐ 692.9 Dermatitis, Allergic
- ☐ 250.01 Diabetes Mellitus, ID
- ☐ 250.00 Diabetes Mellitus, NID
- ☐ 558.9 Diarrhea
- ☐ 562.11 Diverticulitis
- ☐ 562.10 Diverticulosis
- ☐ 782.3 Edema
- ☐ 492.8 Emphysema
- ☐ V16.0 Family History Of Diabetes
- ☐ 780.6 Fever of Undetermined Origin
- ☐ 578.9 G.I. Bleeding, Unspecified
- ☐ 727.41 Ganglion of Joint
- ☐ 535.0 Gastritis, Acute
- ☐ V72.3 Arythmia, NOS
- ☐ 748.0 Headache
- ☐ 550.90 Hernia, Inguinal, NOS
- ☐ 054.9 Herpes Simplex
- ☐ 053.9 Herpes Zoster
- ☐ 708.9 Hives/Urticaria
- ☐ 401.1 Hypertension, Benign
- ☐ 401.0 Hypertension, Malignant
- ☐ 402.90 Hypertension, W/O CHF
- ☐ 244.9 Hypothyroidism, Primary
- ☐ 380.4 Impacted Cerumen
- ☐ 487.1 Influenza
- ☐ 564.1 Irritable Bowel Syndrome
- ☐ 464.0 Laryngitis, Acute
- ☐ 454.9 Leg Varicose Veins
- ☐ 424.0 Mitral Valve Prolapse
- ☐ 412 Myocardial Infarction, Old
- ☐ 715.90 Osteoarthritis, Unspec. Site
- ☐ 620.2 Ovarian Cyst
- ☐ 614.9 Pelvic Inflammatory Disease
- ☐ 685.1 Pilonidal Cyst
- ☐ 462 Pharyngitis, Acute
- ☐ 627.1 Postmenopausal Bleeding
- ☐ 625.4 Premenstrual Tension
- ☐ 782.1 Rash
- ☐ 569.3 Rectal Bleeding
- ☐ 398.90 Rheumatic Heart Disease, NOS
- ☐ 431.9 Sinusitis, Acute, NOS
- ☐ 782.1 Skin Eruption, Rash
- ☐ 845.00 Sprain, Ankle
- ☐ 848.9 Sprain, Muscle, Unspec. Site
- ☐ 785.6 Swollen Glands
- ☐ 246.9 Thyroid Disease, Unspecified
- ☐ 463 Tonsillitis, Acute
- ☐ 474.0 Tonsillitis, Chronic
- ☐ 465.9 Upper Respiratory Infection, Acute
- ☐ 599.0 Urinary Tract Infection
- ☐ V03.9 Vaccination/Bacterial Dis.
- ☐ V06.8 Vaccination/Combination
- ☐ V04.8 Vaccination, Influenza
- ☐ 616.10 Vaginitis, Vulvitis, NOS
- ☐ 780.4 Vertigo
- ☐ 787.0 Vomiting, Nausea
- ☐ ____ ____________
- ☐ ____ ____________
- ☐ ____ ____________
- ☐ ____ ____________

RETURN APPOINTMENT

________ Days
________ Weeks
________ Months

Authorization Number:
▶ ______________

BALANCE DUE

DATE OF SERVICE	CPT CODE	DIAGNOSIS CODE(S)	CHARGE

Place of Service:
( ) Office
( ) Emergency Room
( ) Inpatient Hospital
( ) Outpatient Hospital
( ) Nursing Home

TOTAL CHARGE	$
AMOUNT PAID	$
PREVIOUS BAL	$
BALANCE DUE	$

Check #: ______________

(Circle Method of Payment)
CASH CHECK MC VISA

Physician's Signature
▶ ______________________________

Blackburn Primary Care Associates, PC
1990 Turquoise Drive
Blackburn, WI 54937
(608) 459-8857

Howard M. Lawler, MD 11
Joanne R. Hughes, MD 21
Ralph Garcia Lopez, MD 31
TAX ID NO. 00-00000000

GUARANTOR NAME AND ADDRESS	PATIENT NO.	PATIENT NAME		DOCTOR NO.	DATE
	DATE OF BIRTH	TELEPHONE NO.	INSURANCE CODE	INSURANCE DESCRIPTION	INSURANCE CERTIFICATE NO.

OFFICE - NEW

X	CPT	SERVICE	FEE
	99201	Prob Foc/Straight	
	99202	Exp Prob/Straight	
	99203	Detailed/Low	
	99204	Compre/Moderate	
	99205	Compre/High	

OFFICE - ESTABLISHED

X	CPT	SERVICE	FEE
	99211	Nurse/Minimal	
	99212	Prob Foc/Straight	
	99213	Exp Prob/Low	
	99214	Detailed/Moderate	
	99215	Compre/High	

OFFICE - CONSULT

X	CPT	SERVICE	FEE
	99241	Prob/Foc/Straight	
	99242	Exp Prob/Straight	
	99243	Detailed/Low	
	99244	Compre/Moderate	
	99245	Compre/High	

PREVENTIVE CARE - ADULT

X	CPT	SERVICE	FEE
	99385	18-39 Initial	
	99386	40-64 Initial	
	99387	65+ Initial	
	99395	18-39 Periodic	
	99396	40-64 Periodic	
	99397	65+ Periodic	

GASTROENEROLOGY

X	CPT	SERVICE	FEE
	45300	Sigmoidoscopy Rig	
	45305	Sigmoid Rig w/bx	
	45330	Sigmoidoscopy Flex	
	45331	Sigmoid Flex w/bx	
	45378	Colonoscopy Diag	
	45380	Colonoscopy w/bx	
	46600	Anoscopy	

CARDIOLOGY & HEARING

X	CPT	SERVICE	FEE
	93000	EKG (Global)	
	93015	Stress Test (Global)	
	93224	Holter (Global)	
	93225	Holter Hook Up	
	93227	Holter Interpretation	
	94010	Pulm Function Test	
	92551	Audiometry Screen	

INJECTIONS & IMMUNIZATION

X	CPT	SERVICE	FEE
	86585	TB Skin Test	
	90716	Varicella Vaccine	
	90724	Flu Vaccine	
	90732	Pneumovax	
	90718	TD Immunization	
	90782	Injection IM*	
	90788	Injection IM Antibiot*	
		Injection joint*	
	SM	MED MAJOR	
		(circle one)	
FOR ALL INJECTIONS, SUPPLY DRUG			
INFORMATION			

REPAIR & DERMATOLOGY

X	CPT	SERVICE	FEE
	17110	Warts: #	
		Tags: #	
		Lesion Excis	
		Lesion Destruct	
	SIZE CM:	SITE:	
	MALIG:	PREMAL/BEN:	
		(Check One Above)	
		Simple Closure	
		Intermed Closure	
	SIZE CM:	SITE:	
	10060	I&D Abscess	
	10080	I&D Cyst	

OTHER

X	CPT	SERVICE	FEE

SUPPLIES/DRUGS*

DRUG NAME:	
UNIT/MEASURE:	
QUANTITY	

DIAGNOSTIC CODES: ICD-9-CM

- ☐ 789.0 Abdominal Pain
- ☐ 795.0 Abnormal Pap Smear
- ☐ 706.1 Acne Vulgaris
- ☐ 477.0 Allergic Rhinitis
- ☐ 285.9 Anemia, NOS
- ☐ 281.0 Pernicious
- ☐ 411.1 Angina, Unstable
- ☐ 427.9 Arythmia, NOS
- ☐ 440.9 Arteriosclerosis
- ☐ 714.0 Arthritis, Rheumatoid
- ☐ 414.0 ASHD
- ☐ 493.90 Asthma, Bronchial W/O Status Ast.
- ☐ 493.91 Asthma, Bronchial W/Status Ast.
- ☐ 466.1 Bronchiolitis, Acute
- ☐ 466.0 Bronchitis, Acute
- ☐ 727.3 Bursitis
- ☐ 786.50 Chest Pain
- ☐ 574.20 Cholelithiasis
- ☐ 372.30 Conjunctivitis, Unspecified
- ☐ 564.0 Constipation
- ☐ 496 COPD
- ☐ 692.9 Dermatitis, Allergic
- ☐ 250.01 Diabetes Mellitus, ID
- ☐ 250.00 Diabetes Mellitus, NID
- ☐ 558.9 Diarrhea
- ☐ 562.11 Diverticulitis
- ☐ 562.10 Diverticulosis
- ☐ 782.3 Edema
- ☐ 492.8 Emphysema
- ☐ V16.0 Family History Of Diabetes
- ☐ 780.6 Fever of Undetermined Origin
- ☐ 578.9 G.I. Bleeding, Unspecified
- ☐ 727.41 Ganglion of Joint
- ☐ 535.0 Gastritis, Acute
- ☐ V72.3 Arythmia, NOS
- ☐ 748.0 Headache
- ☐ 550.90 Hernia, Inguinal, NOS
- ☐ 054.9 Herpes Simplex
- ☐ 053.9 Herpes Zoster
- ☐ 708.9 Hives/Urticaria
- ☐ 401.1 Hypertension, Benign
- ☐ 401.0 Hypertension, Malignant
- ☐ 402.90 Hypertension, W/O CHF
- ☐ 244.9 Hypothyroidism, Primary
- ☐ 380.4 Impacted Cerumen
- ☐ 487.1 Influenza
- ☐ 564.1 Irritable Bowel Syndrome
- ☐ 464.0 Laryngitis, Acute
- ☐ 454.9 Leg Varicose Veins
- ☐ 424.0 Mitral Valve Prolapse
- ☐ 412 Myocardial Infarction, Old
- ☐ 715.90 Osteoarthritis, Unspec. Site
- ☐ 620.2 Ovarian Cyst
- ☐ 614.9 Pelvic Inflammatory Disease
- ☐ 685.1 Pilonidal Cyst
- ☐ 462 Pharyngitis, Acute
- ☐ 627.1 Postmenopausal Bleeding
- ☐ 625.4 Premenstrual Tension
- ☐ 782.1 Rash
- ☐ 569.3 Rectal Bleeding
- ☐ 398.90 Rheumatic Heart Disease, NOS
- ☐ 431.9 Sinusitis, Acute, NOS
- ☐ 782.1 Skin Eruption, Rash
- ☐ 845.00 Sprain, Ankle
- ☐ 848.9 Sprain, Muscle, Unspec. Site
- ☐ 785.6 Swollen Glands
- ☐ 246.9 Thyroid Disease, Unspecified
- ☐ 463 Tonsillitis, Acute
- ☐ 474.0 Tonsillitis, Chronic
- ☐ 465.9 Upper Respiratory Infection, Acute
- ☐ 599.0 Urinary Tract Infection
- ☐ V03.9 Vaccination/Bacterial Dis.
- ☐ V06.8 Vaccination/Combination
- ☐ V04.8 Vaccination, Influenza
- ☐ 616.10 Vaginitis, Vulvitis, NOS
- ☐ 780.4 Vertigo
- ☐ 787.0 Vomiting, Nausea
- ☐ _____ ____________
- ☐ _____ ____________
- ☐ _____ ____________
- ☐ _____ ____________

RETURN APPOINTMENT

_______ Days
_______ Weeks
_______ Months

Authorization Number:
▶ ____________________

BALANCE DUE

DATE OF SERVICE	CPT CODE	DIAGNOSIS CODE(S)	CHARGE

Place of Service:		
( ) Office	TOTAL CHARGE	$
( ) Emergency Room	AMOUNT PAID	$
( ) Inpatient Hospital ( ) Outpatient Hospital	PREVIOUS BAL	$
( ) Nursing Home	BALANCE DUE	$

Check #: ______________

(Circle Method of Payment)
CASH CHECK MC VISA

Physician's Signature
▶ ________________________________

Blackburn Primary Care Associates, PC
1990 Turquoise Drive
Blackburn, WI 54937
(608) 459-8857

Howard M. Lawler, MD 11
Joanne R. Hughes, MD 21
Ralph Garcia Lopez, MD 31
TAX ID NO. 00-00000000

GUARANTOR NAME AND ADDRESS	PATIENT NO.	PATIENT NAME		DOCTOR NO.	DATE
	DATE OF BIRTH	TELEPHONE NO.	INSURANCE: CODE	DESCRIPTION	CERTIFICATE NO.

X	CPT	SERVICE	FEE	X	CPT	SERVICE	FEE	X	CPT	SERVICE	FEE	X	CPT	SERVICE	FEE
		OFFICE - NEW				**OFFICE - ESTABLISHED**				**OFFICE - CONSULT**				**PREVENTIVE CARE - ADULT**	
	99201	Prob Foc/Straight			99211	Nurse/Minimal			99241	Prob/Foc/Straight			99385	18-39 Initial	
	99202	Exp Prob/Straight			99212	Prob Foc/Straight			99242	Exp Prob/Straight			99386	40-64 Initial	
	99203	Detailed/Low			99213	Exp Prob/Low			99243	Detailed/Low			99387	65+ Initial	
	99204	Compre/Moderate			99214	Detailed/Moderate			99244	Compre/Moderate			99395	18-39 Periodic	
	99205	Compre/High			99215	Compre/High			99245	Compre/High			99396	40-64 Periodic	
													99397	65+ Periodic	
		GASTROENEROLOGY				**CARDIOLOGY & HEARING**				**INJECTIONS & IMMUNIZATION**				**REPAIR & DERMATOLOGY**	
	45300	Sigmoidoscopy Rig			93000	EKG (Global)			86585	TB Skin Test			17110	Warts: #	
	45305	Sigmoid Rig w/bx			93015	Stress Test (Global)			90716	Varicella Vaccine				Tags: #	
	45330	Sigmoidoscopy Flex			93224	Holter (Global)			90724	Flu Vaccine				Lesion Excis	
	45331	Sigmoid Flex w/bx			93225	Holter Hook Up			90732	Pneumovax				Lesion Destruct	
	45378	Colonoscopy Diag			93227	Holter Interpretation			90718	TD Immunization			SIZE CM:	SITE:	
	45380	Colonoscopy w/bx			94010	Pulm Function Test							MALIG:	PREMAL/BEN:	
	46600	Anoscopy			92551	Audiometry Screen			90782	Injection IM*				(Check One Above)	
									90788	Injection IM Antibiot*				Simple Closure	
		OTHER				**SUPPLIES/DRUGS***				Injection joint*				Intermed Closure	
						DRUG NAME:			SM	MED MAJOR			SIZE CM:	SITE:	
						UNIT/MEASURE:				(circle one)					
						QUANTITY			FOR ALL INJECTIONS, SUPPLY DRUG				10060	I&D Abscess	
									INFORMATION				10080	I&D Cyst	

DIAGNOSTIC CODES: ICD-9-CM

- ☐ 789.0 Abdominal Pain
- ☐ 795.0 Abnormal Pap Smear
- ☐ 706.1 Acne Vulgaris
- ☐ 477.0 Allergic Rhinitis
- ☐ 285.9 Anemia, NOS
- ☐ 281.0 Pernicious
- ☐ 411.1 Angina, Unstable
- ☐ 427.9 Arythmia, NOS
- ☐ 440.9 Arteriosclerosis
- ☐ 714.0 Arthritis, Rheumatoid
- ☐ 414.0 ASHD
- ☐ 493.90 Asthma, Bronchial W/O Status Ast.
- ☐ 493.91 Asthma, Bronchial W/Status Ast.
- ☐ 466.1 Bronchiolitis, Acute
- ☐ 466.0 Bronchitis, Acute
- ☐ 727.3 Bursitis
- ☐ 786.50 Chest Pain
- ☐ 574.20 Cholelithiasis
- ☐ 372.30 Conjunctivitis, Unspecified
- ☐ 564.0 Constipation
- ☐ 496 COPD
- ☐ 692.9 Dermatitis, Allergic
- ☐ 250.01 Diabetes Mellitus, ID
- ☐ 250.00 Diabetes Mellitus, NID
- ☐ 558.9 Diarrhea
- ☐ 562.11 Diverticulitis
- ☐ 562.10 Diverticulosis
- ☐ 782.3 Edema
- ☐ 492.8 Emphysema
- ☐ V16.0 Family History Of Diabetes
- ☐ 780.6 Fever of Undetermined Origin
- ☐ 578.9 G.I. Bleeding, Unspecified
- ☐ 727.41 Ganglion of Joint
- ☐ 535.0 Gastritis, Acute
- ☐ V72.3 Arythmia, NOS
- ☐ 748.0 Headache
- ☐ 550.90 Hernia, Inguinal, NOS
- ☐ 054.9 Herpes Simplex
- ☐ 053.9 Herpes Zoster
- ☐ 708.9 Hives/Urticaria
- ☐ 401.1 Hypertension, Benign
- ☐ 401.0 Hypertension, Malignant
- ☐ 402.90 Hypertension, W/O CHF
- ☐ 244.9 Hypothyroidism, Primary
- ☐ 380.4 Impacted Cerumen
- ☐ 487.1 Influenza
- ☐ 564.1 Irritable Bowel Syndrome
- ☐ 464.0 Laryngitis, Acute
- ☐ 454.9 Leg Varicose Veins
- ☐ 424.0 Mitral Valve Prolapse
- ☐ 412 Myocardial Infarction, Old
- ☐ 715.90 Osteoarthritis, Unspec. Site
- ☐ 620.2 Ovarian Cyst
- ☐ 614.9 Pelvic Inflammatory Disease
- ☐ 685.1 Pilonidal Cyst
- ☐ 462 Pharyngitis, Acute
- ☐ 627.1 Postmenopausal Bleeding
- ☐ 625.4 Premenstrual Tension
- ☐ 782.1 Rash
- ☐ 569.3 Rectal Bleeding
- ☐ 398.90 Rheumatic Heart Disease, NOS
- ☐ 431.9 Sinusitis, Acute, NOS
- ☐ 782.1 Skin Eruption, Rash
- ☐ 845.00 Sprain, Ankle
- ☐ 848.9 Sprain, Muscle, Unspec. Site
- ☐ 785.6 Swollen Glands
- ☐ 246.9 Thyroid Disease, Unspecified
- ☐ 463 Tonsillitis, Acute
- ☐ 474.0 Tonsillitis, Chronic
- ☐ 465.9 Upper Respiratory Infection, Acute
- ☐ 599.0 Urinary Tract Infection
- ☐ V03.9 Vaccination/Bacterial Dis.
- ☐ V06.8 Vaccination/Combination
- ☐ V04.8 Vaccination, Influenza
- ☐ 616.10 Vaginitis, Vulvitis, NOS
- ☐ 780.4 Vertigo
- ☐ 787.0 Vomiting, Nausea
- ☐ _____ ____________
- ☐ _____ ____________
- ☐ _____ ____________
- ☐ _____ ____________

RETURN APPOINTMENT

_______ Days
_______ Weeks
_______ Months

Authorization Number:
▶ ____________________

BALANCE DUE

DATE OF SERVICE	CPT CODE	DIAGNOSIS CODE(S)	CHARGE

Place of Service:
( ) Office
( ) Emergency Room
( ) Inpatient Hospital
( ) Outpatient Hospital
( ) Nursing Home

TOTAL CHARGE	$
AMOUNT PAID	$
PREVIOUS BAL	$
BALANCE DUE	$

Check #: ____________

(Circle Method of Payment)
CASH CHECK MC VISA

Physician's Signature
▶ ______________________________

PATIENT LEDGER

BLACKBURN PRIMARY CARE ASSOCIATES, PC
1990 Turquiose Drive
Blackburn, WI 54937
608-459-8857

STATEMENT TO:

				PREVIOUS BALANCE			
DATE	PROFESSIONAL SERVICE	CHARGE	PAYMENT	ADJUST-MENT		NEW BALANCE	

PATIENT LEDGER

BLACKBURN PRIMARY CARE ASSOCIATES, PC
1990 Turquiose Drive
Blackburn, WI 54937
608-459-8857

STATEMENT TO:

				PREVIOUS BALANCE			
DATE	PROFESSIONAL SERVICE	CHARGE	PAYMENT	ADJUST-MENT		NEW BALANCE	

PATIENT LEDGER

BLACKBURN PRIMARY CARE ASSOCIATES, PC
1990 Turquiose Drive
Blackburn, WI 54937
608-459-8857

STATEMENT TO:

				PREVIOUS BALANCE			
DATE	PROFESSIONAL SERVICE	CHARGE	PAYMENT	ADJUST-MENT		NEW BALANCE	

PATIENT LEDGER

BLACKBURN PRIMARY CARE ASSOCIATES, PC
1990 Turquiose Drive
Blackburn, WI 54937
608-459-8857

STATEMENT TO:

				PREVIOUS BALANCE			
DATE	PROFESSIONAL SERVICE	CHARGE	PAYMENT	ADJUST-MENT		NEW BALANCE	

PATIENT LEDGER

BLACKBURN PRIMARY CARE ASSOCIATES, PC
1990 Turquiose Drive
Blackburn, WI 54937
608-459-8857

STATEMENT TO:

			PREVIOUS BALANCE				
DATE	PROFESSIONAL SERVICE	CHARGE	PAYMENT	ADJUST-MENT		NEW BALANCE	

PLACE FIRST PEG HERE

JOURNAL OF DAILY CHARGES, PAYMENTS & DEPOSITS

	DATE	PROFESSIONAL SERVICE	FEE	PAYMENT	ADJUST-MENT	NEW BALANCE	OLD BALANCE	PATIENT'S NAME	
1									1
2									2
3									3
4									4
5									5
6									6
7									7
8									8
9									9
10									10
11									11
12									12
13									13
14									14
15									15
16									16
17									17
18									18
19									19
20									20
21									21
22									22
23									23
24									24
25									25
26									26
27									27
28									28
29									29
30									30
31								TOTALS THIS PAGE	31
32								TOTALS PREVIOUS PAGE	32
33								TOTALS MONTH TO DATE	33
			COLUMN A	COLUMN B	COLUMN C	COLUMN D	COLUMN E		

MEMO ____________________

DAILY-FROM LINE 31

ARITHMETIC POSTING PROOF	
Column E	
Plus Column A	
Sub-Total	
Minus Column B	
Sub-Total	
Minus Column C	
Equals Column D	

Box 1

MONTH-FROM LINE 31

ARITHMETIC POSTING PROOF	
Accts. Receivable Previous Day	$
Plus Column A	
Sub-Total	
Minus Column B	
Sub-Total	
Minus Column C	
Accts. Receivable End of Day	

Box 2

BANK DEPOSIT DETAIL

	PAYMENTS		
BANK NUMBER	BY CHECK OR PMO	BY COIN OR CURRENCY	CREDIT CARD
TOTALS			

CURRENCY	
COIN	
CHECKS	
CREDIT CARDS	
TOTAL RECEIPTS	
LESS CREDIT CARD $	
TOTAL DEPOSITS	

DEPOSIT
DATE: ____________ FIRM: ____________

THIS WORKSHEET IS PROVIDED TO HELP YOU BALANCE YOUR ACCOUNT

1. Go through your register and mark each check, withdrawal, Express ATM transaction, payment, deposit, or other credit listed on this statement. Be sure that your register shows any interest paid into your account, and any service charges, automatic payments, or Express Transfers withdrawn from your account during this statement period.
2. Using the chart below, list any outstanding checks, Express ATM withdrawals, payments, or any other withdrawals (including any from previous months) that are listed in your register but are not shown on this statement.
3. Balance your account by filling in the spaces below.

ITEMS OUTSTANDING		
NUMBER	**AMOUNT**	
TOTAL	**$**	

ENTER

The NEW BALANCE shown on this statement____________________________$

ADD

Any deposits listed in your register $
or transfers into your account $
which are not shown on this $
statement. +$ ______

TOTAL

CALCULATE THE SUBTOTAL______________$

SUBTRACT

The total outstanding checks and withdrawals from the chart at left___________-$

CALCULATE THE ENDING BALANCE

This amount should be the same as the current balance shown in your check register______________________$

1837

DATE ____________

TO ____________

FOR ____________

BALANCE BROUGHT FORWARD		
DEPOSITS		
BALANCE		
AMT THIS CK		
BALANCE CARRIED FORWARD		

1837

BLACKBURN PRIMARY CARE ASSOCIATES, PC
1990 Turquoise Drive
Blackburn, WI 54937
608-459-8857

94-72/1224

DATE ____________

PAY TO THE ORDER OF ____________ $

____________ DOLLARS

DERBYSHIRE SAVINGS
Member FDIC
P.O. BOX 8923
Blackburn, WI 54937

FOR ____________

⑈055003⑈ 44678201⑉ 678800470

1838

DATE ____________

TO ____________

FOR ____________

BALANCE BROUGHT FORWARD		
DEPOSITS		
BALANCE		
AMT THIS CK		
BALANCE CARRIED FORWARD		

1838

BLACKBURN PRIMARY CARE ASSOCIATES, PC
1990 Turquoise Drive
Blackburn, WI 54937
608-459-8857

94-72/1224

DATE ____________

PAY TO THE ORDER OF ____________ $

____________ DOLLARS

DERBYSHIRE SAVINGS
Member FDIC
P.O. BOX 8923
Blackburn, WI 54937

FOR ____________

⑈055003⑈ 44678201⑉ 678800470

1839

DATE ____________

TO ____________

FOR ____________

BALANCE BROUGHT FORWARD		
DEPOSITS		
BALANCE		
AMT THIS CK		
BALANCE CARRIED FORWARD		

1839

BLACKBURN PRIMARY CARE ASSOCIATES, PC
1990 Turquoise Drive
Blackburn, WI 54937
608-459-8857

94-72/1224

DATE ____________

PAY TO THE ORDER OF ____________ $

____________ DOLLARS

DERBYSHIRE SAVINGS
Member FDIC
P.O. BOX 8923
Blackburn, WI 54937

FOR ____________

⑈055003⑈ 44678201⑉ 678800470

DISBURSEMENT RECORD

Check No.	Name	Date	Amount	Deposit	Beg.Balance Balance	1 Supplies	2 Salary	3 Rent	4 Misc.

Procedure 36-1: Preparing Charge Slips for the Day's Patients

Performance Objective

Task: Prepare charge slips for patients using the day's schedule

Conditions: Blank charge slips, patient ledger cards, daily patient schedule, and medical record for each patient scheduled

Standards: Complete the procedure in 20 minutes, and achieve a satisfactory score on the procedure performance checklist

Scoring Key: (**S**)*atisfactory,* (**U**)*nsatisfactory,* (**NA**) *Not Applicable*
◆ *Denotes a critical element for a satisfactory score on the procedure*

Procedure Steps	1st trial	2nd trial	3rd trial
1. Place patients' medical records in order of appointment time, referring to appointment schedule.			
2. If using a pegboard accounting system, pull the ledger card for each patient from the ledger file and place in appointment order.			
or 2A. If using a computerized accounting system, print a charge slip for each patient that contains the patient information.			
3. For each patient, write the patient's name (for pegboard system only) and any previous balance on the charge slip.			
4. If preauthorization is required for the service anticipated, call the insurance provider and enter the preauthorization number on the charge slip.			
5. Attach the correct charge slip (and ledger card) to the front of each patient's medical record with a paper clip.			
6. Complete the procedure within 20 minutes. ◆			

Evaluator Comments:

Score Calculation:

For each procedural step marked U (Unsatisfactory) deduct 6 points
For each procedural step (◆) marked U (Unsatisfactory) deduct 20 points

Score calculation	100 points			
	− ____ points missed	1st	2nd	3rd
	Total score			

Satisfactory score: 85 or above

Procedure 36-2: Completing an Encounter Form (Superbill) for a Patient

Performance Objective

Task: Complete an encounter form (superbill) with information from the charge slip and/or the fee schedule after a patient visit

Conditions: Charge slip, encounter form, fee schedule, pen

Standards: Complete the procedure in 5 minutes, and achieve a satisfactory score on the procedure performance checklist

Scoring Key: (**S**)*atisfactory,* (**U**)*nsatisfactory,* (**NA**) *Not Applicable*
◆ *Denotes a critical element for a satisfactory score on the procedure*

Procedure Steps	1st trial	2nd trial	3rd trial
1. Using a charge slip that contains the patient's name, date, previous balance, and services provided, or a superbill with procedures checked off, add fees for each procedure using the fee schedule.			
2. Total the charges and enter the amount in the correct box.			
3. Record any payment made by the patient.			
4. Calculate the new balance.			
5. Check the correct place of service.			
6. Set the superbill (encounter form) aside if one or more diagnosis codes must be looked up.			
7. The new balance is the same as that obtained by the evaluator. ◆			
8. Complete the procedure within 5 minutes. ◆			

Evaluator Comments:

Score Calculation:

For each procedural step marked U (Unsatisfactory) deduct 6 points
For each procedural step (◆) marked U (Unsatisfactory) deduct 20 points

Score calculation 100 points

		1st	2nd	3rd
	− points missed			
	Total score			

Satisfactory score: 85 or above

Procedure 36-3: Posting Charges to the Patient Ledger

Performance Objective

Task: Post charges to a patient ledger

Conditions: Completed patient charge slip or superbill, patient ledger, calculator or adding machine, pen or computer

Standards: Complete the procedure in 5 minutes, and achieve a satisfactory score on the procedure performance checklist

Scoring Key: (**S**)*atisfactory,* (**U**)*nsatisfactory,* (**NA**) *Not Applicable*
◆ *Denotes a critical element for a satisfactory score on the procedure*

Procedure Steps	1st trial	2nd trial	3rd trial
1. Remove charge slip from chart after patient visit.			
2. Check name on charge slip against name on ledger card or computer account.			
3. Post all charges from one day on patient ledger using one line. **or**			
3A. In computerized systems, enter the procedure code in the screen for posting charges and the usual charge is automatically generated. Accept the charge (or change if directed by the physician.)			
4. Add any new charges to any previous balance.			
5. Record the new balance due.			
6. The charge posted and balance due is the same as that of the evaluator. ◆			
7. Complete the procedure within 5 minutes. ◆			

Evaluator Comments:

Score Calculation:

For each procedural step marked U (Unsatisfactory) deduct 6 points
For each procedural step (◆) marked U (Unsatisfactory) deduct 20 points

Score calculation	100 points			
	− ____ points missed	1st	2nd	3rd
	Total score			

Satisfactory score: 85 or above

Procedure 36-4: Posting Payments and/or Adjustments

Performance Objective

Task: Post payments and/or adjustments to a patient account

Conditions: Patient ledger card or computer, check or cash from the patient, or check from an insurance carrier, calculator or adding machine

Standards: Complete the procedure in 5 minutes, and achieve a satisfactory score on the procedure performance checklist

Scoring Key: (**S**)*atisfactory*, (**U**)*nsatisfactory*, (**NA**) *Not Applicable*
◆ *Denotes a critical element for a satisfactory score on the procedure*

Procedure Steps	1st trial	2nd trial	3rd trial
1. When payment has been made, select the correct patient ledger card or locate the patient account in the computer database.			
2. Compare the amount of payment against the total owed.			
3. Record payment in column labeled payment.			
4. Identify payment as cash or check.			
5. Identify payment as coming from patient or insurance company.			
6. Identify charge to which payment is applied.			
7. Subtract the payment from any previous balance.			
8. Record the new balance due.			
9. Enter any adjustments in the adjustments column.			
10. Add or subtract the amount of the adjustment.			
11. Record the new balance due.			
12. Place cash or check in designated drawer or money box.			
13. The payment or adjustment posted and balance due is the same as that of the evaluator. ◆			
14. Complete the procedure within 5 minutes. ◆			

Evaluator Comments:

Score Calculation:

For each procedural step marked U (Unsatisfactory) deduct 6 points
For each procedural step (◆) marked U (Unsatisfactory) deduct 20 points

Score calculation	100 points			
	– ____ points missed	1st	2nd	3rd
	Total score			

Satisfactory score: 85 or above

Procedure 36-5: Recording a Patient Visit on the Day Sheet

Performance Objective

Task: Post charges and payments on a day sheet using information from the superbill, ledger, and charge slip

Conditions: Day sheet or accounts receivable record, encounter form, charge slip (if separate from encounter form), patient ledger, patient medical record, pen

Standards: Complete the procedure in 5 minutes, and achieve a satisfactory score on the procedure performance checklist

Scoring Key: (**S**)*atisfactory,* (**U**)*nsatisfactory,* (**NA**) *Not Applicable*
◆ *Denotes a critical element for a satisfactory score on the procedure*

Procedure Steps	1st trial	2nd trial	3rd trial
1. Prepare the day sheet by reviewing appointment schedule.			
2. If using pegboard, set up the pegboard with the day sheet on the bottom, and shingled charge slips aligned with the lines of the day sheet.			
3. As each patient completes his or her appointment, complete charge slip, encounter form (if separate), and patient ledger card.			
4. When these forms are properly positioned on the pegboard, the identical information appears as a carbon copy on the day sheet.			
5. Enter the charge in the space marked "Fee."			
6. Enter any payment made by the patient in the space marked "Payment."			
7. Enter any adjustment in the space marked "adjustment."			
8. Calculate the new balance and enter in the space marked "Balance."			
9. Record each payment on the deposit slip when it is received.			
10. If necessary, verify that entries have been copied on the ledger card and/or day sheet in the correct spaces.			
11. The posting(s) and balance due are the same as those posted by the evaluator. ◆			
12. Complete the procedure within 5 minutes. ◆			

Evaluator Comments:

Score Calculation:

For each procedural step marked U (Unsatisfactory) deduct 6 points
For each procedural step (◆) marked U (Unsatisfactory) deduct 20 points

Score calculation	100 points			
	– points missed	1st	2nd	3rd
	Total score			

Satisfactory score: 85 or above

Procedure 36-6: Balancing the Day Sheet

Performance Objective

Task: Verify accounts receivable daily by balancing the day sheet entries

Conditions: Completed day sheet, calculator or adding machine, pencil, pen

Standards: Complete the procedure in 30 minutes, and achieve a satisfactory score on the procedure performance checklist

Scoring Key: (**S**)*atisfactory,* (**U**)*nsatisfactory,* (**NA**) *Not Applicable*
◆ *Denotes a critical element for a satisfactory score on the procedure*

Procedure Steps	**1st trial**	**2nd trial**	**3rd trial**
1. Determine if all entries have been made for the day.			
2. Add up each column with a calculator and place the total in pencil in the bottom row labeled "Total This Page."			
3. Add the totals from the current day to totals from the previous page to obtain the total for the month to date.			
4. Verify correctness of entries by adding the total of the column labeled "old balance" or "previous balance" plus the total of the column labeled "fees" or "charges" minus the total of the column labeled "payments" and the total of the column labeled "adjustments." Enter these figures in the Daily Arithmetic Posting Proof at the bottom of the day sheet.			
5. Complete the same type of proof for the monthly figures (Monthly Arithmetic Posting Proof).			
6. When the day sheet balances, rewrite the totals with a pen.			
7. Complete the procedure within 30 minutes. ◆			

Evaluator Comments:

Score Calculation:

For each procedural step marked U (Unsatisfactory) deduct 6 points
For each procedural step (◆) marked U (Unsatisfactory) deduct 20 points

Score calculation	100 points			
	− ___ points missed	1st	2nd	3rd
	Total score			

Satisfactory score: 85 or above

Procedure 36-7: Preparing a Bank Deposit

Performance Objective

Task: Prepare a bank deposit

Conditions: Deposit slip, cash and checks received as payments, calculator or adding machine, envelope or bank deposit envelope or bag

Standards: Complete the procedure in 20 minutes, and achieve a satisfactory score on the procedure performance checklist

Scoring Key: (**S**)*atisfactory,* (**U**)*nsatisfactory,* (**NA**) *Not Applicable*
◆ *Denotes a critical element for a satisfactory score on the procedure*

Procedure Steps	1st trial	2nd trial	3rd trial
1. Obtain a practice deposit slip and place today's date on it or use the deposit slip to the right on the day sheet.			
2. Total all the currency, using calculator or adding machine.			
3. Place the total on the line that says "Currency."			
4. Total all coins by counting.			
5. Place the total on the line that says "Coin."			
6. Insert the amount of each check on the bank deposit detail, with a reference number (usually the ABA number).			
7. Total all the checks and place the total where it indicates for checks.			
8. Add the total cash to the total for checks to achieve the total amount of the bank deposit.			
9. Add the total bank deposit and total amount received from credit cards and compare to total payments on the day sheet to be sure that they are the same.			
10. Copy the deposit slip if a duplicate deposit record has not been made when creating the day sheet.			
11. Place deposit slip, checks, and cash in envelope, bank deposit envelope, or deposit bag for transporting to bank.			
12. The amount of the total deposit matches that of the evaluator. ◆			
13. Complete the procedure within 20 minutes. ◆			

Evaluator Comments:

Score Calculation:

For each procedural step marked U (Unsatisfactory) deduct 6 points
For each procedural step (◆) marked U (Unsatisfactory) deduct 20 points

Score calculation	100 points			
	− ____ points missed	1st	2nd	3rd
	Total score			

Satisfactory score: 85 or above

Procedure 36-8: Reconciling a Bank Statement

Performance Objective

Action: Reconcile a bank statement

Conditions: Monthly bank statement, checkbook and/or disbursement record, pen, calculator

Standards: Complete the procedure in 30 minutes, and achieve a satisfactory score on the procedure performance checklist

Scoring Key: (S)atisfactory, (U)nsatisfactory, (NA) Not Applicable
◆ *Denotes a critical element for a satisfactory score on the procedure*

Procedure Steps	1st trial	2nd trial	3rd trial
1. Examine the record of disbursements or checkbook ledger, and determine which portion applies to the current bank statement.			
2. Open the current bank statement and locate the ending balance and list of checks deposited.			
3. Match items from checkbook register or disbursement record against bank statement.			
4. Place a check mark next to each check number and deposit amount on your record that has been recorded on the bank statement.			
5. Note those checks or deposits in your record that have not appeared on the bank statement.			
6. Note any additional service charges, and record them in your checkbook register or disbursement record.			
7. Total any outstanding checks, withdrawals, or charges.			
8. Reconcile the account. Enter the bank's ending balance on the worksheet.			
9. Add any deposits listed on your register but not on the bank statement.			
10. Find the subtotal.			
11. Subtract the total of items outstanding.			
12. Verify that the ending balance matches the current balance shown in your checkbook register.			
13. If the balances do not match, recalculate the balance in your checkbook until you locate the error.			
14. Complete the procedure within 30 minutes. ◆			

Evaluator Comments:

Score Calculation:

For each procedural step marked U (Unsatisfactory) deduct 6 points
For each procedural step (◆) marked U (Unsatisfactory) deduct 20 points

Score calculation	100 points			
	– ___ points missed	1st	2nd	3rd
	Total score			

Satisfactory score: 85 or above

Procedure 36-9: Writing Checks to Pay Bills

Performance Objective

Task: Write a check and record it in the checkbook register and the disbursement record

Conditions: Checkbook, bill, cash disbursement record, pen

Standards: Complete the procedure in 5 minutes, and achieve a satisfactory score on the procedure performance checklist

Scoring Key: (**S**)*atisfactory,* (**U**)*nsatisfactory,* (**NA**) *Not Applicable*
◆ *Denotes a critical element for a satisfactory score on the procedure*

Procedure Steps	1st trial	2nd trial	3rd trial
1. Assemble supplies and bill.			
2. Write the name of the person or company to whom the check is being paid on the line of the check that says "Pay to the order of."			
3. Write the date on the line that says "Date."			
4. If the check does not have a pre-printed number, write the number of the check in the top right-hand corner. Refer to the check register to find the last number used.			
5. Write the amount of the check in numbers next to the dollar sign.			
6. Write the amount in words on the line below.			
7. Do not leave blank spaces between the dollar sign and number or at the beginning of the line when writing in words.			
8. Write the invoice number or account number, and the reason for the check on the line marked "For," "Reference," or "Note."			
9. Record the date, payee, account, and reason for the check on the check stub in the checkbook or in the check register.			
10. Record the information about the check on the cash disbursement record as it was recorded on the check.			
11. Subtract the amount of the check from the balance in the check register.			
12. The balance in the check register is the same as the evaluator's. ◆			
13. Complete the procedure within 5 minutes. ◆			

Evaluator Comments:

Score Calculation:

For each procedural step marked U (Unsatisfactory) deduct 6 points
For each procedural step (◆) marked U (Unsatisfactory) deduct 20 points

Score calculation 100 points

− points missed

Total score	1st	2nd	3rd

Satisfactory score: 85 or above

SELF-EVALUATION

Chapter 37

Coding

CHAPTER FOCUS

Numerical codes are used in various ways in the medical office, but primarily as a standard means of identifying diagnoses and procedures for insurance companies. Although the subject of coding is complex enough to be studied on its own, medical assistants must have a basic understanding of how it is done, especially for the most common procedures done in the medical office. In this chapter you learned how to look up and use ICD-9-CM diagnostic codes, as well as CPT-4 and HCPCS procedure codes.

TERMINOLOGY REVIEW

Vocabulary Matching: Match each term with its definition.

___ 1. morphology

___ 2. evaluation and management

___ 3. panel

___ 4. coordination of care

___ 5. starred procedure

___ 6. nonessential modifiers

___ 7. comprehensive

___ 8. established patient

A. Includes complete medical history and physical examination

B. A level of E/M service involving planning with other providers

C. A patient who has had services performed by the provider within the last three years

D. The section where CPT codes for office visits provided by primary-care doctors and specialists are found

E. Includes the affected body system as well as other symptomatic or affected body systems

F. Words that may occur in the diagnosis, but are not required

G. A two- or five-digit addition to a CPT code

H. Structure and form

___	9. surgery package	I.	Abnormal growth of tissue
___	10. neoplasm	J.	Group of laboratory tests usually ordered together
___	11. problem focused	K.	History or physical examination that only addresses the chief complaint
___	12. expanded problem focused	L.	A surgical procedure that is not bundled and submitted as a surgery package
___	13. modifier	M.	A group of bundled services, including the surgery, anesthesia, and normal, uncomplicated follow-up
___	14. new patient	N.	A patient who has not had services performed by the provider in the previous three years

Abbreviations: Expand each abbreviation to its complete form.

1. CPT-4 ______________________________
2. E/M ______________________________
3. HCFA ______________________________
4. HCPCS ______________________________
5. NEC ______________________________
6. NOS ______________________________
7. ICD-9-CM ______________________________
8. WHO ______________________________

Matching: Choose the letter of the type of code for which each of the following descriptions is true. Each answer may be used more than once.

___ 1. Consists only of five numbers without a decimal
___ 2. Used to code the patient's diagnosis
___ 3. Contains three levels of codes
___ 4. A two-digit modifier added to the code, gives more information
___ 5. Consists of three digits, often followed by a decimal point and one to two digits
___ 6. Contains codes describing evaluation and management
___ 7. Used to bill Medicare for supplies, materials, and injections
___ 8. E codes are used to classify external causes of injuries and poisoning

A. ICD-9-CM
B. CPT-4
C. HCPCS

CONTENT REVIEW QUESTIONS

1. Describe the history of the International Classification of Disease coding system

___

___

___

2. Describe how and when the Current Procedural Terminology and HCPCS coding systems developed.

___

___

___

3. What types of services are covered in the Evaluation and Management section of the CPT-4 coding system?

___

___

___

4. Identify the seven factors that affect the level of service when identifying E/M codes.

   a. ___

   b. ___

   c. ___

   d. ___

   e. ___

   f. ___

   g. ___

5. Give a general statement that identifies when a code can be chosen that will provide more reimbursement for a patient visit.

___

___

___

6. What is a modifier for a CPT code and how is it used? What is its format?

___

___

___

7. When is a single code used to indicate a surgery package (including routine preoperative and postoperative care)? When is the office allowed to bill separately for surgery, anesthesia, and follow-up?

8. What are the four subsections of the Radiology section of the CPT manual?

   a.

   b.

   c.

   d.

9. When coding for chemistry screens such as an SMA-12 or SMA-24, can the coder use a separate code for each test in the screen (i.e., 12 codes or 24 codes)? Why or why not?

10. What types of procedures are included in the Medicine section of the CPT manual?

11. Describe the steps to look up a procedure code properly.

12. Describe the three levels of HCPCS codes.

    a.

    b.

    c.

13. Give several examples of services that require HCPCS codes.

14. What is the format of ICD-9-CM codes?

15. Identify what types of diagnosis codes begin with the following letters:

    a. V-codes

    b. E-codes

    c. M-codes

16. Describe the steps to look up a diagnosis code properly.

CRITICAL THINKING QUESTIONS

1. Identify a general guideline for coding the patient's diagnosis from a patient medical record.

2. Insurance companies often refuse to pay for medical services when the procedures are not justified by the diagnosis. Discuss what this means in your own words. What is the role of the medical assistant in avoiding this situation?

3. Discuss the benefits to the medical practice if coding is done accurately and carefully. Discuss the pitfalls if codes are used that are not justified by information contained in the medical record (even if they accurately reflect service given).

____

____

____

____

____

____

PRACTICAL APPLICATIONS

ICD-9-CM Codes: Identify the correct codes for the following diagnoses to at least four-digit specificity.

1. Viral pneumonia ______________________________
2. Benign prostatic hypertrophy with post-void dribbling (2 codes)

   ______________________________ ______________________________
3. Chronic otitis media ______________________________
4. Osteoarthritis of the left hip ______________________________
5. Acute pyelonephritis ______________________________
6. Acute appendicitis ______________________________
7. Morbid obesity ______________________________
8. Closed fracture of shaft of the third metacarpal of the left hand ______________________________ caused by accidentally striking a table ______________________________
9. Normal pregnancy visit, first pregnancy ______________________________
10. Abscess of Bartholin's gland ______________________________
11. Nontoxic multinodular goiter ______________________________
12. Left hemiplegia ______________________________
13. First-degree atrioventricular heart block ______________________________
14. Chronic obstructive asthma ______________________________
15. Bunion of right foot ______________________________

CPT-4 Codes: Identify the correct procedure codes.

1. New patient seen in the office for gradual onset of joint pain (polyarthralgia), reddened areas on face covering the nose and surrounding cheek area, and decreased circulation to fingers, especially in cold weather. The physician performed a complete history and review of systems and an extended examination of the patient's musculoskeletal, cardiovascular, and integumentary systems.

   Management of the patient required moderate decision-making.

   ____

2. Follow-up visit in the office for a patient with asthma requiring minor adjustment of medication, although the patient is generally doing well.

____

3. Office visit for an established patient with arteriosclerotic heart disease who is now complaining of increasing frequency of chest tightness during and after exercise. The cardiovascular history was reviewed and the cardiovascular system was examined, with referral to a cardiologist.

____

4. An established patient is seen in the office for the second in a series of three hepatitis B injections given by the nurse.

____

5. A family practice physician requests a consult for a 30-year-old woman with a large and uncomfortable bunion on her right foot. The orthopedic surgeon performs a problem-focused history and problem-focused physical examination, and recommends outpatient bunionectomy at the patient's convenience.

____

6. A new patient is seen in the office for a sore throat with fever. The history is problem focused, the examination is problem focused, and the decision-making is straightforward. __________
7. A patient receives a 12-lead EKG in the medical office. __________
8. The physician performs a flexible sigmoidoscopy on a patient in the special procedure room of the office suite. No problems are identified. __________
9. The medical assistant performs a dipstick urinalysis. __________
10. The medical assistant performs a rapid strep test. __________
11. The patient receives a chest x-ray with two views (AP and lateral). __________
12. The patient receives a urine culture and colony count. __________
13. Blood is drawn during the office visit and sent to the hospital laboratory. __________
14. The patient has a wart frozen with liquid nitrogen (4 mm). __________
15. The patient receives an intramuscular injection of antibiotic. __________

HCPCS Codes

1. The patient receives a pair of wooden underarm crutches. __________
2. Injection of ceftriaxone sodium 250 mg. __________
3. The patient receives an electric heating pad, moist. __________
4. Trimming of dystrophic toenails. __________
5. Injection iron dextran, 50 mg. __________

PROCEDURE PERFORMANCE CHECKLISTS

Procedure 37-1: Looking Up a CPT-4 Code

Performance Objective

Task: Look up the proper CPT-4 code

Conditions: Patient's medical record, charge slip, CPT-4 manual

Standards: Complete the procedure in 5 minutes, and achieve a satisfactory score on the procedure performance checklist

Scoring Key: (**S**)*atisfactory,* (**U**)*nsatisfactory,* (**NA**) *Not Applicable*
◆ *Denotes a critical element for a satisfactory score on the procedure*

Procedure Steps	1st trial	2nd trial	3rd trial
1. Find the name of the procedure to look up, and information about the procedure (if necessary) using patient charge slip.			
2. For evaluation and management (E/M) services, identify if the patient is a new or established patient.			
3. For E/M services, identify if patient was seen in the office or at another location.			
4. Using the index at the back of the manual, locate the section in which the category of codes is found.			
5. Look in the manual at the code or range of codes to find the description of the service.			
6. If the service is unusual or does not seem to fit the description of the code completely, check the list of modifiers.			
7. Enter the correct code(s) on the charge slip or encounter form.			
8. The code entered is the same as that identified by the evaluator. ◆			
9. Complete the procedure within 5 minutes. ◆			

Evaluator Comments:

Score Calculation:

For each procedural step marked U (Unsatisfactory) deduct 6 points
For each procedural step (◆) marked U (Unsatisfactory) deduct 20 points

Score calculation	100 points			
	− points missed	1st	2nd	3rd
	Total score			

Satisfactory score: 85 or above

Procedure 37-2: Looking Up a HCPCS Code

Performance Objective

Task: Look up the proper HCPCS code for a service or piece of equipment

Conditions: Patient medical record, charge slip, HCPCS manual

Standards: Complete the procedure in 5 minutes, and achieve a satisfactory score on the procedure performance checklist

Scoring Key: (**S**)*atisfactory,* (**U**)*nsatisfactory,* (**NA**) *Not Applicable*
◆ *Denotes a critical element for a satisfactory score on the procedure*

Procedure Steps	1st trial	2nd trial	3rd trial
1. Refer to the charge slip and/or medical record to locate the service, supplies, or equipment requiring a HCPCS code.			
2. Using the index at the back of the manual, locate the section in which the category of codes is found.			
3. Look in the manual at the code, or range of codes, to find the description and determine the correct code.			
4. If the service is unusual or does not seem to fit the description of the code completely, check the list of modifiers.			
5. Enter the correct code(s) on the charge slip or encounter form.			
6. The code entered is the same as that identified by the evaluator. ◆			
7. Complete the procedure within 5 minutes. ◆			

Evaluator Comments:

Score Calculation:

For each procedural step marked U (Unsatisfactory) deduct 6 points
For each procedural step (◆) marked U (Unsatisfactory) deduct 20 points

Score calculation 100 points
− points missed

	1st	2nd	3rd
Total score			

Satisfactory score: 85 or above

Notes

Procedure 37-3: Looking Up an ICD-9-CM Code

Performance Objective

Task: Look up the proper ICD-9-CM code to describe a patient's diagnosis

Conditions: Medical record, charge slip, ICD-9-CM manual

Standards: Complete the procedure in 5 minutes, and achieve a satisfactory score on the procedure performance checklist

Scoring Key: (**S**)*atisfactory,* (**U**)*nsatisfactory,* (**NA**) *Not Applicable*
◆ *Denotes a critical element for a satisfactory score on the procedure*

Procedure Steps	1st trial	2nd trial	3rd trial
1. Refer to the patient charge slip and/or medical record to identify the diagnosis.			
2. Decide on the key word or phrase to look for the code in the list of diseases (Volume 2).			
3. Locate the key word and look for the body part or other distinguishing factors.			
4. Identify all possible code number(s).			
5. Locate all number(s) in the tabular list (Volume 1).			
6. Review the information given in the tabular list and select the correct four-digit code.			
7. Add a fifth digit if required.			
8. Enter the correct code(s) on the charge slip or encounter form.			
9. The code entered is the same as that identified by the evaluator. ◆			
10. Complete the procedure within 5 minutes. ◆			

Evaluator Comments:

Score Calculation:

For each procedural step marked U (Unsatisfactory) deduct 6 points
For each procedural step (◆) marked U (Unsatisfactory) deduct 20 points

Score calculation 100 points

− points missed

Total score

1st	2nd	3rd

Satisfactory score: 85 or above

SELF-EVALUATION

Chapter 38

Health Insurance

CHAPTER FOCUS

In this chapter you learned about health insurance and how to submit insurance claim forms. Although this is a highly complex topic, medical assistants need to understand how insurance claims are generated and processed, because many decisions about medical care are based on how care will be reimbursed and what types of services patients are eligible for. Proper submission of insurance claims and management of outstanding claims is vital for the economic health of the medical practice.

TERMINOLOGY REVIEW

Vocabulary Matching: Match each term with its definition.

___ 1. CHAMPVA

___ 2. exclusive provider organization (EPO)

___ 3. independent practice association (IPA)

___ 4. Medicaid

A. A private insurance policy purchased in addition to Medicare that pays medical costs not covered by Medicare

B. An HMO in which the health plan hires the doctors directly and pays them a salary for providing health care to members

C. Insurance to cover lost wages and the cost of medical treatment for workers injured on the job, or who fall ill due to workplace hazards

D. The federally financed health insurance program that pays for medical services provided to dependent spouses and children of military veterans with service-connected disabilities

___ 5. Medicare	E. A plan in which an organization of doctors pays providers on a fee-for-service basis and maintains contracts with a network of providers-similar to network HMO
___ 6. Medigap	F. The health insurance program that pays for medical services provided to the poor
___ 7. network model HMO	G. The federally financed health insurance program to provide medical care in the private sector for dependent spouses and children of active-duty military personnel—formerly CHAMPUS
___ 8. staff model HMO	H. An organization in which the doctors work independently in the community, but formally organize a physician association
___ 9. TRICARE	I. An HMO in which the health plan contracts with two or more group practices to provide health care services
___ 10. workers' compensation	J. The federally financed health insurance program that pays for medical services provided to the elderly, disabled, and those with end-stage kidney disease

Abbreviations: Expand each abbreviation to its complete form

1. DRG ______________________________
2. EOB ______________________________
3. SOF ______________________________
4. POS ______________________________
5. PPO ______________________________
6. RBRVS ______________________________

Definitions: Insert the correct word to complete the sentence

1. If a patient is covered by both Medicare and Medicaid, Medicare is the primary insurer. The type of claim that is automatically sent to Medicaid after processing by Medicare is called a ______________ ______________.
2. The insurance company that writes the medical insurance policy is called the insurance ______________.
3. A private insurance company that processes Medicare and/or Medicaid claims for the Health Care Financing Agency is called a ______________ ______________.
4. ______________ ______ ______________ allows the medical provider to bill the insurance company and receive payment directly rather than having the patient pay for the service and then seek reimbursement.

5. The small, fixed-dollar amount, which must be paid by a patient under managed care each time he or she visits a doctor's office or fills a prescription is called a ____________________.
6. When the insurance company pays the primary care provider a set amount of money for managing all of an individual's health care needs in a given time period, the payment method is called ____________________.
7. The individual who is the beneficiary of a medical insurance policy is called the ____________________.
8. The rules insurance companies use to coordinate the payments for medical services so that no more than 100 percent of the charge is paid for an insurance claim is called ____________________ ________ ____________________.
9. The money paid to purchase health insurance is called the ____________________.
10. When the insurance company pays the provider all or part of the charge(s) for service(s) provided, as long as the charge is usual, customary, and reasonable, the payment method is called ____________________ ________ ____________________.
11. Various types of health maintenance organizations are known collectively as ____________________ ____________________.
12. An amount of money that must be paid for services provided every year before insurance begins to pay for services is called a ____________________.
13. ____________________ is an insurance policy held by a spouse or partner that pays for any portion of charges not covered by a person's primary insurance.
14. A percentage of the doctor's fee or allowable charge paid by the patient after a deductible has been met is called ____________________.
15. The ____________________ ____________________ determines whether the insurance of the father or the mother covers the child if both parents obtain insurance through their employers.

CONTENT REVIEW QUESTIONS

1. Identify three ways for individuals and families to obtain health insurance coverage.
   a. ____
   b. ____
   c. ____
2. What is the tax advantage to obtaining health insurance through the employer?

   ____

   ____

   ____

3. If both parents have health insurance through their employers, what determines which parent's insurance is primary for their children? Is it the same if the parents are divorced?

____

____

____

4. What are three ways that fee-for-service insurance plans determine the amount they will pay for services?

   a. ____

   b. ____

   c. ____

5. The primary insured person under a fee-for-service insurance plan is called a _______________; if the person belongs to an HMO, he or she is called a _______________.

6. What is the function of the primary care provider under a health maintenance organization?

____

____

____

7. Describe four types of HMOs.

   a. ____

   ____

   b. ____

   ____

   c. ____

   ____

   d. ____

   ____

8. Describe three types of managed care that combine features of HMOs and traditional insurance plans.

   a. ____

   ____

   b. ____

   ____

   c. ____

   ____

9. Identify three differences between Medicare Part A and Medicare Part B.

a. ______________________________

b. ______________________________

c. ______________________________

10. What are Medicare Part B payments based on and how is the allowable charge calculated?

____

____

____

11. What part of the bill for services is the patient covered by Medicare Part B responsible for if the physician participates in the Medicare program? If the physician does not participate?

____

____

____

12. If a patient is covered by Medicaid insurance, what portion of the bill is the patient responsible for?

____

____

13. What additional services are covered by Medicaid that other health insurance is usually not responsible for?

____

____

14. Why do some physicians refuse to accept Medicaid patients?

____

____

15. What are CHIPS?

____

____

16. Describe who purchases workers' compensation insurance and when claims must be filed to this program.

____

____

____

17. Why is a separate medical record established for a patient who is being treated for a work-related injury or illness?

____

____

18. Describe who receives benefits under the government TRICARE plan, and describe the three levels of service briefly.

____

____

____

19. What group of people is covered by CHAMPVA?

____

____

20. Identify the three boxes on the HCFA-1500 form that require signatures, who must sign, and what each signature authorizes. What can replace the signature for each?

a. _______________

b. _______________

c. _______________

21. What are recommendations for completing insurance forms to facilitate optical scanning?

____

____

____

22. Describe the two basic types of reimbursement from insurance companies:

a. _______________

____

b. _______________

____

PRACTICAL APPLICATIONS

1. In the Swann family, the mother has insurance from her own employment (individual plan) and the father has insurance from his employment (family plan). The mother's birthday is January 31 and her husband's birthday is May 10. Whose insurance is the primary insurance and whose is the secondary insurance (if any) for each of the following family members?

a. mother primary insurance: _______________

secondary insurance: _______________

b. father primary insurance: _______________

secondary insurance: _______________

c. son primary insurance: _______________

secondary insurance: _______________

d. daughter primary insurance: _______________

secondary insurance: _______________

2. In the McGrath family, the mother has insurance from her own employment (family plan) and the father has insurance from his employment (family plan). The mother's birthday is January 31 and her husband's birthday is May 10. Whose insurance is the primary insurance and whose is the secondary insurance (if any) for each of the following family members?

   a. mother — primary insurance: ______________________

   secondary insurance: ______________________

   b. father — primary insurance: ______________________

   secondary insurance: ______________________

   c. son — primary insurance: ______________________

   secondary insurance: ______________________

   d. daughter — primary insurance: ______________________

   secondary insurance: ______________________

3. Eleanor Whitby is 68 and her husband, Jeremy Whitby, is 69. Eleanor is a retired office worker with Medicare (Part A and Part B) and a Medigap insurance policy, which she purchases on her own. Jeremy is covered by Medicare Part A since he is over 65, but he is still employed full-time and has health insurance from his employer (individual policy). Which is the primary and which is the secondary insurance (if any) for each?

   a. Eleanor — primary insurance: ______________________

   secondary insurance: ______________________

   b. Jeremy (hospital charges) — primary insurance: ______________________

   secondary insurance: ______________________

   c. Jeremy (office charges) — primary insurance: ______________________

   secondary insurance: ______________________

4. Using the five encounter forms you prepared in Chapter 36, add diagnosis codes using the following information:

June St. Cyr	Arteriosclerosis Wound, open, on hand, piercing skin
Robert Ricigliano	Angina pectoris on exertion Hypertension, benign Benign prostatic hypertrophy (hyperplasia of the prostate) Post void dribbling
Marie Richards	Inflammatory polyarthritis Erythema of face Raynaud's syndrome R/O rheumatoid arthritis R/O systemic lupus erythematosis
Mary Ann St. Cyr	Asthma
James Winston	Atrioventricular heart block, first degree Angina pectoris on exertion

5. After completing the encounter forms, use them and the ledger cards if necessary to complete insurance forms for each of the above patients, manually using the forms at the end of this section.

6. Enter the diagnosis information into the Lytec computer program on the CD-ROM for these patients using the tutorial in Appendix B, and print an insurance form for each patient to check your work.

7. Use the CD-ROM and complete an insurance form for each of the case studies presented in Cases 3 and 4 and the Administrative Skills section from the main menu. You may also complete these forms manually using forms in Appendix A of this book

PLEASE DO NOT STAPLE IN THIS AREA

APPROVED OMB-0938-0008

CARRIER

PICA

HEALTH INSURANCE CLAIM FORM

PICA

1. MEDICARE (Medicare #) MEDICAID (Medicaid #) CHAMPUS (Sponsor's SSN) CHAMPVA (VA File #) GROUP HEALTH PLAN (SSN or ID) FECA BLK LUNG (SSN) OTHER (ID)

1a. INSURED'S I.D. NUMBER (FOR PROGRAM IN ITEM 1)

2. PATIENT'S NAME (Last Name, First Name, Middle Initial)

3. PATIENT'S BIRTH DATE MM DD YY SEX M F

4. INSURED'S NAME (Last Name, First Name, Middle Initial)

5. PATIENT'S ADDRESS (No., Street)

6. PATIENT RELATIONSHIP TO INSURED Self Spouse Child Other

7. INSURED'S ADDRESS (No., Street)

CITY STATE

8. PATIENT STATUS Single Married Other

CITY STATE

ZIP CODE TELEPHONE (Include Area Code) ( )

Employed Full-Time Student Part-Time Student

ZIP CODE TELEPHONE (INCLUDE AREA CODE) ( )

9. OTHER INSURED'S NAME (Last Name, First Name, Middle Initial)

10. IS PATIENT'S CONDITION RELATED TO:

11. INSURED'S POLICY GROUP OR FECA NUMBER

a. OTHER INSURED'S POLICY OR GROUP NUMBER

a. EMPLOYMENT? (CURRENT OR PREVIOUS) YES NO

a. INSURED'S DATE OF BIRTH MM DD YY SEX M F

b. OTHER INSURED'S DATE OF BIRTH MM DD YY SEX M F

b. AUTO ACCIDENT? PLACE (State) YES NO

b. EMPLOYER'S NAME OR SCHOOL NAME

c. EMPLOYER'S NAME OR SCHOOL NAME

c. OTHER ACCIDENT? YES NO

c. INSURANCE PLAN NAME OR PROGRAM NAME

d. INSURANCE PLAN NAME OR PROGRAM NAME

10d. RESERVED FOR LOCAL USE

d. IS THERE ANOTHER HEALTH BENEFIT PLAN? YES NO *If yes,* return to and complete item 9 a-d.

READ BACK OF FORM BEFORE COMPLETING & SIGNING THIS FORM.

12. PATIENT'S OR AUTHORIZED PERSON'S SIGNATURE I authorize the release of any medical or other information necessary to process this claim. I also request payment of government benefits either to myself or to the party who accepts assignment below.

SIGNED ______ DATE ______

13. INSURED'S OR AUTHORIZED PERSON'S SIGNATURE I authorize payment of medical benefits to the undersigned physician or supplier for services described below.

SIGNED ______

PATIENT AND INSURED INFORMATION

14. DATE OF CURRENT: MM DD YY ILLNESS (First symptom) OR INJURY (Accident) OR PREGNANCY(LMP)

15. IF PATIENT HAS HAD SAME OR SIMILAR ILLNESS. GIVE FIRST DATE MM DD YY

16. DATES PATIENT UNABLE TO WORK IN CURRENT OCCUPATION FROM MM DD YY TO MM DD YY

17. NAME OF REFERRING PHYSICIAN OR OTHER SOURCE

17a. I.D. NUMBER OF REFERRING PHYSICIAN

18. HOSPITALIZATION DATES RELATED TO CURRENT SERVICES FROM MM DD YY TO MM DD YY

19. RESERVED FOR LOCAL USE

20. OUTSIDE LAB? YES NO $ CHARGES

21. DIAGNOSIS OR NATURE OF ILLNESS OR INJURY. (RELATE ITEMS 1,2,3 OR 4 TO ITEM 24E BY LINE)

1. ___ . ___ 3. ___ . ___

2. ___ . ___ 4. ___ . ___

22. MEDICAID RESUBMISSION CODE ORIGINAL REF. NO.

23. PRIOR AUTHORIZATION NUMBER

24.	A DATE(S) OF SERVICE From MM DD YY To MM DD YY	B Place of Service	C Type of Service	D PROCEDURES, SERVICES, OR SUPPLIES (Explain Unusual Circumstances) CPT/HCPCS MODIFIER	E DIAGNOSIS CODE	F $ CHARGES	G DAYS OR UNITS	H EPSDT Family Plan	I EMG	J COB	K RESERVED FOR LOCAL USE
1											
2											
3											
4											
5											
6											

25. FEDERAL TAX I.D. NUMBER SSN EIN

26. PATIENT'S ACCOUNT NO.

27. ACCEPT ASSIGNMENT? (For govt. claims, see back) YES NO

28. TOTAL CHARGE $

29. AMOUNT PAID $

30. BALANCE DUE $

31. SIGNATURE OF PHYSICIAN OR SUPPLIER INCLUDING DEGREES OR CREDENTIALS (I certify that the statements on the reverse apply to this bill and are made a part thereof.)

SIGNED DATE

32. NAME AND ADDRESS OF FACILITY WHERE SERVICES WERE RENDERED (If other than home or office)

33. PHYSICIAN'S, SUPPLIER'S BILLING NAME, ADDRESS, ZIP CODE & PHONE #

PIN# GRP#

PHYSICIAN OR SUPPLIER INFORMATION

(APPROVED BY AMA COUNCIL ON MEDICAL SERVICE 8/88)

PLEASE PRINT OR TYPE

FORM HCFA-1500 (12-90) FORM OWCP-1500 FORM RRB-1500

PLEASE DO NOT STAPLE IN THIS AREA

APPROVED OMB-0938-0008

CARRIER

PICA

HEALTH INSURANCE CLAIM FORM

PICA

1. MEDICARE (Medicare #) MEDICAID (Medicaid #) CHAMPUS (Sponsor's SSN) CHAMPVA (VA File #) GROUP HEALTH PLAN (SSN or ID) FECA BLK LUNG (SSN) OTHER (ID)

1a. INSURED'S I.D. NUMBER (FOR PROGRAM IN ITEM 1)

2. PATIENT'S NAME (Last Name, First Name, Middle Initial)

3. PATIENT'S BIRTH DATE MM DD YY SEX M F

4. INSURED'S NAME (Last Name, First Name, Middle Initial)

5. PATIENT'S ADDRESS (No., Street)

6. PATIENT RELATIONSHIP TO INSURED Self Spouse Child Other

7. INSURED'S ADDRESS (No., Street)

CITY STATE

8. PATIENT STATUS Single Married Other Employed Full-Time Student Part-Time Student

CITY STATE

ZIP CODE TELEPHONE (Include Area Code) ( )

ZIP CODE TELEPHONE (INCLUDE AREA CODE) ( )

9. OTHER INSURED'S NAME (Last Name, First Name, Middle Initial)

10. IS PATIENT'S CONDITION RELATED TO:

11. INSURED'S POLICY GROUP OR FECA NUMBER

a. OTHER INSURED'S POLICY OR GROUP NUMBER

a. EMPLOYMENT? (CURRENT OR PREVIOUS) YES NO

a. INSURED'S DATE OF BIRTH MM DD YY SEX M F

b. OTHER INSURED'S DATE OF BIRTH MM DD YY SEX M F

b. AUTO ACCIDENT? PLACE (State) YES NO

b. EMPLOYER'S NAME OR SCHOOL NAME

c. EMPLOYER'S NAME OR SCHOOL NAME

c. OTHER ACCIDENT? YES NO

c. INSURANCE PLAN NAME OR PROGRAM NAME

d. INSURANCE PLAN NAME OR PROGRAM NAME

10d. RESERVED FOR LOCAL USE

d. IS THERE ANOTHER HEALTH BENEFIT PLAN? YES NO *If yes*, return to and complete item 9 a-d.

READ BACK OF FORM BEFORE COMPLETING & SIGNING THIS FORM.

12. PATIENT'S OR AUTHORIZED PERSON'S SIGNATURE I authorize the release of any medical or other information necessary to process this claim. I also request payment of government benefits either to myself or to the party who accepts assignment below.

SIGNED DATE

13. INSURED'S OR AUTHORIZED PERSON'S SIGNATURE I authorize payment of medical benefits to the undersigned physician or supplier for services described below.

SIGNED

PATIENT AND INSURED INFORMATION

14. DATE OF CURRENT: MM DD YY ILLNESS (First symptom) OR INJURY (Accident) OR PREGNANCY(LMP)

15. IF PATIENT HAS HAD SAME OR SIMILAR ILLNESS. GIVE FIRST DATE MM DD YY

16. DATES PATIENT UNABLE TO WORK IN CURRENT OCCUPATION FROM MM DD YY TO MM DD YY

17. NAME OF REFERRING PHYSICIAN OR OTHER SOURCE

17a. I.D. NUMBER OF REFERRING PHYSICIAN

18. HOSPITALIZATION DATES RELATED TO CURRENT SERVICES FROM MM DD YY TO MM DD YY

19. RESERVED FOR LOCAL USE

20. OUTSIDE LAB? YES NO $ CHARGES

21. DIAGNOSIS OR NATURE OF ILLNESS OR INJURY. (RELATE ITEMS 1,2,3 OR 4 TO ITEM 24E BY LINE)

1. ___ . __

2. ___ . __

3. ___ . __

4. ___ . __

22. MEDICAID RESUBMISSION CODE ORIGINAL REF. NO.

23. PRIOR AUTHORIZATION NUMBER

24. A DATE(S) OF SERVICE From MM DD YY To MM DD YY	B Place of Service	C Type of Service	D PROCEDURES, SERVICES, OR SUPPLIES (Explain Unusual Circumstances) CPT/HCPCS MODIFIER	E DIAGNOSIS CODE	F $ CHARGES	G DAYS OR UNITS	H EPSDT Family Plan	I EMG	J COB	K RESERVED FOR LOCAL USE
1										
2										
3										
4										
5										
6										

25. FEDERAL TAX I.D. NUMBER SSN EIN

26. PATIENT'S ACCOUNT NO.

27. ACCEPT ASSIGNMENT? (For govt. claims, see back) YES NO

28. TOTAL CHARGE $

29. AMOUNT PAID $

30. BALANCE DUE $

31. SIGNATURE OF PHYSICIAN OR SUPPLIER INCLUDING DEGREES OR CREDENTIALS (I certify that the statements on the reverse apply to this bill and are made a part thereof.)

SIGNED DATE

32. NAME AND ADDRESS OF FACILITY WHERE SERVICES WERE RENDERED (If other than home or office)

33. PHYSICIAN'S, SUPPLIER'S BILLING NAME, ADDRESS, ZIP CODE & PHONE #

PIN# GRP#

PHYSICIAN OR SUPPLIER INFORMATION

(APPROVED BY AMA COUNCIL ON MEDICAL SERVICE 8/88)

PLEASE PRINT OR TYPE

FORM HCFA-1500 (12-90) FORM OWCP-1500 FORM RRB-1500

PLEASE DO NOT STAPLE IN THIS AREA

APPROVED OMB-0938-0008

CARRIER

PICA

HEALTH INSURANCE CLAIM FORM

PICA

1. MEDICARE (Medicare #) MEDICAID (Medicaid #) CHAMPUS (Sponsor's SSN) CHAMPVA (VA File #) GROUP HEALTH PLAN (SSN or ID) FECA BLK LUNG (SSN) OTHER (ID)

1a. INSURED'S I.D. NUMBER (FOR PROGRAM IN ITEM 1)

2. PATIENT'S NAME (Last Name, First Name, Middle Initial)

3. PATIENT'S BIRTH DATE MM DD YY SEX M F

4. INSURED'S NAME (Last Name, First Name, Middle Initial)

5. PATIENT'S ADDRESS (No., Street)

6. PATIENT RELATIONSHIP TO INSURED Self Spouse Child Other

7. INSURED'S ADDRESS (No., Street)

CITY STATE

8. PATIENT STATUS Single Married Other

CITY STATE

ZIP CODE TELEPHONE (Include Area Code) ( )

Employed Full-Time Student Part-Time Student

ZIP CODE TELEPHONE (INCLUDE AREA CODE) ( )

9. OTHER INSURED'S NAME (Last Name, First Name, Middle Initial)

10. IS PATIENT'S CONDITION RELATED TO:

11. INSURED'S POLICY GROUP OR FECA NUMBER

a. OTHER INSURED'S POLICY OR GROUP NUMBER

a. EMPLOYMENT? (CURRENT OR PREVIOUS) YES NO

a. INSURED'S DATE OF BIRTH MM DD YY SEX M F

b. OTHER INSURED'S DATE OF BIRTH MM DD YY SEX M F

b. AUTO ACCIDENT? PLACE (State) YES NO

b. EMPLOYER'S NAME OR SCHOOL NAME

c. EMPLOYER'S NAME OR SCHOOL NAME

c. OTHER ACCIDENT? YES NO

c. INSURANCE PLAN NAME OR PROGRAM NAME

d. INSURANCE PLAN NAME OR PROGRAM NAME

10d. RESERVED FOR LOCAL USE

d. IS THERE ANOTHER HEALTH BENEFIT PLAN? YES NO *If yes*, return to and complete item 9 a-d.

READ BACK OF FORM BEFORE COMPLETING & SIGNING THIS FORM.

12. PATIENT'S OR AUTHORIZED PERSON'S SIGNATURE I authorize the release of any medical or other information necessary to process this claim. I also request payment of government benefits either to myself or to the party who accepts assignment below.

SIGNED DATE

13. INSURED'S OR AUTHORIZED PERSON'S SIGNATURE I authorize payment of medical benefits to the undersigned physician or supplier for services described below.

SIGNED

PATIENT AND INSURED INFORMATION

14. DATE OF CURRENT: MM DD YY ILLNESS (First symptom) OR INJURY (Accident) OR PREGNANCY(LMP)

15. IF PATIENT HAS HAD SAME OR SIMILAR ILLNESS. GIVE FIRST DATE MM DD YY

16. DATES PATIENT UNABLE TO WORK IN CURRENT OCCUPATION FROM MM DD YY TO MM DD YY

17. NAME OF REFERRING PHYSICIAN OR OTHER SOURCE

17a. I.D. NUMBER OF REFERRING PHYSICIAN

18. HOSPITALIZATION DATES RELATED TO CURRENT SERVICES FROM MM DD YY TO MM DD YY

19. RESERVED FOR LOCAL USE

20. OUTSIDE LAB? YES NO $ CHARGES

21. DIAGNOSIS OR NATURE OF ILLNESS OR INJURY. (RELATE ITEMS 1,2,3 OR 4 TO ITEM 24E BY LINE)

1. ___ . __

2. ___ . __

3. ___ . __

4. ___ . __

22. MEDICAID RESUBMISSION CODE ORIGINAL REF. NO.

23. PRIOR AUTHORIZATION NUMBER

24. A DATE(S) OF SERVICE From MM DD YY To MM DD YY	B Place of Service	C Type of Service	D PROCEDURES, SERVICES, OR SUPPLIES (Explain Unusual Circumstances) CPT/HCPCS MODIFIER	E DIAGNOSIS CODE	F $ CHARGES	G DAYS OR UNITS	H EPSDT Family Plan	I EMG	J COB	K RESERVED FOR LOCAL USE
1										
2										
3										
4										
5										
6										

25. FEDERAL TAX I.D. NUMBER SSN EIN

26. PATIENT'S ACCOUNT NO.

27. ACCEPT ASSIGNMENT? (For govt. claims, see back) YES NO

28. TOTAL CHARGE $

29. AMOUNT PAID $

30. BALANCE DUE $

31. SIGNATURE OF PHYSICIAN OR SUPPLIER INCLUDING DEGREES OR CREDENTIALS (I certify that the statements on the reverse apply to this bill and are made a part thereof.)

SIGNED DATE

32. NAME AND ADDRESS OF FACILITY WHERE SERVICES WERE RENDERED (If other than home or office)

33. PHYSICIAN'S, SUPPLIER'S BILLING NAME, ADDRESS, ZIP CODE & PHONE #

PIN# GRP#

PHYSICIAN OR SUPPLIER INFORMATION

(APPROVED BY AMA COUNCIL ON MEDICAL SERVICE 8/88)

PLEASE PRINT OR TYPE

FORM HCFA-1500 (12-90) FORM OWCP-1500 FORM RRB-1500

PLEASE DO NOT STAPLE IN THIS AREA

APPROVED OMB-0938-0008

CARRIER

PICA

HEALTH INSURANCE CLAIM FORM

PICA

PATIENT AND INSURED INFORMATION

1. MEDICARE (Medicare #) MEDICAID (Medicaid #) CHAMPUS (Sponsor's SSN) CHAMPVA (VA File #) GROUP HEALTH PLAN (SSN or ID) FECA BLK LUNG (SSN) OTHER (ID)

1a. INSURED'S I.D. NUMBER (FOR PROGRAM IN ITEM 1)

2. PATIENT'S NAME (Last Name, First Name, Middle Initial)

3. PATIENT'S BIRTH DATE MM DD YY SEX M F

4. INSURED'S NAME (Last Name, First Name, Middle Initial)

5. PATIENT'S ADDRESS (No., Street)

6. PATIENT RELATIONSHIP TO INSURED Self Spouse Child Other

7. INSURED'S ADDRESS (No., Street)

CITY STATE

8. PATIENT STATUS Single Married Other

CITY STATE

ZIP CODE TELEPHONE (Include Area Code) ( )

Employed Full-Time Student Part-Time Student

ZIP CODE TELEPHONE (INCLUDE AREA CODE) ( )

9. OTHER INSURED'S NAME (Last Name, First Name, Middle Initial)

10. IS PATIENT'S CONDITION RELATED TO:

11. INSURED'S POLICY GROUP OR FECA NUMBER

a. OTHER INSURED'S POLICY OR GROUP NUMBER

a. EMPLOYMENT? (CURRENT OR PREVIOUS) YES NO

a. INSURED'S DATE OF BIRTH MM DD YY SEX M F

b. OTHER INSURED'S DATE OF BIRTH MM DD YY SEX M F

b. AUTO ACCIDENT? PLACE (State) YES NO

b. EMPLOYER'S NAME OR SCHOOL NAME

c. EMPLOYER'S NAME OR SCHOOL NAME

c. OTHER ACCIDENT? YES NO

c. INSURANCE PLAN NAME OR PROGRAM NAME

d. INSURANCE PLAN NAME OR PROGRAM NAME

10d. RESERVED FOR LOCAL USE

d. IS THERE ANOTHER HEALTH BENEFIT PLAN? YES NO *If yes*, return to and complete item 9 a-d.

READ BACK OF FORM BEFORE COMPLETING & SIGNING THIS FORM.

12. PATIENT'S OR AUTHORIZED PERSON'S SIGNATURE I authorize the release of any medical or other information necessary to process this claim. I also request payment of government benefits either to myself or to the party who accepts assignment below.

SIGNED ______ DATE ______

13. INSURED'S OR AUTHORIZED PERSON'S SIGNATURE I authorize payment of medical benefits to the undersigned physician or supplier for services described below.

SIGNED ______

PHYSICIAN OR SUPPLIER INFORMATION

14. DATE OF CURRENT: MM DD YY ILLNESS (First symptom) OR INJURY (Accident) OR PREGNANCY(LMP)

15. IF PATIENT HAS HAD SAME OR SIMILAR ILLNESS. GIVE FIRST DATE MM DD YY

16. DATES PATIENT UNABLE TO WORK IN CURRENT OCCUPATION FROM MM DD YY TO MM DD YY

17. NAME OF REFERRING PHYSICIAN OR OTHER SOURCE

17a. I.D. NUMBER OF REFERRING PHYSICIAN

18. HOSPITALIZATION DATES RELATED TO CURRENT SERVICES FROM MM DD YY TO MM DD YY

19. RESERVED FOR LOCAL USE

20. OUTSIDE LAB? YES NO $ CHARGES

21. DIAGNOSIS OR NATURE OF ILLNESS OR INJURY. (RELATE ITEMS 1,2,3 OR 4 TO ITEM 24E BY LINE)

1. ___ . __ 3. ___ . __

2. ___ . __ 4. ___ . __

22. MEDICAID RESUBMISSION CODE ORIGINAL REF. NO.

23. PRIOR AUTHORIZATION NUMBER

24. A DATE(S) OF SERVICE From MM DD YY	To MM DD YY	B Place of Service	C Type of Service	D PROCEDURES, SERVICES, OR SUPPLIES (Explain Unusual Circumstances) CPT/HCPCS MODIFIER	E DIAGNOSIS CODE	F $ CHARGES	G DAYS OR UNITS	H EPSDT Family Plan	I EMG	J COB	K RESERVED FOR LOCAL USE
1											
2											
3											
4											
5											
6											

25. FEDERAL TAX I.D. NUMBER SSN EIN

26. PATIENT'S ACCOUNT NO.

27. ACCEPT ASSIGNMENT? (For govt. claims, see back) YES NO

28. TOTAL CHARGE $

29. AMOUNT PAID $

30. BALANCE DUE $

31. SIGNATURE OF PHYSICIAN OR SUPPLIER INCLUDING DEGREES OR CREDENTIALS (I certify that the statements on the reverse apply to this bill and are made a part thereof.)

SIGNED DATE

32. NAME AND ADDRESS OF FACILITY WHERE SERVICES WERE RENDERED (If other than home or office)

33. PHYSICIAN'S, SUPPLIER'S BILLING NAME, ADDRESS, ZIP CODE & PHONE #

PIN# GRP#

(APPROVED BY AMA COUNCIL ON MEDICAL SERVICE 8/88)

PLEASE PRINT OR TYPE

FORM HCFA-1500 (12-90)
FORM OWCP-1500 FORM RRB-1500

PLEASE DO NOT STAPLE IN THIS AREA

APPROVED OMB-0938-0008

CARRIER

PICA

HEALTH INSURANCE CLAIM FORM

PICA

1. MEDICARE (Medicare #) MEDICAID (Medicaid #) CHAMPUS (Sponsor's SSN) CHAMPVA (VA File #) GROUP HEALTH PLAN (SSN or ID) FECA BLK LUNG (SSN) OTHER (ID)

1a. INSURED'S I.D. NUMBER (FOR PROGRAM IN ITEM 1)

2. PATIENT'S NAME (Last Name, First Name, Middle Initial)

3. PATIENT'S BIRTH DATE MM DD YY SEX M F

4. INSURED'S NAME (Last Name, First Name, Middle Initial)

5. PATIENT'S ADDRESS (No., Street)

6. PATIENT RELATIONSHIP TO INSURED Self Spouse Child Other

7. INSURED'S ADDRESS (No., Street)

CITY STATE

8. PATIENT STATUS Single Married Other

CITY STATE

ZIP CODE TELEPHONE (Include Area Code) ( )

Employed Full-Time Student Part-Time Student

ZIP CODE TELEPHONE (INCLUDE AREA CODE) ( )

9. OTHER INSURED'S NAME (Last Name, First Name, Middle Initial)

10. IS PATIENT'S CONDITION RELATED TO:

11. INSURED'S POLICY GROUP OR FECA NUMBER

a. OTHER INSURED'S POLICY OR GROUP NUMBER

a. EMPLOYMENT? (CURRENT OR PREVIOUS) YES NO

a. INSURED'S DATE OF BIRTH MM DD YY SEX M F

b. OTHER INSURED'S DATE OF BIRTH MM DD YY SEX M F

b. AUTO ACCIDENT? PLACE (State) YES NO

b. EMPLOYER'S NAME OR SCHOOL NAME

c. EMPLOYER'S NAME OR SCHOOL NAME

c. OTHER ACCIDENT? YES NO

c. INSURANCE PLAN NAME OR PROGRAM NAME

d. INSURANCE PLAN NAME OR PROGRAM NAME

10d. RESERVED FOR LOCAL USE

d. IS THERE ANOTHER HEALTH BENEFIT PLAN? YES NO ***If yes,*** return to and complete item 9 a-d.

READ BACK OF FORM BEFORE COMPLETING & SIGNING THIS FORM.

12. PATIENT'S OR AUTHORIZED PERSON'S SIGNATURE I authorize the release of any medical or other information necessary to process this claim. I also request payment of government benefits either to myself or to the party who accepts assignment below.

SIGNED ______ DATE ______

13. INSURED'S OR AUTHORIZED PERSON'S SIGNATURE I authorize payment of medical benefits to the undersigned physician or supplier for services described below.

SIGNED ______

PATIENT AND INSURED INFORMATION

14. DATE OF CURRENT: MM DD YY ILLNESS (First symptom) OR INJURY (Accident) OR PREGNANCY(LMP)

15. IF PATIENT HAS HAD SAME OR SIMILAR ILLNESS. GIVE FIRST DATE MM DD YY

16. DATES PATIENT UNABLE TO WORK IN CURRENT OCCUPATION FROM MM DD YY TO MM DD YY

17. NAME OF REFERRING PHYSICIAN OR OTHER SOURCE

17a. I.D. NUMBER OF REFERRING PHYSICIAN

18. HOSPITALIZATION DATES RELATED TO CURRENT SERVICES FROM MM DD YY TO MM DD YY

19. RESERVED FOR LOCAL USE

20. OUTSIDE LAB? YES NO $ CHARGES

21. DIAGNOSIS OR NATURE OF ILLNESS OR INJURY. (RELATE ITEMS 1,2,3 OR 4 TO ITEM 24E BY LINE)

1. ___ . __

3. ___ . __

2. ___ . __

4. ___ . __

22. MEDICAID RESUBMISSION CODE ORIGINAL REF. NO.

23. PRIOR AUTHORIZATION NUMBER

24. A DATE(S) OF SERVICE From MM DD YY To MM DD YY	B Place of Service	C Type of Service	D PROCEDURES, SERVICES, OR SUPPLIES (Explain Unusual Circumstances) CPT/HCPCS MODIFIER	E DIAGNOSIS CODE	F $ CHARGES	G DAYS OR UNITS	H EPSDT Family Plan	I EMG	J COB	K RESERVED FOR LOCAL USE
1										
2										
3										
4										
5										
6										

25. FEDERAL TAX I.D. NUMBER SSN EIN

26. PATIENT'S ACCOUNT NO.

27. ACCEPT ASSIGNMENT? (For govt. claims, see back) YES NO

28. TOTAL CHARGE $

29. AMOUNT PAID $

30. BALANCE DUE $

31. SIGNATURE OF PHYSICIAN OR SUPPLIER INCLUDING DEGREES OR CREDENTIALS (I certify that the statements on the reverse apply to this bill and are made a part thereof.)

SIGNED DATE

32. NAME AND ADDRESS OF FACILITY WHERE SERVICES WERE RENDERED (If other than home or office)

33. PHYSICIAN'S, SUPPLIER'S BILLING NAME, ADDRESS, ZIP CODE & PHONE #

PIN# GRP#

PHYSICIAN OR SUPPLIER INFORMATION

(APPROVED BY AMA COUNCIL ON MEDICAL SERVICE 8/88)

PLEASE PRINT OR TYPE

FORM HCFA-1500 (12-90) FORM OWCP-1500 FORM RRB-1500

PROCEDURE PERFORMANCE CHECKLISTS

Procedure 38-1: Completing the HCFA-1500 Form for Insurance Reimbursement

Performance Objective

Task: Complete a HCFA-1500 form

Conditions: Patient information, patient account or ledger card, copy of patient insurance card, claim form, typewriter or computer

Standards: Complete the procedure in 15 minutes, and achieve a satisfactory score on the procedure performance checklist

*Scoring Key: (**S**)atisfactory, (**U**)nsatisfactory, (**NA**) Not Applicable*
◆ *Denotes a critical element for a satisfactory score on the procedure*

Procedure Steps	1st trial	2nd trial	3rd trial
1. Assemble information needed to prepare insurance claim.			
2. Enter information as required on the HCFA-1500 form, using capital letters and no punctuation.			
3. Enter the name and address of the insurance company to whom the claim is being sent on top of the form, above the words "Health Insurance Claim Form."			
4. Complete the patient portion of the insurance form using information on the new patient registration form, or from the patient's computerized information form (Boxes 2–6, 8, 10, 12, 13).			
5. Complete the subscriber (insured) portion of the claim form using information found on the copy of the patient's insurance card and/or the new patient information sheet (Boxes 1, 1a, 4, 7, 9, 11).			
6. Complete the physician information on the bottom half of the form using information from the patient's ledger card or computer account (Boxes 14–24).			
7. Complete the remainder of the form using information about the medical practice and information from the patient's ledger card or computer account (Boxes 25–33).			
8. Copy and proofread the form before mailing.			
9. All necessary information is complete and accurate compared to the form filled out by the evaluator or computer program. ◆			
10. Complete the procedure within 15 minutes. ◆			

Evaluator Comments:

Score Calculation:

For each procedural step marked U (Unsatisfactory) deduct 6 points
For each procedural step (◆) marked U (Unsatisfactory) deduct 20 points

Score calculation		100 points	1st	2nd	3rd
	−	points missed			
		Total score			

Satisfactory score: 85 or above

SELF-EVALUATION

Chapter 39

Billing and Collections

CHAPTER FOCUS

Although most doctors' offices request that payment be made at the time a medical service is provided, it is still necessary for the office to send regular bills for services not covered by insurance and to initiate collection activities when bills are not paid promptly. The medical assistant must understand how to determine how long balances have remained unpaid and how to collect an unpaid balance without violating the legal rights of the person who owes money.

TERMINOLOGY REVIEW

Vocabulary Matching: Match each term with its definition.

__ 1. account aging record

__ 2. aging of accounts

__ 3. bankruptcy

__ 4. balance due

__ 5. billing

__ 6. collection agency

__ 7. credit

A. A company that collects overdue bills for other companies

B. Dividing up the total number of bills and sending a portion of them at regular intervals

C. Determining how long specific accounts/balances have been outstanding

D. Civil courts where lawsuits involving small amounts of money are heard

E. The process of sending bills for money that is owed to the practice by individual patients for services provided

F. An account where there is no billing information or incorrect billing information

G. The agreement that allows a patient to set up a schedule of payments of bills, as long as they make a specified monthly payment

__ 8. cycle billing

__ 9. small claims court

__ 10. skip

H. The amount left on a bill after a portion has been paid

I. The record in which accounts that are overdue are recorded

J. A means for an individual or business to "get out from under" a crushing load of debt, either by reorganizing the debts or by liquidating assets and dividing the funds among creditors

CONTENT REVIEW QUESTIONS

1. What information should be on any bill sent to a patient?

____

____

____

2. What are three ways that bills can be produced?

   a. ____

   b. ____

   c. ____

3. If the medical office bills every week, how are patient accounts usually divided?

____

____

____

4. What is the advantage to the office of weekly cycle billing?

____

____

____

5. When is a patient account considered overdue?

____

____

____

6. What are the usual categories of overdue accounts when an account aging record is created?

____

____

7. What is the usual progression in collection activity when a patient's account is overdue?

____

____

____

8. Why is it recommended to place a telephone call regarding an overdue account in addition to placing claim messages on the bill?

____

____

____

9. When does the office need to have a written credit arrangement with a patient?

____

____

____

10. What does a truth-in-lending statement include and when should it be sent to a patient?

____

____

____

11. Identify three methods to try to trace a patient whose bill is returned with the notation "address unknown."

a. _______________

b. _______________

c. _______________

12. If the three methods identified in the previous question fail to locate a "skip," what should the medical office do to try to collect a bill?

____

____

____

13. How should a collection agency payment be entered on the patient's ledger card and on the day sheet?

____

____

____

14. If a patient has died, how and when should the bill for services rendered prior to death be sent?

____

____

____

15. If the bill of a deceased individual is not paid promptly, how should the medical assistant follow up?

____

____

____

16. What is the status of outstanding medical bills if a person declares bankruptcy under Chapter VII? Under Chapter XIII?

____

____

____

CRITICAL THINKING QUESTIONS

1. Discuss the advantages and disadvantages of pursuing unpaid patient accounts in small claims courts. If possible, survey offices in your area and determine how frequently they do this.

____

____

____

____

____

____

2. Describe how you would feel if you were asked to call 12 patients with overdue accounts to discuss payment. What are some techniques you might use to do this professionally? What would you want to avoid saying? How do you feel about individuals who do not pay their medical bills?

____

____

____

____

____

____

3. There is a trend in many parts of the country for medical offices to employ a billing service instead of processing bills and insurance claims in the office. The billing service usually charges a percentage of the accounts receivable (assuming that the larger the amount billed, the more

work is necessary to collect it). What are some of the factors that influence the choice of billing from the office or having the billing done by an outside service?

____

____

____

____

____

____

PRACTICAL APPLICATIONS

1. Create a patient aging report based on information from the accounts of the following patients. Assume that you are creating the report on 11/24 for bills that were sent on 8/1, 9/1, 10/1, and 11/1.

Daryl P. Saitta

Date	Professional Service	Fee	Payment	Adjustment	New Balance
9/4/XX	99202, ROA cash	55.00	20.00		35.00
10/2/XX	ROA ck #219		20.00		15.00

Lloyd Ridlon

Date	Professional Service	Fee	Payment	Adjustment	New Balance
7/15/XX	99204, 93000, ROA ck #664	95.00	15.00		135.00
7/28/00	Ins ck #604 (for 6/15)		128.00		7.00
10/8/XX	99212	48.00	15.00		40.00

Maria Rivera Santos

Date	Professional Service	Fee	Payment	Adjustment	New Balance
10/6/XX	99204, ROA ck #259	135.00	27.00		108.00

Thomas Maxwell

Date	Professional Service	Fee	Payment	Adjustment	New Balance
9/1/XX	99213, 81002, 93000, ROA ck #322	122.00	50.00		72.00
10/12	99212, ROA ck #602	48.00	15.00		105.00
10/15	Ins ck #2298 (for 9/1)		56.00	16.00	33.00

2. Based on the information from the Accounts Aging Record, determine what you should do for each of the following accounts. If a telephone call is warranted, simulate the call with a classmate, then compose a follow-up letter. If a letter demanding collection is needed, compose a letter demanding payment, using the information from the patient ledger card that you created in Chapter 36. Identify how you would send the collection letter.

   Daryl Saitta ______________________________

   Lloyd Ridlon ______________________________

   Marie Rivera Santos ______________________________

   Thomas Maxwell ______________________________

3. Using the Lytec billing program on the CD-ROM, print patient statements for the following patients for their visits on 10/12/XX. Instructions are found in Appendix C.

   June St. Cyr
   Robert Ricigliano
   Marie Richards
   Mary Ann St. Cyr
   James Winston

4. Create an accounts aging report using the Lytec program following the instructions in Appendix C.

Blackburn Primary Care Associates
Patient Account Aging Report

		Current	Past	Past	Past	Past	Total Balance
Patient Name	**Last Payment**	0 - 30	31 - 60	61 - 90	91 -120	121+	

Procedure 39-1: Creating and Examining an Accounts Aging Record

Performance Objective

Task: Create and examine an accounts aging record

Conditions: Patient account ledgers, accounts aging record analysis form, pen or computer

Standards: Complete the procedure in 20 minutes, and achieve a satisfactory score on the procedure performance checklist

Scoring Key: (**S**)*atisfactory,* (**U**)*nsatisfactory,* (**NA**) *Not Applicable*
◆ *Denotes a critical element for a satisfactory score on the procedure*

Procedure Steps	1st trial	2nd trial	3rd trial
1. Assemble all ledgers with outstanding balances.			
2. For each account with an outstanding balance, record the amount still owed (in the column that describes the length of time it has been owed since the first bill was sent).			
3. If the office uses computerized accounting, request that the program print out a report on accounts aging for patients and one for insurance companies.			
4. Separate accounts with unpaid insurance claims from bills that insurance has already paid, and disregard those with unpaid claims.			
5. For accounts that are 31–60 days old, attach a note or sticker to the bill to remind the patient that payment is due.			
6. For accounts that are 61–90 days old, telephone the patient and discuss how and when the patient will pay the bill (or part of the bill).			
7. For bills that are 91–120 days old, set aside to send a collection letter demanding payment unless there are special circumstances that warrant a delay.			
8. Review accounts over 120 days old, and unless there are special circumstances that warrant a delay, set them aside to send a collection letter stating that the account will be turned over to a collection agency unless paid promptly.			
9. Review actions with the doctor or billing manager before mailing letters.			

Procedure Steps	1st trial	2nd trial	3rd trial
10. Complete the procedure within 20 minutes. ◆			
11. Write follow-up letters including letters to document in writing any agreements made during telephone conversations.			
12. Record all action taken on the back of the ledger card.			

Charting

DATE	

Evaluator Comments:

Score Calculation:

For each procedural step marked U (Unsatisfactory) deduct 6 points
For each procedural step (◆) marked U (Unsatisfactory) deduct 20 points

Score calculation 100 points

− points missed

Total score

1st	2nd	3rd

Satisfactory score: 85 or above

Procedure 39-2: Writing a Collection Letter

Performance Objective

Action: Compose a collection letter

Conditions: Accounts aging record, patient ledgers for patients with accounts that are 91–120 days old, letterhead stationery, envelope, computer or typewriter

Standards: Complete the procedure in 20 minutes, and achieve a satisfactory score on the procedure performance checklist

Scoring Key: (**S**)*atisfactory,* (**U**)*nsatisfactory,* (**NA**) *Not Applicable*
◆ *Denotes a critical element for a satisfactory score on the procedure*

Procedure Steps	1st trial	2nd trial	3rd trial
1. After the account record has been created, determine which accounts need letters.			
2. Review each account for the amount due, how long it has been due, any previous activity, and special circumstances.			
3. Prepare a letter for each outstanding account, except those due from a patient's estate, an insurance company, or a patient who has special circumstances.			
4. State the amount due in the letter.			
5. Include how long the balance has been due in the letter.			
6. Identify a date (usually 10 days from the date of the letter) when the balance should be paid in full.			
7. State the substance of any discussions you have had with the person who owes the balance and/or any agreements you have made.			
8. Prepare an envelope.			
9. The letter contains all information, is formatted as a business letter and does not contain any typographical or spelling errors. ◆			
10. The envelope is formatted correctly and does not contain any typographical or spelling errors. ◆			
11. Have the doctor sign the letter.			
12. Make a copy of the letter for the patient's file and a copy for the collection follow-up file.			
13. Complete the procedure within 20 minutes. ◆			

Evaluator Comments:

Score Calculation:

For each procedural step marked U (Unsatisfactory) deduct 6 points
For each procedural step (◆) marked U (Unsatisfactory) deduct 20 points

Score calculation	100 points			
	− points missed	1st	2nd	3rd
	Total score			

Satisfactory score: 85 or above

SELF-EVALUATION

J

K

M

G

E
F

N
A
S
P

international law

administrative law

common law

criminal law

statutory law

UNIT 9

From Student to Professional Medical Assistant

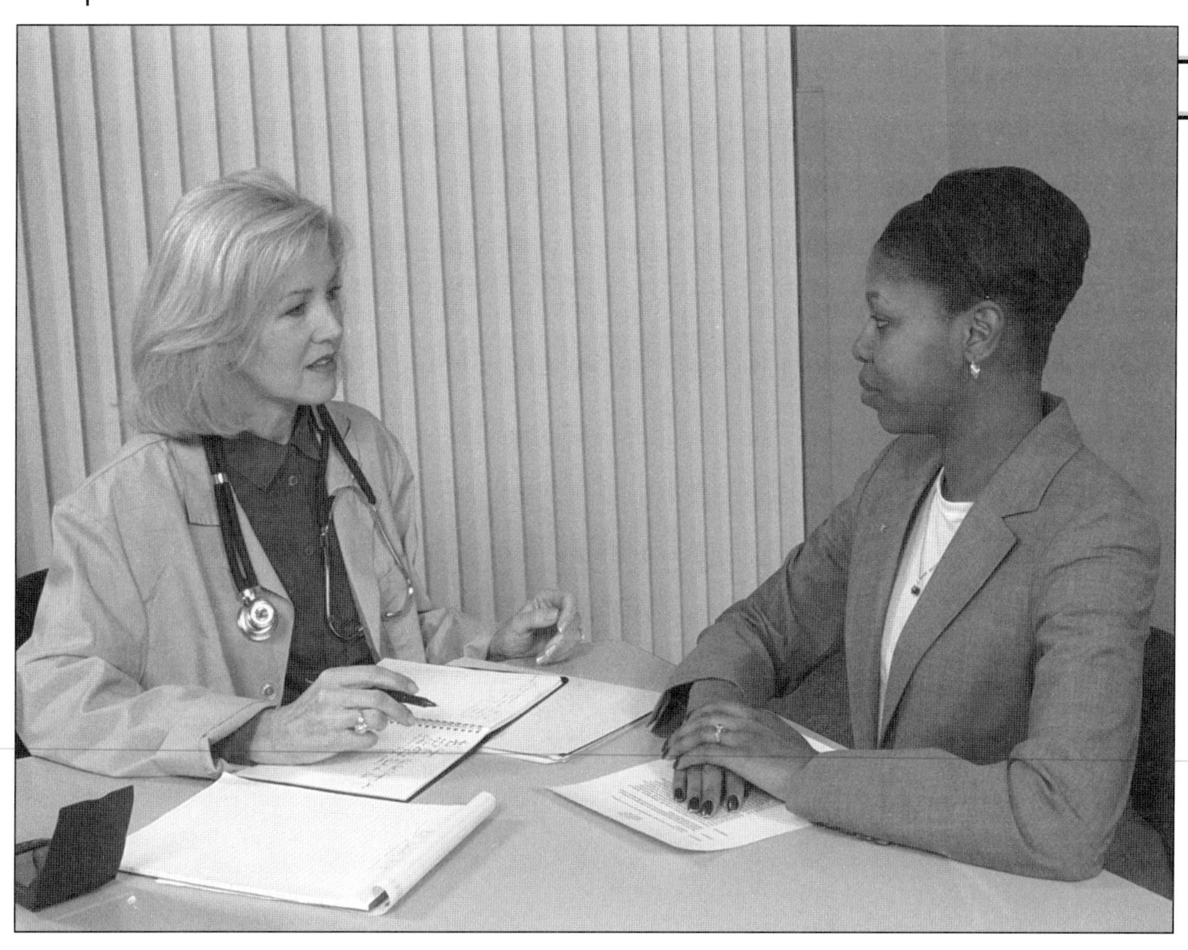

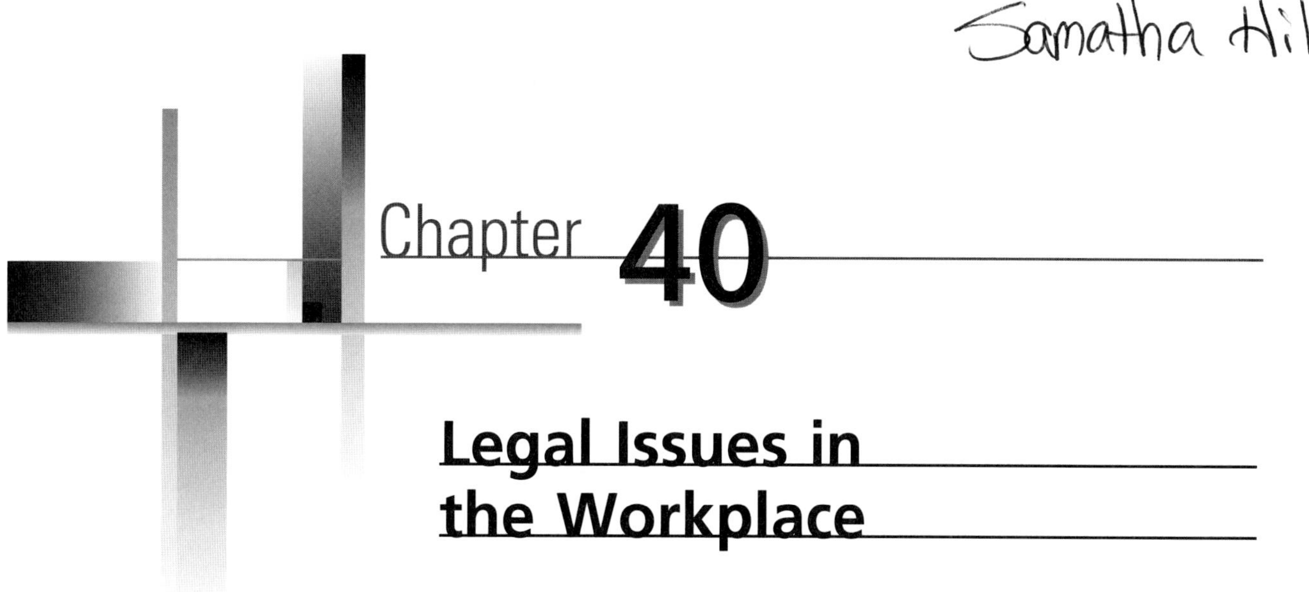

Chapter 40

Legal Issues in the Workplace

CHAPTER FOCUS

Although the law and how it influences the medical assistant have already been discussed earlier in this book, as a medical assistant you should still know more as you prepare to enter the workplace. This chapter provides additional information about the American legal system, litigation, and legal issues that relate to the medical office as a business.

TERMINOLOGY REVIEW

Vocabulary Matching: Match each term with its definition.

____ 1. precedent

____ 2. litigation

____ 3. revocation

____ 4. discovery

____ 5. arbitration

____ 6. statute of limitations

____ 7. appeal

____ 8. *res ipsa loquitur*

____ 9. complaint

A. A court order requiring an individual to make himself or herself available to be deposed or testify in court

B. A request for a hearing from a higher court, usually on the basis that the legal process in the lower court was faulty

C. A process where a neutral party attempts to settle a legal dispute

D. A written statement listing the claims against a person or facility

E. An attorney's fee, paid only if a plaintiff collects a damage award.

F. When an injured person has played a part in causing his or her injury

G. The party against whom a lawsuit is brought

H. Oral testimony taken, under oath, by a court reporter at a location outside the courtroom

I. The process of gathering information to prepare for a trial

J 10. expert witness

K 11. interrogatory

M 12. subpoena *duces tecum*

G 13. defendant

E 14. contingency

F 15. contributory negligence

H 16. deposition

N 17. plaintiff

A 18. subpoena

S 19. statute

P 20. privilege

J. An uninvolved expert who is hired to give a professional opinion

K. A written set of questions that must be answered, under oath, within a specific time period.

L. The process of taking a lawsuit or criminal case through the courts

M. A court order requiring that documents or other physical evidence be made available to the court

N. The party bringing a legal action

O. A decision made by a court in the past that is used as the basis for a decision in the present

P. A special right or permission granted to a certain group of individuals

Q. "The thing speaks for itself"

R. Permanent cancellation

S. An individual law or group of related laws

T. The time limit during which a person can initiate a lawsuit

Definitions: Insert the correct words to complete the sentence.

1. The law based on treaties and other agreements between and among two or more counties is called international law.
2. administrative law establishes administrative agencies of the federal government, and describes their powers and procedures.
3. common law is based on the individual decisions of a court, rather than on specific statutes.
4. The branch of statutory law that deals with offenses against the public welfare is called criminal law.
5. The body of laws enacted by a legislative body with the power to make laws is called statutory law.

Civil or criminal law? Enter the letter of the type of law to which the term is most likely to refer. Each letter can be used more than once.

C 1. crime

C 2. misfeasance

A 3. misdemeanor

C 4. malpractice

B 5. nonfeasance

A 6. tort

B 7. embezzlement

A 8. felony

B 9. fraud

A. Criminal

B. Civil

C. Both civil and criminal

___ 10. manslaughter
___ 11. malfeasance
___ 12. negligence
___ 13. larceny
___ 14. assault and battery

CONTENT REVIEW QUESTIONS

1. Are decisions in court cases based on statutory law, common law, or a combination of both? Explain your answer.

____
____
____
____
____
____

2. Describe two classifications of crimes.
   a. Felony - which is a serious crime / death or imprisonment
   b. misdemeanor - less serious crime / Fine or imprisonment for less than a year

3. Give four examples of mandated reports.
   a. ____
   b. ____
   c. ____
   d. ____

4. If a physician is convicted of a crime such as fraud, how may it affect the physician's license to practice medicine?

____
____
____
____

5. Describe each of the following crimes, and identify how each might occur in a medical office.
   a. Wrongful death ____
   ____
   b. Embezzlement Appropriating funds from client, customer or employer
   c. Fraud deliberate deception carried out to secure unlawful gain

6. Give an example of breach of contract that might occur in the medical office.

7. When a person initiates a civil lawsuit for a tort or breach of contract, what is the usual purpose of the lawsuit?

8. What is the major difference between an intentional tort and an unintentional tort?

9. Describe the following defenses against a charge of an intentional tort.

   a. Privilege

   b. Consent

   c. Self-defense

   d. Error

10. Describe how each of the following can be used as a defense against a charge of negligence.

    a. Statute of limitations

    b. Contributory or comparative negligence

    c. Assumption of risk

11. If a patient initiates a lawsuit against a physician or group practice, why must the patient sign a document releasing the doctor from the requirement of patient confidentiality?

____

____

____

12. What should a physician do promptly when notified that an attorney is requesting medical records?

____

____

____

13. Describe the following steps in the process of a civil lawsuit.

a. Filing a complaint _______________

____

b. Formal discovery _______________

____

c. Pretrial conference _______________

____

d. Trial _______________

____

e. Judgment _______________

____

f. Appeal _______________

____

14. Describe three types of damages that may be awarded in a civil lawsuit.

a. _______________

b. _______________

c. _______________

15. Describe two additional ways of settling a dispute in addition to using the court system.

a. _______________

____

b. _______________

____

16. If a patient is unsatisfied with the care he or she receives from an HMO, can the patient sue the doctor? The HMO? Why or why not?

____

____

____

____

17. Identify one advantage and one disadvantage for each of the following business forms for a medical practice.

a. Sole proprietorship

Advantage ______________________________

Disadvantage ______________________________

b. Partnership

Advantage ______________________________

Disadvantage ______________________________

c. Corporation

Advantage ______________________________

Disadvantage ______________________________

18. Describe three ways that doctors may be paid for their work.

a. ______________________________

____

b. ______________________________

____

c. ______________________________

____

19. How are medical assistants usually paid for their work? Describe common benefits.

____

____

____

20. Identify six types of insurance that the medical practice may purchase to protect the business and employees.

a. ______________________________

b. ______________________________

c. ______________________________

d. ______________________________

e. ___

f. ___

21. What employee rights are protected by the following laws?

a. Equal Opportunity Employment laws

___

___

b. Americans with Disabilities Act

___

___

c. Family and Medical Leave Act

___

___

d. Fair Labor Standards Act

___

___

e. Employee Retirement Income Security Act

Regulates employee benefit plans

___

CRITICAL THINKING QUESTIONS

1. If a patient suffers an injury while hospitalized, the patient may initiate a lawsuit against the physician or other person who caused the injury, and against the hospital, under legal precedent. There is an underlying assumption that the hospital is responsible for ensuring that the care provided by physicians and staff is not negligent. A patient is not allowed to sue his or her HMO if the doctor failed to provide adequate care or if the HMO itself refused to pay for care that the physician recommended. Discuss this issue and its implications for the cost of insurance and for patient care.

___

___

___

___

___

___

___

___

2. Discuss the possibility of a patient bringing a lawsuit against a medical assistant and the consequences of such a lawsuit. Include a discussion of the types of injury that might occur from a medical assistant's actions, the standard of care that the medical assistant might be held to, the expenses the medical assistant might incur during and after the legal case, and the implications for the medical assistant's financial status and career.

3. Discuss how a medical office might implement measures to be sure that sexual harassment is minimized and that it is correctly responded to if an allegation of sexual harassment occurs.

SELF-EVALUATION

Chapter 41

Managing the Office

CHAPTER FOCUS

Although a medical assistant may not have management responsibilities in an entry-level position, he or she must still understand the role and duties of the manager in the medical office. Effective management sets the tone and creates an environment in which employees can work effectively as team members.

TERMINOLOGY REVIEW

Vocabulary Matching: Match each term with its definition.

___	1. minutes	A. Person who works for a business or professional service practice, such as a medical office
___	2. net pay	B. Covered by insurance to reimburse the employer in the event of unforeseen financial loss because of an employee's actions
___	3. policy	C. A guiding principle for management of an office or business
___	4. bonded	D. A description of the steps needed to handle a specific situation or perform a certain task
___	5. agenda	E. A list of specific items of business to be covered in a meeting
___	6. Social Security	F. A meeting scheduled with a departing employee to achieve a sense of closure
___	7. employee	G. The national program of retirement benefits into which non-government workers pay a percentage of their income

___ 8. procedure	H. The salary or wage paid during a pay period, before taxes and withholdings for benefits are taken out
___ 9. gross pay	I. The salary or wage paid during a pay period, after taxes and withholdings for benefits are taken out
___ 10. memorandum	J. Written summaries of meeting discussions and recommendations
___ 11. exit interview	K. The form of written communication usually used within an organization instead of letters

CONTENT REVIEW QUESTIONS

1. Identify six management functions of the individual who supervises personnel in the medical office.

   a. ______________________________

   b. ______________________________

   c. ______________________________

   d. ______________________________

   e. ______________________________

   f. ______________________________

2. How can staff meetings help create an environment for teamwork?

   ____

   ____

   ____

   ____

3. Describe two methods used to prepare meeting participants, keep a meeting running smoothly, and keep track of decisions made during the meeting.

   a. ______________________________

   ____

   b. ______________________________

   ____

4. Identify three methods to recruit new staff when a medical office has a job vacancy.

   a. ______________________________

   b. ______________________________

   c. ______________________________

5. Identify six types of information that should be included in any job posting.

a. ____________________

b. ____________________

c. ____________________

d. ____________________

e. ____________________

f. ____________________

6. Identify four topics that should be discussed at a job interview.

a. ____________________

b. ____________________

c. ____________________

d. ____________________

7. Describe how and when a specific salary is offered for a position.

____

____

____

8. After one candidate has accepted a position, how should the person in charge of hiring follow up with other applicants?

____

____

____

9. What must the supervisor do when a new employee begins work?

____

____

____

____

10. When should employees receive performance evaluations and what should they consist of?

____

____

____

11. Describe how an organization might document an ongoing pattern of unsatisfactory job performance before terminating an employee.

____

____

____

____

12. When preparing payroll checks for employees, what five items of information must be recorded in the payroll record for each employee?

a. ______

b. ______

c. ______

d. ______

e. ______

13. Differentiate between a policy and a procedure.

______

______

______

14. Identify three reasons that it is important for organizations to have procedure manuals available.

a. ______

b. ______

c. ______

15. Describe the medical assistant's role if an office is involved in clinical trials or other research.

______

______

______

16. How might a medical assistant assist a physician to prepare a presentation?

______

______

______

______

CRITICAL THINKING QUESTIONS

1. If you think you would like to move into medical office management, discuss how you would try to prepare yourself to assume increasing responsibility in the area of management.

______

______

______

______

______

______

2. Discuss the reasons that preparation of payroll might be contracted to an outside service instead of being done within an organization. Are the reasons the same or different from those resulting in the use of an outside billing company?

PRACTICAL APPLICATIONS

1. Find advertisements for medical assistants and/or other office personnel in your local newspaper. How are each of the following described in the advertisement that most appeals to you?

   a. Job title

   b. Type of medical office

   c. Duties

   d. Full- or part-time

   e. Type of benefits

   f. Hours of work

   g. Qualifications

   h. Method of contacting the employer

2. Write a newspaper advertisement to find a part-time medical assistant to assist one of the physicians at Blackburn Primary Care Associates on Tuesdays and Thursdays from 10:30 AM until the office closes (usually around 6:00 PM). You would prefer a candidate with experience and certification.

____

____

____

3. If a recent graduate of a medical assisting program was one of the best-qualified candidates for the position described in Question 2, identify four questions that would be important to ask during a job interview.

   a. ____

   b. ____

   c. ____

   d. ____

4. Create a memorandum on a word processor or computer to inform office staff that the following topics will be discussed at the weekly staff meeting on Thursday, March 16: the proposed change from cloth to paper gowns and drapes, and vacation requests for the summer. Staff meetings are regularly held in the break room at 9:00 AM before patients are scheduled.

SELF-EVALUATION

Chapter 42

Biomedical Ethics

CHAPTER FOCUS

Biomedical ethics examines issues that guide how scientific research is carried out and how medicine is practiced. Although ethics is an abstract discipline, the ability to make moral and responsible choices is vital for a medical assistant. This ability is based on an understanding of historical factors, science, and social thinking about ethical choices.

TERMINOLOGY REVIEW

Vocabulary Matching: Match each term with its definition.

___ 1. deontological

___ 2. biomedical ethics

___ 3. veracity

___ 4. autonomy

___ 5. etiquette

___ 6. fidelity

___ 7. teleological

A. The right to make decisions about one's health care according to individual values and concerns, without constraint or coercion

B. The concept of doing the best possible

C. Ethical theories that require the individual to make ethical decisions largely without respect to the consequences

D. An attempt to establish what is right and what is wrong through the use of systematic thinking

E. The standards or customs of a culture or social group

F. Being faithful; in the case of medical practice, faithful to reasonable expectations

G. The concept that means doing no harm in any medical treatment given

___ 8. ethics	H. Theories of ethics that begin by considering the consequences of choices (rather than absolute principles)
___ 9. utilitarianism	I. The ethical theory that defines the best action as the one that does the most good for the largest number of people
___ 10. beneficence	J. The concept of sharing truthful information without having to be asked
___ 11. nonmalfeasance	K. The examination of issues related to how biomedical research is carried out and how medical care is provided

CONTENT REVIEW QUESTIONS

1. Identify four reasons why medical assisting students can benefit from studying about ethics and bioethics.

   a. ______________________________

   b. ______________________________

   c. ______________________________

   d. ______________________________

2. What do deontological ethical theories try to provide? Give an example.

   ____

   ____

   ____

   ____

3. What do teleological ethical theories try to provide? Give an example.

   ____

   ____

   ____

   ____

4. What is the advantage of a combination theory of ethics?

   ____

   ____

   ____

   ____

5. What is the relationship between law and ethics in a democracy?

______

______

______

______

6. Identify five sources of beliefs about the rights and duties of individuals and society as a whole in the United States.

a. ______

b. ______

c. ______

d. ______

e. ______

7. Describe briefly what is included in each of the following rights:

a. Right to life ______

______

b. Right to privacy ______

______

c. Right to autonomy ______

______

d. Right to the means to sustain life ______

______

8. Identify five duties of a health professional.

a. ______

b. ______

c. ______

d. ______

e. ______

9. When does ethical conflict arise?

______

______

______

10. Identify six steps that can be used to make ethical decisions when different choices carry moral weight.

a. ______

b. ______

c. ______

d. ______________________________

e. ______________________________

f. ______________________________

11. When is it important for more than one person to agree about a decision that has ethical connotations? Give an example.

12. If a medical assistant is thinking about reporting a coworker to the supervisor because the coworker is drinking excessive amounts of alcohol during the lunch hour, what rights and values are in conflict? What duties may the medical assistant have trouble meeting if the situation is not resolved?

13. If patients participate in medical research, what guidelines should be followed?

14. Identify several ways that ethical controversy has arisen about genetic engineering.

15. How are the options for abortion expanded with the introduction of mifepristone (RU-486)?

16. What issues are raised for society as a whole by *in vitro* fertilization techniques?

17. What is the basis for ethical conflict regarding assisted suicide?

____

____

____

____

18. Briefly discuss four areas in which decisions must be made about the best use of scarce medical resources.

a. _______________

b. _______________

c. _______________

d. _______________

CRITICAL THINKING QUESTIONS

1. Select one of the following statements for investigation. Do research about the topic to obtain information. Write a short paper giving information to support or disagree with the statement and using the results of your research to back up your position. With your instructor's approval, you may identify a different topic. Be sure to give credit for ideas and/or statistics that you have obtained from a book, journal article, or Internet article.

   a. The Food and Drug Administration should allow the production of genetically engineered food if it is demonstrated to be safe for human consumption, but all products containing genetically engineered material should be clearly labeled.

   b. The government should pass laws to prohibit further experiments in human cloning.

   c. Medical research and financial investment should remain separate. Universities and foundations should not allow research in situations where professors or researchers have a financial interest in companies supporting the research.

   d. Larger fines and stronger penalties should be imposed on drug companies that do not publish information about harmful side effects of medications, because these companies may think it is worth concealing problems resulting in injury to people taking the medications.

   e. Mifepristone (RU-486) should not have been approved for use in the United States.

2. Describe what you would consider the ethical action in each of the following situations and give reasons for your choice.

   a. You find your brother, who is 12 years old, smoking a cigarette in the backyard.

   ____

   ____

   ____

   ____

b. You are raped and become pregnant at the age of 18.

____

____

____

____

c. A relative with whom you are very close has a chronic condition causing muscle weakness. He begs you to help him "end everything."

____

____

____

____

d. Your sister has been married for eight years and has not been able to become pregnant using artificial insemination. She and her husband both want children more than anything. She suggests, only half joking, that you might want to be a surrogate for her.

____

____

____

____

SELF-EVALUATION

Chapter 43

Professionalism: From Externship to Employment

CHAPTER FOCUS

The final step in your training is to apply what you have learned during an externship in a physician's office or clinic. This is an opportunity for you to perform a medical assisting role with help and supervision. At the end of the externship, you may take a certification examination (if your educational program is accredited) and prepare to look for a job. This chapter provides information to help you carry out these final steps of your education process.

TERMINOLOGY REVIEW

Vocabulary Matching: Match each term with its definition.

___ 1. Certified Medical Assistant (CMA)

___ 2. networking

___ 3. Registered Medical Assistant (RMA)

___ 4. burnout

___ 5. resume

___ 6. internship

A. A letter accompanying a resume that explains briefly why the resume is being sent

B. Practical experience a student receives in an facility other than the educational institution

C. Practical experience a student receives within a learning institution

D. Using people you know to explore job opportunities

E. A summary of information about a person that describes education, work experience, and other information an employer wants to know

F. A medical assistant who has passed the certification examination given by the American Association of Medical Assistants

___ 7. continuing education unit (CEU)

___ 8. cover letter

___ 9. externship

G. A medical assistant who has passed the examination given by the American Medical Technologists

H. Disillusionment with work or school and loss of interest or enthusiasm

I. The classes and other educational programs attended regularly in order to maintain licensure or certification

CONTENT REVIEW QUESTIONS

1. What is a medical assisting externship?

____

____

____

____

2. Because the student in a medical assisting externship is not an employee, what are the implications for the student and the office providing the externship?

____

____

____

____

3. List seven ways that a student can work to ensure a successful externship experience.

   a. ____

   b. ____

   c. ____

   d. ____

   e. ____

   f. ____

   g. ____

4. What is the difference between a certificate, certification, and licensure?

____

____

____

____

5. Identify two organizations that validate the knowledge of a medical assistant and the credentials that the medical assistant can use if each organization's certification exam is passed.

   a. Organization ______________________ Credential ______________________

   b. Organization ______________________ Credential ______________________

6. Identify four benefits for members of a national professional organization.

   a. ____

   b. ____

   c. ____

   d. ____

7. Describe three styles of resumes.

   a. ____

   b. ____

   c. ____

8. List in order the steps you would use (or have used) to prepare a resume.

____

____

____

____

9. What is the advantage to a medical assisting student of using a category labeled RELATED HEALTH CARE EXPERIENCE instead of WORK EXPERIENCE on a resume?

____

____

____

10. What is the purpose of a cover letter when sending out resumes?

____

____

____

11. What are the advantages and disadvantages of faxing a resume?

____

____

____

12. In addition to a resume, what information should the medical assistant bring when applying for a job?

____

____

____

13. Identify six specific ways that the medical assistant can make a favorable impression during a job interview.

a. ______________________________

b. ______________________________

c. ______________________________

d. ______________________________

e. ______________________________

f. ______________________________

14. What kinds of questions might a medical assistant ask during a job interview?

____

____

____

15. What kind of follow-up is appropriate after a job interview?

____

____

____

16. Identify three specific actions you can take if you think that you may be experiencing job burnout?

a. ______________________________

b. ______________________________

c. ______________________________

17. In what areas may medical assistants need continuing education to keep their skills current?

____

____

____

18. Identify four routes that a medical assistant may take to advance his or her career.

a. ______________________________

b. ______________________________

c. ______________________________

d. ______________________________

CRITICAL THINKING QUESTIONS

1. Discuss potential problems and possible actions by the student if the following situations occur in a medical office where the student is on externship.

   a. Two staff members are making negative comments about a patient out of range of the patient's hearing but so that the medical assisting student can overhear the conversation. The patient is a relative of the student.

   b. While eating lunch in the break room of the medical office, the medical assisting student expresses to an employee of the office that she feels like the office takes advantage of her for "free work."

   c. The medical assisting student is told by the office manager not to use gloves for phlebotomy or injections because the physician doesn't want the patients to feel like the office staff thinks they may be infected with AIDS.

   d. The student is assigned to spend about half the time in the office, where she does her externship filing reports and charts. The student feels frustrated because she wants a more varied experience.

2. Prepare a personalized and thoughtful response to each of the following questions, which you might be asked during a job interview.

   a. Where do you see yourself in five years?

   b. Describe a difficult situation you have had at work and how you handled it.

   c. What could you contribute to our office?

   d. What are some of your weaknesses or areas you need to work on?

   e. What would your medical assisting instructor say about you if I were to call her for a reference?

PRACTICAL APPLICATIONS

1. Identify the Web site address for the following organizations, and determine if and when you will be eligible to take their certification examinations.

   American Association of Medical Assistants ______________________

   American Medical Technologists ______________________

2. Complete the following information worksheet to prepare your resume.

   a. Identify the kind of job(s) you are looking for:

   First choice

   ____

   Second choice

   ____

   b. Summarize your education, beginning with your most recent:

   Name of school

   ____

   City ____________ State ____________

   Dates attended: ______/ ______/ ______ to ______/ ______/ ______

   Degree: ____________ Date: ______/ ______/ ______

   Major (or courses completed if you did not graduate):

   ____

   ____

   Awards, GPA (if over 3.0), Dean's list (dates):

   ____

   Previous education (beyond high school)

   Name of school

   ____

   City ____________ State ____________

   Dates attended: ______/ ______/ ______ to ______/ ______/ ______

   Degree: ____________ Date: ______/ ______/ ______

   Major (or courses completed if you did not graduate):

   ____

   ____

Awards, GPA (if over 3.0), Dean's list (dates):

____

Other relevant training and dates of completion including first aid training, CPR training, and computer training.

____

____

____

Other skills including foreign languages spoken and skills you have learned but never practiced in an externship or work setting.

____

____

____

c. Summarize your experience in the health care field, beginning with your most recent. Include your medical assisting externship.

Name of organization or physician:

____

City ____________________ State ____________________

Dates of experience: ______/ ______/ ______ to ______/ ______/ ______

Type of experience or job title: ______________________________

Indicate if the following apply: Externship/Coop ________ Volunteer ________

Part-time ________ Summer ________

Identify your duties and responsibilities, one per line. Use a consistent form (i.e., "prepared patients for examinations," or "responsible for preparing patients for examinations").

____

____

____

____

____

____

Identify any special accomplishments, promotions, or other positive outcomes from this position.

____

____

Next most recent health-related experience:

Name of organization or physician:

____

City ____________________ State ____________________

Dates of experience: _______/ _______/ _______ to _______/ _______/ _______

Type of experience or job title: ______________________________________

Indicate if the following apply: Externship/Coop _______ Volunteer _______

Part-time _______ Summer _______

Identify your duties and responsibilities, one per line. Use a consistent form (i.e., "prepared patients for examinations" or "responsible for preparing patients for examinations").

____

____

____

____

____

____

Identify any special accomplishments, promotions, or other positive outcomes from this position.

____

____

Next most recent health-related experience:

Name of organization or physician:

____

City ____________________ State ____________________

Dates of experience: _______/ _______/ _______ to _______/ _______/ _______

Type of experience or job title: ______________________________________

Indicate if the following apply: Externship/Coop _______ Volunteer _______

Part-time _______ Summer _______

Identify your duties and responsibilities, one per line. Use a consistent form (i.e., "prepared patients for examinations" or "responsible for preparing patients for examinations").

____

____

____

____

____

____

Identify any special accomplishments, promotions, or other positive outcomes from this position.

____

____

d. Identify work experience that is not related to health care. Include all full-time jobs, but if you have not been employed consistently, include part-time and/or summer employment, volunteer experience, or time spent as a homemaker.

Employer (or organization):

____

City ____________ State ____________

Dates of experience: _____/ _____/ _____ to _____/ _____/ _____

Type of experience or job title: ____________

Indicate if the following apply: Externship/Coop _____ Volunteer _____

Part-time _____ Summer _____

Identify your duties and responsibilities, one per line. Use a consistent form (i.e., "prepared weekly reports" or "responsible for preparing weekly reports").

____

____

____

____

____

____

Identify any special accomplishments, promotions, or other positive outcomes from this position.

____

____

Next most recent experience:

Employer (or organization):

____

City ________________ State ________________

Dates of experience: _____/ _____/ _____ to _____/ _____/ _____

Type of experience or job title: ___________________________________

Indicate if the following apply: Externship/Coop ________ Volunteer ________

Part-time ________ Summer ________

Identify your duties and responsibilities, one per line. Use a consistent form (i.e., "prepared weekly reports" or "responsible for preparing weekly reports").

Identify any special accomplishments, promotions, or other positive outcomes from this position.

Next most recent experience:

Employer (or organization):

____

City ________________ State ________________

Dates of experience: _____/ _____/ _____ to _____/ _____/ _____

Type of experience or job title: ___________________________________

Indicate if the following apply: Externship/Coop ________ Volunteer ________

Part-time ________ Summer ________

Identify your duties and responsibilities, one per line. Use a consistent form (i.e., "prepared weekly reports" or "responsible for preparing weekly reports").

Identify any special accomplishments, promotions, or other positive outcomes from this position.

3. Complete the following information to help you prepare a cover letter to accompany your resume when you look for a job.

   a. Describe in one sentence the reason that you are currently seeking a job.

   b. Describe the type of position you seek (job title, full-time and/or part-time) and when you will be available to begin working.

   c. Describe your personal qualifications in a few sentences focusing on your strengths as a person as well as your skills.

4. Complete the following information to help you prepare a list of at least three references. If possible, include a supervisor from employment and/or externship and an instructor or coach from your educational program. Indicate whether you have already obtained permission from the person to use him or her as a reference.

   a. Name ______________________ Permission Requested: __________

   This person's relationship to you ______________________

   Contact information:

   Employer: ______________________ Job Title: __________

   Address: ______________________

   ____

   Telephone Number: ______________________

   b. Name ______________________ Permission Requested: __________

   This person's relationship to you ______________________

Contact information:

Employer: ______________________ Job Title: ______________________

Address: ____

____

Telephone Number: ____

c. Name ______________________ Permission Requested: __________

This person's relationship to you ______________________________

Contact information:

Employer: ______________________ Job Title: ______________________

Address: ____

____

Telephone Number: ____

d. Name ______________________ Permission Requested: __________

This person's relationship to you ______________________________

Contact information:

Employer: ______________________ Job Title: ______________________

Address: ____

____

Telephone Number: ____

SELF-EVALUATION

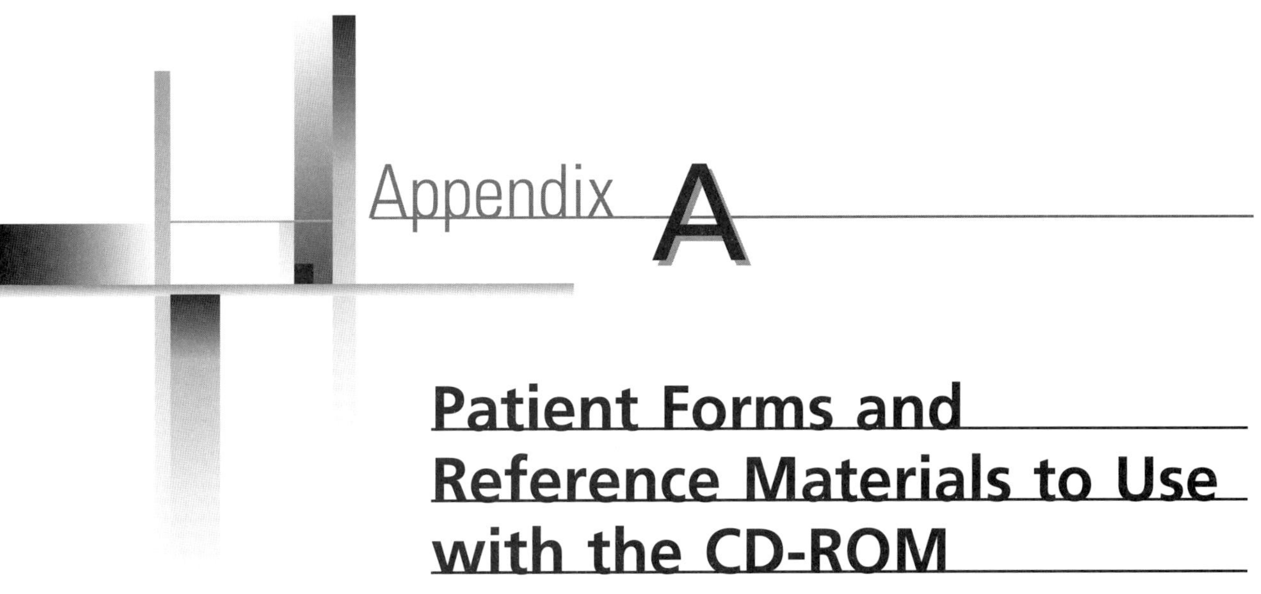

Appendix A

Patient Forms and Reference Materials to Use with the CD-ROM

The following forms are available for students to use in order to reference information or complete forms manually when using the *Virtual Medical Office Challenge* program. Instructions for installing and using the program are found in Appendix E of the textbook: *Saunders Fundamentals of Medical Assisting.*

CASE ONE FORMS:

Form 1: Telephone Message Form
Form 2: Appointment Schedule for Blackburn Primary Care Associates
Form 3: Health History Questionnaire for Ivan Shapiro
Form 4: Patient Information Form for Ivan Shapiro
Form 5: Patient Encounter Form for Ivan Shapiro
Form 6: Blackburn Primary Care Associates Physician's Fee Schedule
Form 7: Blank HCFA-1500 Form for billing Ivan Shapiro's visit

CASE TWO FORM:

Form 8: Progress Note Form for documenting Raymond Johnson's visit

CASE THREE FORMS:

Form 9: Infant Growth and Development Chart for documenting Robin Soto's height and weight
Form 10: Progress Note Form for documenting Robin Soto's visit
Form 11: Patient Information Form for Robin Soto
Form 12: Patient Encounter Form for Robin Soto
Form 13: Blackburn Primary Care Associates Physician's Fee Schedule
Form 14: Blank HCFA-1500 Form for billing Robin Soto's visit

CASE FOUR FORMS:

Form 15: Appointment Schedule for Blackburn Primary Care Associates
Form 16: Health History Questionnaire for Lucille Ferguson
Form 17: Patient Information Form for Lucille Ferguson
Form 18: Patient Encounter Form for Lucille Ferguson
Form 19: Blackburn Primary Care Associates Physician's Fee Schedule
Form 20: Blank HCFA-1500 Form for billing Lucille Ferguson's visit

ADMINISTRATIVE SKILLS FORMS:

Form 21: Patient Information Form for Charles Latham
Form 22: Patient Encounter Form for Charles Latham
Form 23: Blackburn Primary Care Associates Physician's Fee Schedule
Form 24: Blank HCFA-1500 Form for billing Charles Latham's visit
Form 25: Patient Information Form for Marrion Jordon
Form 26: Patient Encounter Form for Marrion Jordon
Form 27: Blackburn Primary Care Associates Physician's Fee Schedule
Form 28: Blank HCFA-1500 Form for billing Marrion Jordon's visit
Form 29: Patient Information Form for Prinnie Minnowitz
Form 30: Patient Encounter Form for Prinnie Minnowitz
Form 31: Blackburn Primary Care Associates Physician's Fee Schedule
Form 32: Blank HCFA-1500 Form for billing Prinnie Minnowitz's visit

Case One, Form 1

Telephone Message Log

NAME OF CALLER | PATIENT'S NAME | AGE | TEMP. | TIME

TELEPHONE NUMBER | PHARMACY | TELEPHONE | CALLED BY: | DATE

COMPLAINT / MESSAGE ☐ PLEASE RETURN THE CALL ☐ WILL CALL AGAIN ☐ RETURNED YOUR CALL ☐ OTHER (SPECIFY) | DOCTOR

INSTRUCTIONS/REPLY:

☐ URGENT
☐ MEDICATION ALLERGY

CALLED BACK: BY: DATE OTHER (SPECIFY)

NAME OF CALLER | PATIENT'S NAME | AGE | TEMP. | TIME

TELEPHONE NUMBER | PHARMACY | TELEPHONE | CALLED BY: | DATE

COMPLAINT / MESSAGE ☐ PLEASE RETURN THE CALL ☐ WILL CALL AGAIN ☐ RETURNED YOUR CALL ☐ OTHER (SPECIFY) | DOCTOR

INSTRUCTIONS/REPLY:

☐ URGENT
☐ MEDICATION ALLERGY

CALLED BACK: BY: DATE OTHER (SPECIFY)

NAME OF CALLER | PATIENT'S NAME | AGE | TEMP. | TIME

TELEPHONE NUMBER | PHARMACY | TELEPHONE | CALLED BY: | DATE

COMPLAINT / MESSAGE ☐ PLEASE RETURN THE CALL ☐ WILL CALL AGAIN ☐ RETURNED YOUR CALL ☐ OTHER (SPECIFY) | DOCTOR

INSTRUCTIONS/REPLY:

☐ URGENT
☐ MEDICATION ALLERGY

CALLED BACK: BY: DATE OTHER (SPECIFY)

Case One, Form 2

Appointment Schedule

DAY: Mon. | Tue. | Wed. | Thu. | Fri. | Sat.

DATE		HUGHES, M.D.	LAWLER, M.D.	LOPEZ, M.D.
8	00			
	10		NO ACUTE	NO NEW
	20		OR	OB
	30		NEW PATIENTS	
9	00	Sx-Blackburn	Johnson, Marvin	
	10	Hosp.	555-921-3195	
	20	Smith,	CPE	
	30	Mariane		
10	00		Seeburn, Kate	Richards, Mary
	10		INFLUENZA 555-817-	↓ PAP 619-3191
	20		↓ FLU 3615	Scheeler, Virginia
	30		Butler, Carl	↓ PAP 721-9951
	40		NEURO ✓ UP	
	50		↓ 555-331-9195	
11	00	Jefferson, Martha	Doyle, Mike 555-	Longfellow, Wilma
	10	NEW OB 555-245-1790	↓ PROSTATE ✓ 277-	PAP, PE
	20		Doyle, Hanah 1965	555-317-2198
	30		↓ ✓ UP	
12	00	Davis, Marvin 555-	HOSPITAL	
	10	↓ ALLERGY 241-9200	ROUNDS	
	20	Martin, Darlene 555-		LUNCH MTG
	30	↓ SUT REM 917-1909		
	40	Sorbin, John 555-		
	50	↓ VACCINES 914-3190		
1	00			Simpson, Lisa
	10			3 MO PRENATAL
	20			↓ 555-129-3190
	30			Schmidt, Cindy
	40			STD 555-377-
	50			↓ 2198
2	00	Docker, Millie 555-219-		
	10	CHEST PAIN 7191		
3	00	Starvey, Jill 555-	AMA Mtg	Jessup, Carl 719-
	10	↓ VACCINES 319-2191	Convention	↓ STRESS EKG 3307
	20		Center	Lawson, Milton 331-
	30		3:30 pm	↓ PROSTATE 9900
4	00	HOSPITAL		Geary, Leon 555-
	10	ROUNDS		↓ VACCINE 498-3150
5	00			MED SOCIETY
	10			MTG
	20			5-7 pm

Form No. 56-7310 © 1977 Bibbero Systems, Inc., Petaluma, CA
Courtesy of Bibbero Systems, Inc., Petaluma, California.

Case One, Form 3

ANDRUS/CLINI-REC® HEALTH HISTORY QUESTIONNAIRE

Chart No. ________

Identification Information

Today's Date ________

Name Shapiro, Ivan   Date of Birth 3/6/45

Occupation Carpenter   Marital Status Married

PART A – PRESENT HEALTH HISTORY

I. CURRENT MEDICAL PROBLEMS

Please list the medical problems for which you came to see the doctor. About when did they begin?

Problems	Date Began
Chest pain when exercising	

What concerns you most about these problems?

If you are being treated for any other illness or medical problems by another physician, please describe the problems and write the name of the physician or medical facility treating you.

Illness or Medical Problem	Physician or Medical Facility	City

II. MEDICATIONS

Please list all medications you are now taking, including those you buy without a doctor's prescription (such as aspirin, cold tablets or vitamin supplements).

III. ALLERGIES AND SENSITIVITIES

List anything that you are allergic to such as certain foods, medications, dust, chemicals or soaps, household items, pollens, bee stings, etc., and indicate how each affects you.

Allergic To:	Effect	Allergic To:	Effect
Penicillin	Hives		

IV. GENERAL HEALTH, ATTITUDE AND HABITS

How is your overall health now? .... Health now: Poor ____ Fair ____ Good X Excellent ____

How has it been most of your life? .... Health has been: Poor ____ Fair ____ Good X Excellent ____

In the past year:

Has your appetite changed? .... Appetite: Decreased ____ Increased ____ Stayed same X

Has your weight changed? .... Weight: Lost ____ lbs. Gained 10 lbs. No change ____

Are you thirsty much of the time? .... Thirsty: No X Yes ____

Has your overall 'pep' changed? .... Pep: Decreased ____ Increased ____ Stayed same X

Do you usually have trouble sleeping? .... Trouble sleeping: No ____ Yes X

How much do you exercise? .... Exercise: Little or none ____ Less than I need ____ All I need X

Do you smoke? .... Smokes: No X Yes ____ If yes, how many years? ____

How many each day? .... ____ Cigarettes ____ Cigars ____ Pipesfull

Have you ever smoked? .... Smoked: No ____ Yes X If yes, how many years? 15

How many each day? .... 20 Cigarettes ____ Cigars ____ Pipesfull

Do you drink alcoholic beverages? .... Alcohol: No ____ Yes X I drink ____ Beers ____ Glasses of wine ____ Drinks of hard liquor - per day Socially

Have you ever had a problem with alcohol? .... Prior problem: No X Yes ____

How much coffee or tea do you usually drink? .... Coffee/Tea: 2 cups of coffee or tea a day

Do you regularly wear seatbelts? .... Seatbelts: No ____ Yes X

DO YOU:	Rarely/ Never	Occasionally	Frequently
Feel nervous?	X		
Feel depressed?	X		
Find it hard to make decisions?	X		
Lose your temper?		X	
Worry a lot?	X		
Tire easily?		X	
Have trouble relaxing?		X	
Have any sexual problems?	X		

DO YOU:	Rarely/ Never	Occasionally	Frequently
Ever feel like committing suicide?	X		
Feel bored with your life?	X		
Use marijuana?	X		
Use "hard drugs"?	X		

Do you want to talk to the doctor about a personal matter? No X Yes ____

C O N F I D E N T I A L

STOCK NO. 19-742-4 8/95

Page 1

Case One, Form 3

PART A – PRESENT HEALTH HISTORY (continued)

IV. GENERAL HEALTH, ATTITUDE AND HABITS (continued)

Have you recently had any changes in your: — If yes, please explain:

	No	Yes	If yes, please explain
Marital status?	X		
Job or work?		X	Self employed
Residence?		X	Moved from LA CA
Financial status?	X		
Are you having any legal problems or trouble with the law?	X		

PART B – PAST HISTORY

I. FAMILY HEALTH

Please give the following information about your immediate family:

Relationship	Age, if Living	Age At Death	State of Health Or Cause of Death
Father		78	Lung cancer
Mother		45	Heart disease
Brothers and Sisters	38		good
Spouse	51		good
Children	22		good
	25		good

Have any **blood relatives** had any of the following illnesses? If so, indicate relationship (mother, brother, etc.)

Illness	Family Members
Asthma	
Diabetes	
Cancer	Father
Blood Disease	
Glaucoma	
Epilepsy	
Rheumatoid Arthritis	Aunt
Tuberculosis	
Gout	
High Blood Pressure	Mother
Heart Disease	Mother
Mental Problems	
Suicide	
Stroke	Grandmother
Alcoholism	
Rheumatic Fever	

II. HOSPITALIZATIONS, SURGERIES, INJURIES

Please list all times you have been hospitalized, operated on, or seriously injured.

Year	Operation, Illness, Injury	Hospital and City
1990	Appendix removed	LA CA

III. ILLNESS AND MEDICAL PROBLEMS

Please mark with an (X) any of the following illnesses and medical problems you have or have had and indicate the year when each started. If you are not certain when an illness started, write down an approximate year.

Illness	(x)	(Year)	Illness	(x)	(Year)
Eye or eye lid infection			Hernia		
Glaucoma			Hemorrhoids		
Other eye problems			Kidney or bladder disease		
Ear trouble			Prostate problem (male only)		
Deafness or decreased hearing			Mental problems		
Thyroid trouble			Headaches		
Strep throat			Head injury		
Bronchitis			Stroke		
Emphysema			Convulsions, seizures		
Pneumonia			Arthritis		
Allergies, asthma or hay fever			Gout		
Tuberculosis			Cancer or tumor		
Other lung problems			Bleeding tendency		
High blood pressure			Diabetes		
Heart attack			Measles/Rubeola		
High cholesterol			German measles/Rubella		
Arteriosclerosis			Polio		
(Hardening of arteries)			Mumps		
Heart murmur			Scarlet fever		
Other heart condition			Chicken pox		
Stomach/duodenal ulcer			Mononucleosis		
Diverticulosis			Eczema		
Colitis			Psoriasis		
Other bowel problems			Venereal disease		
Hepatitis			Genital herpes		
Liver trouble			HIV test		
Gallbladder trouble			AIDS		

CONFIDENTIAL

Case One, Form 3

PART C – BODY SYSTEMS REVIEW

Please answer all of the following questions.

Circle any questions you find difficult to answer.

MEN: Please answer questions 1 through 12, then skip to question 18.

WOMEN: Please start on question 6.

MEN ONLY

	No	Yes
1. Have you had or do you have prostate trouble?	X	
2. Do you have any sexual problems or a problem with impotency?	X	
3. Have you ever had sores or lesions on your penis?	X	
4. Have you ever had any discharge from your penis?	X	
5. Do you ever have pain, lumps or swelling in your testicles?	X	

Check here if you wish to discuss any special problems with the doctor ☐

MEN & WOMEN

	Rarely/ Never	Occasionally	Frequently
6. Is it sometimes hard to start your urine flow?	X		
7. Is urination ever painful?	X		
8. Do you have to urinate more than 5 times a day?	X		
9. Do you get up at night to urinate?	X		
10. Has your urine ever been bloody or dark colored?	X		
11. Do you ever lose urine when you strain, laugh, cough or sneeze?	X		
12. Do you ever lose urine during sleep?	X		

WOMEN ONLY

Do you:

	Rarely/ Never	Occasionally	Frequently
13. a. Have any menstrual problems?			
b. Feel rather tense just before your period?			
c. Have heavy menstrual bleeding?			
d. Have painful menstrual periods?			
e. Have any bleeding between periods?			
f. Have any unusual vaginal discharge or itching?			
g. Ever have tender breasts?			
h. Have any discharge from your nipples?			
i. Have any hot flashes?			

14. How many times, if any, have you been pregnant? ______

15. How many children born alive? ______

16. Are you taking birth control pills? No____ Yes____

17. Do you examine your breasts monthly for lumps? No____ Yes____

17a. What was the date of your last menstrual period? Date ______

Check here if you wish to discuss any special problem with the doctor ☐

MEN & WOMEN

18. In the past year have you had any:

	Rarely/ Never	Occasionally	Frequently
a. Severe shoulder pain?	X		
b. Severe back pain?	X		
c. Muscle or joint stiffness or pain due to sports, exercise or injury?		X	
d. Pain or swelling in any joints not due to sports, exercise or injury?	X		

	No	Yes
19. Do you have dry skin or brittle fingernails?	X	
20. Do you bruise easily?	X	
21. Do you have any moles that have changed in color or in size?	X	
22. Do you have any other skin problems?	X	
23. In the last 3 months have you had:		
a. A fever that lasted more than one day?	X	
b. Sores or cuts that were hard to heal?	X	
c. Any cold sores (fever blisters)?	X	
d. Any lumps in your neck, armpits or groin?	X	
e. Do you ever have chills or sweat at night?	X	
24. Have you traveled out of the country in the last 2 years?	X	Yes, Traveled in: ______

25. Write in the dates for the shots you have had: Measles ____ Mumps ____ Polio ____ Smallpox ____ Tetanus ____ Typhoid ____

26. Have you had a tuberculin (TB) skin test? No____ Yes X Date 2003
If so, was it negative or positive? Neg X Pos____

27. Have you had an HIV test for AIDS? No X Yes____ Date ______
If so, was it negative or positive? Neg____ Pos____

CONFIDENTIAL

 PLEASE TURN THIS PAGE STOCK NO. 19-742-4 8/95 Page 3

REMOVE THIS PAGE AFTER COMPLETING QUESTIONNAIRE

					VISION / HEARING
28.	Do you wear eyeglasses?	No X	Yes___		Wears eyeglasses
29.	Do you wear contact lenses?	No X	Yes___		Wears contacts
30.	Has your vision changed in the last year?	No X	Yes___		Vision changes in last year
		Rarely/ Never	**Occasionally**	**Frequently**	
31.	How often do you have:				
	a. Double vision?	X			Double vision
	b. Blurry vision?	X			Blurred vision
	c. Watery or itchy eyes?	X			Watery/itchy eyes
32.	Do you ever see colored rings around lights?	X			Sees halos
33.	Do others tell you you have a hearing problem?	X			Hearing problem
34.	Do you have trouble keeping your balance?	X			Loses balance
35.	Do you have any discharge from your ears?	X			Discharge from ears
36.	Do you ever feel dizzy or have motion sickness?	X			Dizzy / motion sickness
37.	Do you have any problems with your hearing?	No X	Yes___	Hearing Problems	
38.	Do you ever have ringing in your ears?	No X	Yes___	Ringing in ears	
		Rarely/ Never	**Occasionally**	**Frequently**	**NOSE / THROAT / RESPIRATORY**
39.	How often do you have:				
	a. Head colds?		X		Head colds
	b. Chest colds?		X		Chest colds
	c. Runny nose?		X		Runny nose
	d. Stuffed up nose?		X		Head congestion
	e. Sore/hoarse throat?	X			Sore / hoarse throat
	f. Bad coughing spells?	X			Coughing spells
	g. Sneezing spells?	X			Sneezing spells
	h. Trouble breathing?	X			Trouble breathing
	i. Nose bleeds?	X			Nose bleeds
	j. Cough blood?	X			Cough blood
40.	Have you ever worked or spent time:				
	a. On a farm?	No___	Yes X	Worked on a farm	
	b. In a mine?	No X	Yes___	Worked in a mine	
	c. In a laundry or mill?	No X	Yes___	Worked in a laundry/mill	
	d. In very dusty places?	No X	Yes___	Worked in high dust concentrations	
	e. With or near toxic chemicals?	No X	Yes___	Exposed to toxic chemicals	
	f. With or near radioactive materials?	No X	Yes___	Exposed to radioactive materials	
	g. With or near asbestos?	No X	Yes___	Exposed to asbestos	
		Rarely/ Never	**Occasionally**	**Frequently**	**CARDIOVASCULAR**
41.	Do you get out of breath easily when you are active (like climbing stairs)?	X			Out of breath quickly when exercising
42.	Do you ever feel light-headed or dizzy?		X		Dizziness
43.	Have you ever fainted or passed out?	X			Fainted
44.	Do you sometimes feel your heart is racing or beating too fast?		X		Rapid heartbeat
45.	When you exercise do you ever get pains in your chest or shoulders?			X	Chest/shoulder pains in exercise
46.	Do you have any leg cramps or pain in your thighs or legs when walking?	X			Pain in thighs or legs when walking
47.	Do you ever have to sit up at night to breathe easier?	X			Sits up at night to breathe easier
48.	Do you use two pillows at night to help you breathe easier?	X			Breathing problems during sleep
49.	Would you say you are a restless sleeper?		X		Restless sleeper
50.	Are you bothered by leg cramps at night?	X			Leg cramps at night
51.	Do you sometimes have swollen ankles or feet?	X			Swollen ankles/feet
		Rarely/ Never	**Occasionally**	**Frequently**	**DIGESTIVE**
52.	How often, if ever:				
	a. Are you nauseated (sick to your stomach)?	X			Nauseated
	b. Do you have stomach pains?	X			Stomach pains
	c. Do you burp a lot after eating?	X			Burps after eating
	d. Do you have heartburn?		X		Heartburn
	e. Do you have trouble swallowing your food?	X			Trouble swallowing food
	f. Have you vomited blood?	X			Vomited blood
	g. Are you constipated?	X			Constipated
	h. Do you have diarrhea (watery stools)?	X			Diarrhea
	i. Are your bowel movements painful?	X			Painful bowel movements
	j. Are your bowel movements bloody?	X			Bloody bowel movements
	k. Are your bowel movements dark or black?	X			Dark bowel movements
53.	Have you ever had a sigmoidoscopy?	No X	Yes___	Date___	Date of last sigmoidoscopy?

PLEASE TURN TO BACK PAGE AND COMPLETE QUESTIONS ON NUTRITION.

Case One, Form 3

Andrus/Clini-Rec®
BIBBERO SYSTEMS, INC.

COMPREHENSIVE
PHYSICAL EXAMINATION
MALE OR FEMALE
NEW OR ESTABLISHED PATIENT
CPT # 99201 - 99215

(For Office Use Only)

NAME Shapiro, Ivan AGE 59 YRS. OLD TODAY'S DATE 1/5/05 DATE OF BIRTH 3/6/45

Key: [O] Neg. Findings [+] Positive Findings [X] Omitted [✔] See Notes/CIRCLE WORDS OF IMPORTANCE & EXPLAIN

1	GEN. APPEARANCE	[ ]	Apparent Age/Nutrition/Development/Mental & Emotional Status/Gait/Posture/Distress/Speech –
2	HEAD / SCALP	[ ]	Size/Shape/Tender over Sinuses/Hair/Alopecia/Eruption/Masses/Bruit –
3	EYES	[ ]	Conjunct/Sclerae/Cornea/Pupils/EOM'S/Arcus/Ptosis/Fundi/Tension/Eyelids/Pallor/Light/Bruit –
4	EARS	[ ]	Ext. Canal/TM's/Perforation/Discharge/Tophi/Hearing Problem/Weber/Rinne –
5	NOSE / SINUSES	[ ]	Septum/Obstruction/Turbinates/Discharge –
6	MOUTH / THROAT	[ ]	Odor/Lips/Tongue/Tonsils/Teeth/Dentures/Gums/Pharynx –
7	NECK	[ ]	Adenopathy/Thyroid/Carotids/Trachea/Veins/Masses/Spine/Motion/Bruit –
8	BACK	[ ]	Kyphosis/Scoliosis/Lordosis/Mobility/CVA/Bone/Tenderness –
9	THORAX	[ ]	Symmetry/Movement/Contour/Tender –
10	BREASTS	[ ]	Size/Size-Consistency/Nipples/Areolar/Palpable Mass/Discharge/Tenderness/Nodes/Scars –
11	HEART	[ ]	Rate/Rhythm/Apical Impulse/Thrills/Quality of Sound/Intensity/Splitting/Extra Sounds/ Murmurs –
12	CHEST / LUNGS	[ ]	Excursion/Dullness or Hyperresonance to Percussion/Quality of Breath Sounds/Rales/Wheezing/ Rhonchi/Diaphragm/Rubs/Bruit –
13	ABDOMEN	[ ]	Bowel Sounds/Appearance/Liver/Spleen/Masses/Hernias/Murmurs/Contour/Tenderness/Bruit/ ING Nodes –
14	GROIN	[ ]	Hernia/Inguinal Nodes/Femoral Pulses –
15	MALE GENITALIA	[ ]	Penis/Testes/Scrotum Epididymis/Varicocele/Scars/Discharge –
16	FEMALE GENITALIA	[ ]	Vuvla/Vagina/Cervix/Uterus/Adnexae/Rectocele/Cystocele/Bartholin Gland/Urethra/ Discharge – Pap Smear (if done ✔) ☐
17	EXTREMITIES	[ ]	Deformity/Clubbing/Cyanosis/Edema/Nails/Peripheral Pulses/Calf Tenderness/Joints for Swelling/ ROM –
18	SKIN	[ ]	Color/Birthmarks/Scars/Texture/Rash/Eczema/Ulcers –
19	NEUROLOGICAL	[ ]	DTR's/Babinski/Cranial Nerves/Motor Abnormalities/Tremor/Paralysis/Sensory Exam – (touch, pin prick, vibration)/Coordination/Romberg –
20	MUSCULAR SYSTEM	[ ]	Strength/Wasting/Development –
21	RECTAL EXAM	[ ]	Sphincter Tone/Hemorrhoids/Fissures/Masses/Prostate/Stool Guaiac (if done ✔) ☐ Pos ☐ Neg –

Impression: ☐ Check If Normal Physical Examination

Summary: ______________________

____

______________________ Signature ______________________ Date ________

CONFIDENTIAL

Page 4

Case One, Form 3

COMPREHENSIVE PHYSICAL EXAMINATION
(continued)

(For Office Use Only)

Body Area Number	REMARKS: PHYSICIAN'S NOTES:

R L L R

R L

HEIGHT________
WEIGHT________
BUILD ________
PULSE ________
RESP. ________
TEMP. ________

VISION

Without Glasses
Far R 20/ L 20/
Near R 20/ L 20/

With Glasses
R 20/ L 20/
R 20/ L 20/

Tonometry R______ L______
Colorvision____________
Peripheral Fields R____ L____

AUDIOMETRIC TESTING

	250	500	1000
R			
L			
	2000	**4000**	**8000**
R			
L			

Gross Hearing ____________

BLOOD PRESSURE

Sitting
R / L /
Standing
R / L /
Lying
R / L /

Diagnostic Test:	Results:

The space below is provided for additional information when these data are being forwarded to a hospital, insurance company, a referral physician, etc.

Significant Comments / Recommendations:

Physician's Name ____________
Address ____________
Telephone (area code) ____________

CONFIDENTIAL

NUTRITION AND DIET

1. How many meals do you eat each day? .... 3 Meals each day
2. Do you usually eat breakfast? .... ☐ No ☒ Yes Breakfast
3. Do you diet frequently and/or are you now dieting? .... ☒ No ☐ Yes Diets
4. Do you consider yourself .... ☐ Underweight ☐ Overweight ☒ Just right? Weight
5. Do you snack? .... ☐ More than once a day ☒ Usually daily ☐ Rarely? Snacks
6. Do you add salt to your food at the table? ..... ☐ Almost always ☐ Sometimes ☒ Rarely Salts food
7. Check the frequency you eat the following types of foods:

	More than once daily	Daily	3 times weekly	Once weekly	Twice monthly	Less or never
a. Whole grain or enriched bread or cereal	X					
b. Milk, cheese, or other dairy products		X				
c. Eggs				X		
d. Meat, Poultry, Fish			X			
e. Beans, Peas, or other legumes		X				
f. Citrus	X					
g. Dark green or deep yellow vegetables		X				

List any food supplements or vitamins you take regularly: One a day vitamins

Additional Patient Comments: ______________________________

Thanks for completing this questionnaire. Please review for skipped questions, sign your name on the space to the right and return it to the physician or assistant. If you wish to add any information, please write it in the spaces provided above.

Patient's Signature ______________________________

Physician's Notes: ______________________________

CONFIDENTIAL

To order, call or write:
Bibbero Systems, Inc.
1300 N. McDowell Blvd., Petaluma, CA 94954-1180
Toll Free: 800-BIBBERO (800 242-2376)
Or Fax: 800-242-9330
STOCK NO. 19-742-4 8/95

Case One, Form 4

Patient Information Sheet

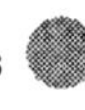

Blackburn Primary Care Associates
1990 Turquoise Drive
Blackburn, WI 54937
(555)555-1234

REGISTRATION
(PLEASE PRINT)

Home Phone: 555-297-1349

Today's Date: 1/5/05

PATIENT INFORMATION

Name: SHAPIRO (Last Name) IVAN (First Name) R. (Initial) Soc. Sec.# 591-23-1971

Address 3242 Kentucky Lane

City Blackburn State WI Zip 54938

Single __ Married ✔ Widowed __ Separated __ Divorced __ Sex M ✔ F __ Age 59 Birthdate 3/6/45

Patient Employed by SELF Occupation CARPENTER

Business Address as above Business Phone as above

By whom were you referred? ________

In case of emergency who should be notified? MARY ANNE SHAPIRO (Name) (wife) (Relation to Patient) Phone 555-297-1349

PRIMARY INSURANCE

Person Responsible for Account SHAPIRO (Last Name) IVAN (First Name) R. (Initial)

Relation to Patient SELF Birthdate 3/6/45 Soc. Sec.# 591-23-1971

Address (if different from patient's) same Phone ________

City ________ State ________ Zip ________

Person Responsible Employed by SELF Occupation CARPENTER

Business Address as above Business Phone ________

Insurance Company Blue Cross / Blue Shield

Contract # none Group # none Subscriber # 591-23-1971A

Name of other dependents covered under this plan MARY ANNE SHAPIRO

ADDITIONAL INSURANCE

Is patient covered by additional insurance? __ Yes ✔ No

Subscriber Name ________ Relation to Patient ________ Birthdate ________

Address (if different from patient's) ________ Phone ________

City ________ State ________ Zip ________

Subscriber Employed by ________ Business Phone ________

Insurance Company ________ Soc. Sec.# ________

Contract # ________ Group # ________ Subscriber # ________

Name of other dependents covered under this plan ________

ASSIGNMENT AND RELEASE

I, the undersigned, certify that I (or my dependent) have insurance coverage with *Blue Cross Blue Shield* (Name of Insurance Company(ies)) and assign directly to Dr. Blackburn Primary Care Associates insurance benefits, if any, otherwise payable to me for services rendered. I understand that I am financially responsible for all charges whether or not paid by insurance. I hereby authorize the doctor to release all information necessary to secure the payment of benefits. I authorize the use of this signature on all insurance submissions.

Ivan Shapiro (Responsible Party Signature) *self* (Relationship) *01/05/05* (Date)

Case One, Form 5

Patient Encounter Form

Blackburn Primary Care Associates
1990 Turquoise Drive
Blackburn, WI 54937
(555) 555-1234

FED. I.D. # 52-1963787

PAT. INFO.

ACCT. NO.	PATIENT'S LAST NAME	FIRST	M.I.	DATE OF BIRTH	SEX	TODAY'S DATE
	SHAPIRO	IVAN	R	3/6/45	☒ M ☐ F	01/05/05

INSURANCE	COPAY	DISABILITY RELATED TO: ☐ ACCIDENT ☐ INDUSTRIAL ☐ ILLNESS ☐ OTHER
BCBS		DATES SYMPTOMS APPEARED, INCEPTION OF PREGNANCY, OR ACCIDENT OCCURRED: / /

✔	DESCRIPTION	CPT/MD	FEE
	OFFICE VISITS-NEW PATIENTS		
	Focused	99201	
	Expanded	99202	
	Detailed	99203	
	Comprehensive	99204	
X	Complex	99205	
	OFFICE VISITS - EST. PATIENTS		
	Minimal	99211	
	Focused	99212	
	Expanded	99213	
	Detailed	99214	
	Comprehensive	99215	
	PREVENTIVE HEALTH CARE NEW PT.	EST. PT	
	Eval./Mgmt. > 1 Yr 99381	99391	
	Early Child 1 - 4 Yrs 99382	99392	
	Late Child 5 - 11 Yrs 99383	99393	
	Adolescent 12 - 17 Yrs 99384	99394	
	Eval./Mgmt. 18 - 39 Yrs 99385	99395	
	Eval./Mgmt. 40 - 64 Yrs 99386	99396	
	Eval./Mgmt. 65 - Over 99387	99397	
	HOSP./SNF/HOME VISITS		
	House Calls	99341	
	ER Visit	9928__	
	Init. Hosp. Care	99222	
	Sub. Hosp. Care	99232	
	SNF, Sub. Care	99312	
	INJECTIONS		
	Allergy	95125	
	B-12	J3420	
	Flu Shot	90724	
	Gamma Globulin	90741	
	Hormone		
	Depo Provera	J1055	
	Kenalog 40-60 mg	J3301	
	Morphine/Demerol	J2270	
	Phenergan	J2550	
	Celestone	J0700	
	Hep B, newborn to 11 years	90744	
	Hep B, 11 - 19 years	90745	
	Hep B, 20 years and above	90746	
	Rocephin/Claforan	J0696	
	Iron	J1760	
	Lidocaine NCL	J2000	
	Admin of INJ	J0110	
	Unlist INJ	90782	
	Drug		
	Dose		

✔	DESCRIPTION	CPT/MD	FEE
	SPECIAL SERVICES		
	Drivers Physical	99214	
	Pelvic/Breast Exam	99214	
	Industrial	99214	
	IMMUNIZATIONS		
	DtaP	90700	
	DPT	90701	
	DT	90702	
	Td (Tetanus Booster)	90703	
	MMR	90707	
	Mumps	90704	
	Pneumococcal	90732	
	Rubella	90706	
	Polio (TOPV)	90712	
	PPD	86580	
	TB Tine Test	86585	
	Hib	90737	
	OFFICE PROCEDURES		
	Audiometry	92551	
	Diathermy (Ultrasound)	97024	
X	EKG Tracing & Interp.	93000	
	Intermed Joint Injection	20605	
	Major Joint Injection	20610	
	Nebulizer TX	94664	
	Rem. Impact. Cer.	69210	
	Spirometry	94010	
	Stress Test	93015	
	Trigger Pt. Inj.	20550	
	Eye Wash	65205*	
	LABORATORY		
	Throat Culture	87060	
	Glucose Blood	82947	
	Glucose Stick	82948	
	UA Pregnancy	81025	
	Occult Blood, Stool	82270	
	Rapid Strep	86588	
	Smear	88150	
X	UA Dip	81002	
	Urinalysis	81000	
	Venipuncture	36415	
	Wet Mount, Smear	87210	
	Wet Mount KOH	87220	
X	Collect/Handling	~~99000~~	36415
	MISCELLANEOUS		
	Pre-OP	993__	
	After Hours	99050	
	Sunday/Holidays	99054	
	Cast Removal	29705	
	Norplant Insertion	11975	
	Norplant Kit	99070	

✔	DESCRIPTION	CPT/MD	FEE
	SURGERY		
	Toenail Removal	11750	
	Cryosurgery	17200	
	I & D	10060	
	Drainage Paronychia	10060	
	Enucleation Ext. Hemorrhoid	46320	
	I & D Abscess/Cyst	10060	
	Podophyllom	17100	
	Removal Foreign Body	10120	
	Wart Removal	17110	
	Destr. Single Lesion Face	17000	
	2nd and 3rd Lesion Face	17001	
	Destr. Single Lesion Body	17106	
	2nd and 3rd Lesion Body	17003	
	Lesion Rem. Excision		
	Anoscopy	46600	
	Flex. Scope with Sig.	45330	
	Vasectomy	55250	
	Therapeutic Abor.	59840	
	Removal Foreign Body of Eye	65205	
	SUPPLIES		
	Ace Wrap	99070	
	Cast Material	99070	
	Cervical Collar	99070	
	Elastic Bandage	99070	
	Splint/Sling	99070	
	Sterile Dressing	99070	
	Surgical Tray	99070	

DIAGNOSIS: ICD-9

☐ Abscess Cellulitis 682.9
☐ Abdominal Pain 789.0
☐ Abrasions 919.0
☐ Acne 706.1
☐ ADD 314.00
☐ Alcoholism 303.90
☐ Allergic Rhinitis 477.9
☐ Allergy, Unsp 995.3
☐ Anemia 285.9
☐ Angina Pectoris 413.9
☐ Anxiety Depression 300.4
☐ Anxiety State 300.00
☐ ASCVD 429.2
☐ Asthma W/O Status Asthma 493.90
☐ Atten Surg. Dressing/Suture V58.3
☐ BCP Consult V25.9
☐ BPH 600
☐ Bronchitis, Acute 466.0
☐ Bronchitis, Chronic 491.9
☐ Burn ____________ 949.0
☐ Bursitis 727.3
☐ C.T.S. 354.0
☐ CAD 746.85
☐ CA-Prostate 185
☐ Cardiac Arrhythmia 427.9
☐ Cataracts 366.9
☐ Chest Pain 786.50
☐ Congestive Heart Failure 428.0
☐ Conjunctivitis 372.30
☐ Constipation 564.0
☐ Consult Vasc. V65.8
☐ Convulsions 780.3
☐ COPD 496
☐ Coronary Atherosclerosis. 414.0
☐ CVA 436
☐ Cyst Sebaceous 706.2
☐ Dermatitis 692.9
☐ Diabetes, Uncomp. Adult 250.00
☐ Diabetes, Complicated . . 250.90
☐ Disc Degeneration 722.6
☐ Duodenal Ulcer 532.90
☐ Dysmenorrhea 625.3
☐ Fatigue 780.7
☐ Flu Shot Only V04.8
☐ Flu Vac V04.8
☐ Flu W/Resp. Manifest . . . 487.1
☐ Folliculitis 704.8
☐ FX ____________
☐ Gallbladder Disease 575.9
☐ Ganglion 727.43
☐ Gastroenteritis 558.9
☐ Gout 274.9
☐ Gyn Exam V72.3
☐ Headache Tension 307.81
☐ Hemorrhoids Ext. 455.3
☐ Hepatitis 573.3
☐ Hernia-Inguinal 550.90
☐ Herpes Zoster 053.9
☐ Hyperlipidemia 272.4
☒ Hypertension 401.9
☐ Hyperthyroidism 242.9
☐ Hypothyroidism 244.9
☐ Impacted Cerumen 380.4
☐ Impetigo 684
☐ Ingrown Toenail 703.0
☐ Internal Derangement Knee . 717.9
☐ Labyrinthitis 386.30
☐ Laceration Open Wound . 879.8__
☐ Levator Scapular Syndrome 726.90
☐ Menopausal Disorder . . . 627.9
☐ Metabolic Diff. 277.8
☐ Migraine 346.90
☐ Mitral Valve Disorder . . . 424.0
☐ Myalgia and Myositis . . . 729.1
☐ Noninf. Gastroenterit. . . . 558.9
☐ Obesity 278.0
☐ Osteoarthrosis 715.00
☐ Osteoporosis 733.00
☐ Otitis Externa 380.10
☐ Otitis Media 382.9
☐ P.I.D. 614.9
☐ Peptic Ulcer 533.90
☐ Pharyngitis, Acute 462
☐ Pneumonia, Viral 480.9
☐ Poison Oak 692.6
☐ Premarital B-Test V70.3
☐ Pregnancy Test, Unconf.. V72.4
☐ Prostatitis 601.9
☐ Psoriasis 696.1
☐ Rheumatoid Arthritis 714.0
☐ Sciatica 724.3
☐ Sacroiliac Sprain 846.1
☐ Sinusitis, Acute 461.9
☐ Smoking Cessation. 305.10
☐ Sprain ____________
☐ SQ. Cell CA-Face. 173.3
☐ Sterilization V25.2
☐ Stye. 373.11
☐ TB Exposure V01.1
☐ Tendonitis 726.90
☐ Tinea. 110.9
☐ Tonsillitis, Acute 463
☐ URI, Acute 465.9
☐ Urine Tract Infection 599.0
☐ Vaginitis. 616.10
☐ Well Adult Medical Exam V70.9
☐ Well Child Health Exam . V20.2

DIAGNOSIS (If not checked above) ICD-9	PHYSICIAN SIGNATURE	TODAY'S FEE	$
Ischemic heart disease, c̄ Coronary occlusion		PAYMENT	
PLEASE REMEMBER THAT PAYMENT IS YOUR OBLIGATION REGARDLESS OF INSURANCE OR OTHER THIRD PARTY INVOLVEMENT.	PAYMENT BY ☐ CASH ☐ CREDIT CARD ☐ CHECK # ________	BALANCE DUE	

Case One, Form 6

FEE SCHEDULE

BLACKBURN PRIMARY CARE ASSOCIATES
1990 TURQUOISE DRIVE
BLACKBURN, WI 54937

Federal Tax ID Number: **52-1963787**

BCBS Group Number: **14982**
Medicare Group Number: **14982**

OFFICE VISIT, NEW PATIENT

Focused, 99201	$ 45.00
Expanded, 99202	$ 53.00
Detailed, 99203	$ 60.00
Comprehensive, 99204	$ 95.00
Complex, 99205	$195.00
Consultation, 99245	$250.00

OFFICE VISIT, ESTABLISHED PATIENT

Minimal, 99211	$ 40.00
Focused, 99212	$ 48.00
Expanded, 99213	$ 55.00
Detailed, 99214	$ 65.00
Comprehensive, 99215	$195.00

OFFICE PROCEDURES

EKG, 12 Lead, 93000	$ 55.00
Stress EKG, Treadmill, 93015	$295.00
Sigmoidoscopy, Flex., 45330	$145.00
Spirometry, 94010	$ 50.00
Cerumen Removal, 69210	$ 40.00
Collection & Handling	
Lab Specimen, 99000	$ 9.00
Venipuncture, 36415	$ 9.00
Urinalysis, 81000	$ 20.00
Urinalysis, 81002 (Dip Only)	$ 12.00
Influenza Injection, 90724	$ 20.00
Pneumococcal Injection, 90732	$ 20.00
Oral Polio, 90712	$ 15.00
DTaP, 90700	$ 20.00
Tetanus Toxoid, 90703	$ 15.00
MMR, 90707	$ 25.00
Hib, 90737	$ 20.00
Hepatitis B, newborn to age 11 years, 90744	$ 60.00
Hepatitis B, 11-19 years, 90745	$ 60.00
Hepatitis B, 20 years and above 90746	$ 60.00
Intramuscular Injection, 90788	
Penicillin	$ 30.00
Ceftriaxone	$ 25.00
Solu-Medrol	$ 23.00
Vitamin B-12	$ 13.00
Subcutaneous Injection, 90782	
Epinephrine	$ 18.00
Sus-Pherine	$ 25.00
Insulin, U-100	$ 15.00

COMMON DIAGNOSIS CODES

Ischemic Heart Disease	414.9
w/o myocardial infarction	411.89
w/ coronary occlusion	411.81
Hypertension, Malignant	401.0
Benign	401.1
Unspecified	401.9
w/ congest. heart failure	402.91
Asthma, Bronchial	493.9
w/ COPD	493.2
allergic, w/ S.A.	493.91
allergic, w/o S.A.	493.90
Kyphosis	737.10
w/ osteoporosis	733.0
Osteoporosis	733.00
Otitis Media, Acute	382.9
Chronic	382.9
Well Child Health Exam	V20.2
Well Adult Medical Exam	V70.9

Case One, Form 7

PLEASE DO NOT STAPLE IN THIS AREA

APPROVED OMB-0938-0008

CARRIER

PICA

HEALTH INSURANCE CLAIM FORM

PICA

1. MEDICARE (Medicare #) MEDICAID (Medicaid #) CHAMPUS (Sponsor's SSN) CHAMPVA (VA File #) GROUP HEALTH PLAN (SSN or ID) FECA BLK LUNG (SSN) OTHER (ID)

1a. INSURED'S I.D. NUMBER (FOR PROGRAM IN ITEM 1)

2. PATIENT'S NAME (Last Name, First Name, Middle Initial)

3. PATIENT'S BIRTHDATE MM DD YY SEX M F

4. INSURED'S NAME (Last Name, First Name, Middle Initial)

5. PATIENT'S ADDRESS (No., Street)

6. PATIENT RELATIONSHIP TO INSURED Self Spouse Child Other

7. INSURED'S ADDRESS (No., Street)

CITY STATE

8. PATIENT STATUS Single Married Other

CITY STATE

ZIP CODE TELEPHONE (Include Area Code) ( )

Employed Full-Time Student Part-Time Student

ZIP CODE TELEPHONE (Include Area Code) ( )

9. OTHER INSURED'S NAME (Last Name, First Name, Middle Initial)

10. IS PATIENT'S CONDITION RELATED TO:

11. INSURED'S POLICY GROUP OR FECA NUMBER

a. OTHER INSURED'S POLICY OR GROUP NUMBER

a. EMPLOYMENT? (CURRENT OR PREVIOUS) YES NO

a. INSURED'S DATE OF BIRTH MM DD YY SEX M F

b. OTHER INSURED'S DATE OF BIRTH MM DD YY SEX M F

b. AUTO ACCIDENT? PLACE (State) YES NO

b. EMPLOYER'S NAME OR SCHOOL NAME

c. EMPLOYER'S NAME OR SCHOOL NAME

c. OTHER ACCIDENT? YES NO

c. INSURANCE PLAN NAME OR PROGRAM NAME

d. INSURANCE PLAN NAME OR PROGRAM NAME

10d. RESERVED FOR LOCAL USE

d. IS THERE ANOTHER HEALTH BENEFIT PLAN? YES NO *If yes, return to and complete item 9a-d.*

PATIENT AND INSURED INFORMATION

READ BACK OF FORM BEFORE COMPLETING & SIGNING THIS FORM.

12. PATIENT'S OR AUTHORIZED PERSON'S SIGNATURE I authorize the release of any medical or other information necessary to process this claim. I also request payment of government benefits either to myself or to the party who accepts assignment below.

SIGNED ______ DATE ______

13. INSURED'S OR AUTHORIZED PERSON'S SIGNATURE I authorize payment of medical benefits to the undersigned physician or supplier for services described below.

SIGNED ______

14. DATE OF CURRENT: MM DD YY ILLNESS (First symptom) OR INJURY (Accident) OR PREGNANCY (LMP)

15. IF PATIENT HAS HAD SAME OR SIMILAR ILLNESS, GIVE FIRST DATE MM DD YY

16. DATES PATIENT UNABLE TO WORK IN CURRENT OCCUPATION FROM MM DD YY TO MM DD YY

17. NAME OF REFERRING PHYSICIAN OR OTHER SOURCE

17a. I.D. NUMBER OF REFERRING PHYSICIAN

18. HOSPITALIZATION DATES RELATED TO CURRENT SERVICES FROM MM DD YY TO MM DD YY

19. RESERVED FOR LOCAL USE

20. OUTSIDE LAB? YES NO $ CHARGES

21. DIAGNOSIS OR NATURE OF ILLNESS OR INJURY. (RELATE ITEMS 1,2,3 OR 4 TO ITEM 24E BY LINE)

1. ___ . ___

2. ___ . ___

3. ___ . ___

4. ___ . ___

22. MEDICAID RESUBMISSION CODE ORIGINAL REF. NO.

23. PRIOR AUTHORIZATION NUMBER

24. A DATE(S) OF SERVICE From MM DD YY To MM DD YY	B Place of Service	C Type of Service	D PROCEDURES, SERVICES, OR SUPPLIES (Explain Unusual Circumstances) CPT/HCPCS MODIFIER	E DIAGNOSIS CODE	F $ CHARGES	G DAYS OR UNITS	H EPSDT Family Plan	I EMG	J COB	K RESERVED FOR LOCAL USE
1										
2										
3										
4										
5										
6										

25. FEDERAL TAX I.D. NUMBER SSN EIN

26. PATIENT'S ACCOUNT NUMBER

27. ACCEPT ASSIGNMENT? (For govt. claims, see back) YES NO

28. TOTAL CHARGE $

29. AMOUNT PAID $

30. BALANCE DUE $

31. SIGNATURE OF PHYSICIAN OR SUPPLIER INCLUDING DEGREES OR CREDENTIALS (I certify that the statements on the reverse apply to this bill and are made a part thereof.)

SIGNED DATE

32. NAME AND ADDRESS OF FACILITY WHERE SERVICES WERE RENDERED (If other than home or office)

33. PHYSICIAN'S, SUPPLIER'S BILLING NAME, ADDRESS, ZIP CODE & PHONE #

PIN # GRP#

PHYSICIAN OR SUPPLIER INFORMATION

(APPROVED BY AMA COUNCIL ON MEDICAL SERVICE 8/88) *PLEASE PRINT OR TYPE* FORM HCFA-1500 (12-90) FORM OWCP-1500 FORM RRB-1500

Form 1240LM

Case Two, Form 8

OUTLINE FORMAT PROGRESS NOTES

Patient Name Johnson, Raymond

Prob. No. or Letter	DATE	S Subjective	O Objective	A Assess	P Plans	Page 3

Start each Progress Note (Subjective, Objective, Assessment and Plans) at the appropriate shaded column to create an outline form. Write through the intervening columns to the right margin of the page.

ANDRUS/CLINI-REC® PRIMARY CARE CHARTING SYSTEM FORM NO. 26-7115, ©1976 BIBBERO SYSTEMS, INC., PETALUMA, CA.

Courtesy of Bibbero Systems, Inc., Petaluma, California.

GIRLS: BIRTH TO 36 MONTHS
PHYSICAL GROWTH
NCHS PERCENTILES*

Case Three, Form 9

NAME ______________________ RECORD # ____________

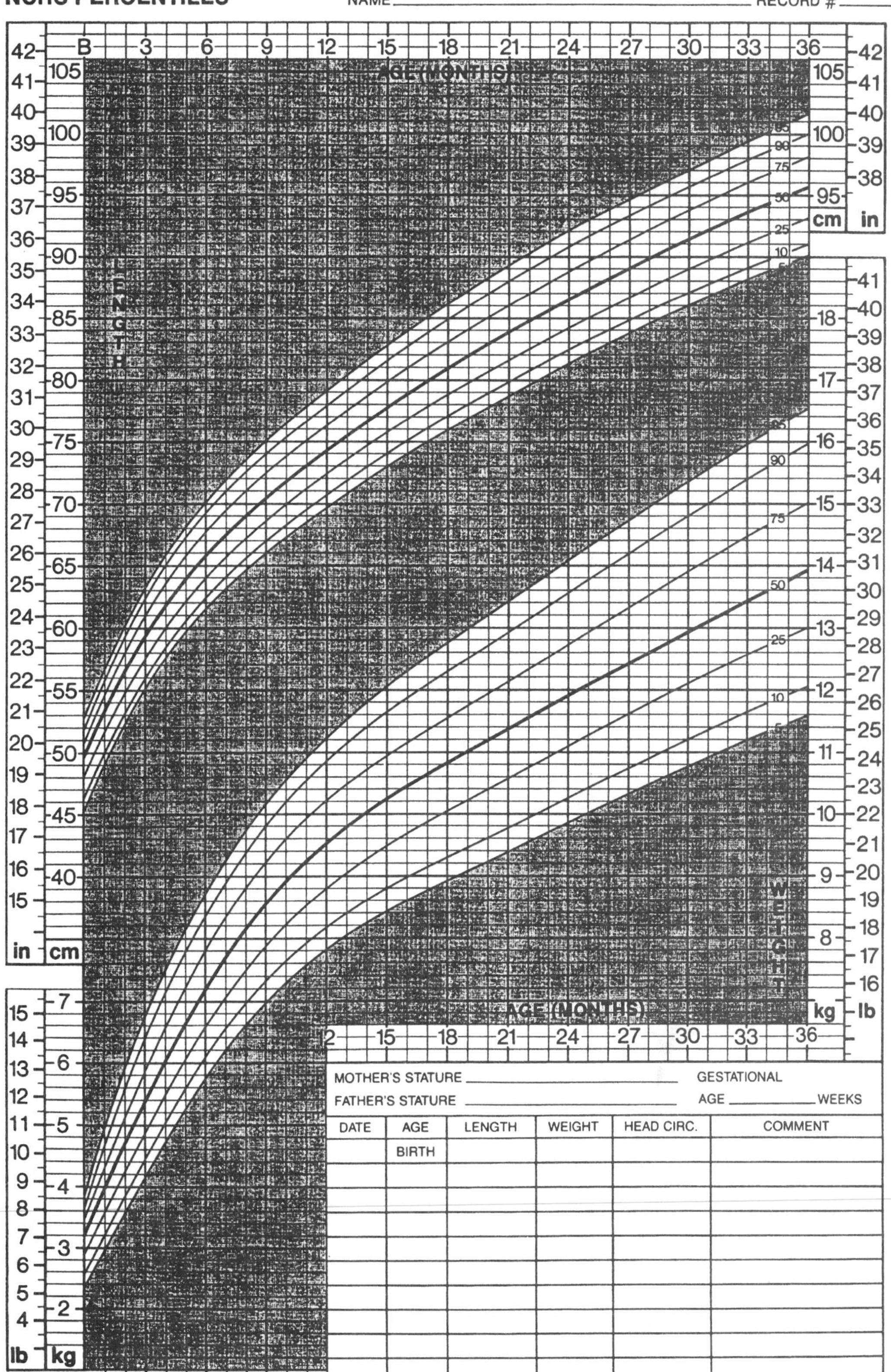

MOTHER'S STATURE ______________ GESTATIONAL
FATHER'S STATURE ______________ AGE ________ WEEKS

DATE	AGE	LENGTH	WEIGHT	HEAD CIRC.	COMMENT
	BIRTH				

*Adapted from: Hamill PVV, Drizd TA, Johnson CL, Reed RB, Roche AF, Moore WM: Physical growth: National Center for Health Statistics percentiles. AM J CLIN NUTR 32:607-629, 1979. Data from the Fels Longitudinal Study, Wright State University School of Medicine, Yellow Springs, Ohio.

Case Three, Form 10

OUTLINE FORMAT PROGRESS NOTES

Patient Name Soto, Robin

Prob. No. or Letter	DATE	S Subjective	O Objective	A Assess	P Plans	Page 2

Start each Progress Note (Subjective, Objective, Assessment and Plans) at the appropriate shaded column to create an outline form. Write through the intervening columns to the right margin of the page.

ANDRUS/CLINI-REC® PRIMARY CARE CHARTING SYSTEM FORM NO. 26-7115, ©1976 BIBBERO SYSTEMS, INC., PETALUMA, CA.

Courtesy of Bibbero Systems, Inc., Petaluma, California.

Case Three, Form 11

Patient Information Sheet

Blackburn Primary Care Associates
1990 Turquoise Drive
Blackburn, WI 54937
(555)555-1234

REGISTRATION
(PLEASE PRINT)

Home Phone: 555-898-6154

Today's Date: 2/25/00

PATIENT INFORMATION

Name: Soto (Last Name) Robin (First Name) A (Initial) Soc. Sec.# 765-19-3190

Address: 28 Lakeland Drive APT 308

City: Blackburn State: WI Zip: 54936

Single ✔ Married ___ Widowed ___ Separated ___ Divorced ___ Sex M ___ F ✔ Age 4 1/2 months Birthdate 10-08-99

Patient Employed by: N/A Occupation: ___

Business Address: ___ Business Phone: ___

By whom were you referred? ___

In case of emergency who should be notified? Janet Soto (Name) Mother (Relation to Patient) Phone 555-898-6154

PRIMARY INSURANCE

Person Responsible for Account: Soto (Last Name) Janet (First Name) M. (Initial)

Relation to Patient: Mother Birthdate: 12-11-62 Soc. Sec.# 219-54-3131

Address (if different from patient's): Same Phone: ___

City: ___ State: ___ Zip: ___

Person Responsible Employed by: W.B.Saunders Occupation: Editor

Business Address: 3500 Barnum Place 54937 Business Phone: 555-263-3500

Insurance Company: Travelers

Contract #: 31965AR21 Group #: TWB198 Subscriber #: 219543131WB

Name of other dependents covered under this plan: none

ADDITIONAL INSURANCE

Is patient covered by additional insurance? ___ Yes ✔ No

Subscriber Name: ___ Relation to Patient: ___ Birthdate: ___

Address (if different from patient's): ___ Phone: ___

City: ___ State: ___ Zip: ___

Subscriber Employed by: ___ Business Phone: ___

Insurance Company: ___ Soc. Sec.# ___

Contract #: ___ Group #: ___ Subscriber #: ___

Name of other dependents covered under this plan: ___

ASSIGNMENT AND RELEASE

I, the undersigned, certify that I (or my dependent) have insurance coverage with *Travelers* (Name of Insurance Company(ies)) and assign directly to Dr. *Blackburn Primary* insurance benefits, if any, otherwise payable to me for services rendered. I understand that I am financially responsible for all charges whether or not paid by insurance. I hereby authorize the doctor to release all information necessary to secure the payment of benefits. I authorize the use of this signature on all insurance submissions.

Janet Soto (Responsible Party Signature) *Mother* (Relationship) 2/25/00 (Date)

Case Three, Form 12

Patient Encounter Form

Blackburn Primary Care Associates

1990 Turquoise Drive
Blackburn, WI 54937
(555) 555-1234

FED. I.D. # 52-1963787

PAT. INFO.	ACCT. NO.	PATIENT'S LAST NAME	FIRST	M.I.	DATE OF BIRTH	SEX	TODAY'S DATE
		SOTO	ROBIN	A	10/8/99	☐ M ☒ F	2/25/00

INSURANCE	COPAY	DISABILITY RELATED TO: ☐ ACCIDENT ☐ INDUSTRIAL ☐ ILLNESS ☐ OTHER
Travelers		DATES SYMPTOMS APPEARED, INCEPTION OF PREGNANCY, OR ACCIDENT OCCURRED: / /

✓	DESCRIPTION	CPT/MD	FEE
	OFFICE VISITS-NEW PATIENTS		
	Focused	99201	
	Expanded	99202	
	Detailed	99203	
	Comprehensive	99204	
	Complex	99205	
	OFFICE VISITS - EST. PATIENTS		
	Minimal	99211	
	Focused	99212	
X	Expanded	99213	
	Detailed	99214	
	Comprehensive	99215	
	PREVENTIVE HEALTH CARE NEW PT.	EST. PT	
	Eval./Mgmt. > 1 Yr 99381	99391	
	Early Child 1 - 4 Yrs 99382	99392	
	Late Child 5 - 11 Yrs 99383	99393	
	Adolescent 12 - 17 Yrs 99384	99394	
	Eval./Mgmt. 18 - 39 Yrs 99385	99395	
	Eval./Mgmt. 40 - 64 Yrs 99386	99396	
	Eval./Mgmt. 65 - Over 99387	99397	
	HOSP./SNF/HOME VISITS		
	House Calls	99341	
	ER Visit	9928__	
	Init. Hosp. Care	99222	
	Sub. Hosp. Care	99232	
	SNF, Sub. Care	99312	
	INJECTIONS		
	Allergy	95125	
	B-12	J3420	
	Flu Shot	90724	
	Gamma Globulin	90741	
	Hormone		
	Depo Provera	J1055	
	Kenalog 40-60 mg	J3301	
	Morphine/Demerol	J2270	
	Phenergan	J2550	
	Celestone	J0700	
	Hep B, newborn to 11 years	90744	
	Hep B, 11 - 19 years	90745	
	Hep B, 20 years and above	90746	
	Rocephin/Claforan	J0696	
	Iron	J1760	
	Lidocaine NCL	J2000	
	Admin of INJ	J0110	
	Unlist INJ	90782	
	Drug		
	Dose		

✓	DESCRIPTION	CPT/MD	FEE
	SPECIAL SERVICES		
	Drivers Physical	99214	
	Pelvic/Breast Exam	99214	
	Industrial	99214	
	IMMUNIZATIONS		
X	DtaP	90700	
	DPT	90701	
	DT	90702	
	Td (Tetanus Booster)	90703	
	MMR	90707	
	Mumps	90704	
	Pneumococcal	90732	
	Rubella	90706	
X	Polio (TOPV)	90712	
	PPD	86580	
	TB Tine Test	86585	
X	Hib	90737	
	OFFICE PROCEDURES		
	Audiometry	92551	
	Diathermy (Ultrasound)	97024	
	EKG Tracing & Interp.	93000	
	Intermed Joint Injection	20605	
	Major Joint Injection	20610	
	Nebulizer TX	94664	
	Rem. Impact. Cer.	69210	
	Spirometry	94010	
	Stress Test	93015	
	Trigger Pt. Inj.	20550	
	Eye Wash	65205*	
	LABORATORY		
	Throat Culture	87060	
	Glucose Blood	82947	
	Glucose Stick	82948	
	UA Pregnancy	81025	
	Occult Blood, Stool	82270	
	Rapid Strep	86588	
	Smear	88150	
	UA Dip	81002	
	Urinalysis	81000	
	Venipuncture	36415	
	Wet Mount, Smear	87210	
	Wet Mount KOH	87220	
	Collect/Handing	99000	
	MISCELLANEOUS		
	Pre-OP	993__	
	After Hours	99050	
	Sunday/Holidays	99054	
	Cast Removal	29705	
	Norplant Insertion	11975	
	Norplant Kit	99070	

✓	DESCRIPTION	CPT/MD	FEE
	SURGERY		
	Toenail Removal	11750	
	Cryosurgery	17200	
	I & D	10060	
	Drainage Paronychia	10060	
	Enucleation Ext. Hemorrhoid	46320	
	I & D Abscess/Cyst	10060	
	Podophyllom	17100	
	Removal Foreign Body	10120	
	Wart Removal	17110	
	Destr. Single Lesion Face	17000	
	2nd and 3rd Lesion Face	17001	
	Destr. Single Lesion Body	17106	
	2nd and 3rd Lesion Body	17003	
	Lesion Rem. Excision		
	Anoscopy	46600	
	Flex. Scope with Sig.	45330	
	Vasectomy	55250	
	Therapeutic Abor.	59840	
	Removal Foreign Body of Eye	65205	
	SUPPLIES		
	Ace Wrap	99070	
	Cast Material	99070	
	Cervical Collar	99070	
	Elastic Bandage	99070	
	Splint/Sling	99070	
	Sterile Dressing	99070	
	Surgical Tray	99070	

DIAGNOSIS: ICD-9	☐ C.T.S. 354.0	☐ Flu Shot Only V04.8	☐ Internal Derangement Knee 717.9	☐ Prostatitis 601.9
☐ Abscess Cellulitis 682.9	☐ CAD 746.85	☐ Flu Vac V04.8	☐ Labyrinthitis 386.30	☐ Psoriasis 696.1
☐ Abdominal Pain 789.0	☐ CA-Prostate 185	☐ Flu W/Resp. Manifest 487.1	☐ Laceration Open Wound 879.8__	☐ Rheumatoid Arthritis 714.0
☐ Abrasions 919.0	☐ Cardiac Arrhythmia 427.9	☐ Folliculitis 704.8	☐ Levator Scapular Syndrome 726.90	☐ Sciatica 724.3
☐ Acne 706.1	☐ Cataracts 366.9	☐ FX ____	☐ Menopausal Disorder 627.9	☐ Sacroiliac Sprain 846.1
☐ ADD 314.00	☐ Chest Pain 786.50	☐ Gallbladder Disease 575.9	☐ Metabolic Diff. 277.8	☐ Sinusitis, Acute 461.9
☐ Alcoholism 303.90	☐ Congestive Heart Failure 428.0	☐ Ganglion 727.43	☐ Migraine 346.90	☐ Smoking Cessation 305.10
☐ Allergic Rhinitis 477.9	☐ Conjunctivitis 372.30	☐ Gastroenteritis 558.9	☐ Mitral Valve Disorder 424.0	☐ Sprain ____
☐ Allergy, Unsp 995.3	☐ Constipation 564.0	☐ Gout 274.9	☐ Myalgia and Myositis 729.1	☐ SQ. Cell CA-Face 173.3
☐ Anemia 285.9	☐ Consult Vasc. V65.8	☐ Gyn Exam V72.3	☐ Noninf. Gastroenterit. 558.9	☐ Sterilization V25.2
☐ Angina Pectoris 413.9	☐ Convulsions 780.3	☐ Headache Tension 307.81	☐ Obesity 278.0	☐ Stye 373.11
☐ Anxiety Depression 300.4	☐ COPD 496	☐ Hemorrhoids Ext. 455.3	☐ Osteoarthrosis 715.00	☐ TB Exposure V01.1
☐ Anxiety State 300.00	☐ Coronary Atherosclerosis 414.0	☐ Hepatitis 573.3	☐ Osteoporosis 733.00	☐ Tendonitis 726.90
☐ ASCVD 429.2	☐ CVA 436	☐ Hernia-Inguinal 550.90	☐ Otitis Externa 380.10	☐ Tinea 110.9
☐ Asthma W/O Status Asthma 493.90	☐ Cyst Sebaceous 706.2	☐ Herpes Zoster 053.9	☐ Otitis Media 382.9	☐ Tonsillitis, Acute 463
☐ Atten Surg. Dressing/Suture V58.3	☐ Dermatitis 692.9	☐ Hyperlipidemia 272.4	☐ P.I.D. 614.9	☐ URI, Acute 465.9
☐ BCP Consult V25.9	☐ Diabetes, Uncomp. Adult 250.00	☐ Hypertension 401.9	☐ Peptic Ulcer 533.90	☐ Urine Tract Infection 599.0
☐ BPH 600	☐ Diabetes, Complicated 250.90	☐ Hyperthyroidism 242.9	☐ Pharyngitis, Acute 462	☐ Vaginitis 616.10
☐ Bronchitis, Acute 466.0	☐ Disc Degeneration 722.6	☐ Hypothyroidism 244.9	☐ Pneumonia, Viral 480.9	☐ Well Adult Medical Exam V70.9
☐ Bronchitis, Chronic 491.9	☐ Duodenal Ulcer 532.90	☐ Impacted Cerumen 380.4	☐ Poison Oak 692.6	☒ Well Child Health Exam V20.2
☐ Burn ____ 949.0	☐ Dysmenorrhea 625.3	☐ Impetigo 684	☐ Premarital B-Test V70.3	
☐ Bursitis 727.3	☐ Fatigue 780.7	☐ Ingrown Toenail 703.0	☐ Pregnancy Test, Unconf. V72.4	

DIAGNOSIS (If not checked above) ICD-9	PHYSICIAN SIGNATURE	TODAY'S FEE	$
	PAYMENT BY	PAYMENT	
PLEASE REMEMBER THAT PAYMENT IS YOUR OBLIGATION REGARDLESS OF INSURANCE OR OTHER THIRD PARTY INVOLVEMENT.	☐ CASH ☐ CREDIT CARD ☐ CHECK # ____	BALANCE DUE	

Case Three, Form 13

FEE SCHEDULE

BLACKBURN PRIMARY CARE ASSOCIATES
1990 TURQUOISE DRIVE
BLACKBURN, WI 54937

Federal Tax ID Number: **52-1963787**

BCBS Group Number: **14982**
Medicare Group Number: **14982**

OFFICE VISIT, NEW PATIENT

Focused, 99201	$ 45.00
Expanded, 99202	$ 53.00
Detailed, 99203	$ 60.00
Comprehensive, 99204	$ 95.00
Complex, 99205	$195.00
Consultation, 99245	$250.00

OFFICE VISIT, ESTABLISHED PATIENT

Minimal, 99211	$ 40.00
Focused, 99212	$ 48.00
Expanded, 99213	$ 55.00
Detailed, 99214	$ 65.00
Comprehensive, 99215	$195.00

OFFICE PROCEDURES

EKG, 12 Lead, 93000	$ 55.00
Stress EKG, Treadmill, 93015	$295.00
Sigmoidoscopy, Flex., 45330	$145.00
Spirometry, 94010	$ 50.00
Cerumen Removal, 69210	$ 40.00
Collection & Handling	
Lab Specimen, 99000	$ 9.00
Venipuncture, 36415	$ 9.00
Urinalysis, 81000	$ 20.00
Urinalysis, 81002 (Dip Only)	$ 12.00
Influenza Injection, 90724	$ 20.00
Pneumococcal Injection, 90732	$ 20.00
Oral Polio, 90712	$ 15.00
DTaP, 90700	$ 20.00
Tetanus Toxoid, 90703	$ 15.00
MMR, 90707	$ 25.00
Hib, 90737	$ 20.00
Hepatitis B, newborn to age 11 years, 90744	$ 60.00
Hepatitis B, 11-19 years, 90745	$ 60.00
Hepatitis B, 20 years and above 90746	$ 60.00
Intramuscular Injection, 90788	
Penicillin	$ 30.00
Ceftriaxone	$ 25.00
Solu-Medrol	$ 23.00
Vitamin B-12	$ 13.00
Subcutaneous Injection, 90782	
Epinephrine	$ 18.00
Sus-Pherine	$ 25.00
Insulin, U-100	$ 15.00

COMMON DIAGNOSIS CODES

Ischemic Heart Disease	414.9
w/o myocardial infarction	411.89
w/ coronary occlusion	411.81
Hypertension, Malignant	401.0
Benign	401.1
Unspecified	401.9
w/ congest. heart failure	402.91
Asthma, Bronchial	493.9
w/ COPD	493.2
allergic, w/ S.A.	493.91
allergic, w/o S.A.	493.90
Kyphosis	737.10
w/ osteoporosis	733.0
Osteoporosis	733.00
Otitis Media, Acute	382.9
Chronic	382.9
Well Child Health Exam	V20.2
Well Adult Medical Exam	V70.9

Case Three, Form 14

PLEASE DO NOT STAPLE IN THIS AREA

APPROVED OMB-0938-0008

PICA

HEALTH INSURANCE CLAIM FORM

PICA

CARRIER

PATIENT AND INSURED INFORMATION

1. MEDICARE (Medicare #) MEDICAID (Medicaid #) CHAMPUS (Sponsor's SSN) CHAMPVA (VA File #) GROUP HEALTH PLAN (SSN or ID) FECA BLK LUNG (SSN) OTHER (ID)

1a. INSURED'S I.D. NUMBER (FOR PROGRAM IN ITEM 1)

2. PATIENT'S NAME (Last Name, First Name, Middle Initial)

3. PATIENT'S BIRTHDATE MM DD YY SEX M F

4. INSURED'S NAME (Last Name, First Name, Middle Initial)

5. PATIENT'S ADDRESS (No., Street)

6. PATIENT RELATIONSHIP TO INSURED Self Spouse Child Other

7. INSURED'S ADDRESS (No., Street)

CITY STATE

8. PATIENT STATUS Single Married Other

CITY STATE

ZIP CODE TELEPHONE (Include Area Code) ( )

Employed Full-Time Student Part-Time Student

ZIP CODE TELEPHONE (Include Area Code) ( )

9. OTHER INSURED'S NAME (Last Name, First Name, Middle Initial)

10. IS PATIENT'S CONDITION RELATED TO:

11. INSURED'S POLICY GROUP OR FECA NUMBER

a. OTHER INSURED'S POLICY OR GROUP NUMBER

a. EMPLOYMENT? (CURRENT OR PREVIOUS) YES NO

a. INSURED'S DATE OF BIRTH MM DD YY SEX M F

b. OTHER INSURED'S DATE OF BIRTH MM DD YY SEX M F

b. AUTO ACCIDENT? PLACE (State) YES NO

b. EMPLOYER'S NAME OR SCHOOL NAME

c. EMPLOYER'S NAME OR SCHOOL NAME

c. OTHER ACCIDENT? YES NO

c. INSURANCE PLAN NAME OR PROGRAM NAME

d. INSURANCE PLAN NAME OR PROGRAM NAME

10d. RESERVED FOR LOCAL USE

d. IS THERE ANOTHER HEALTH BENEFIT PLAN? YES NO *If yes, return to and complete item 9a-d.*

READ BACK OF FORM BEFORE COMPLETING & SIGNING THIS FORM.

12. PATIENT'S OR AUTHORIZED PERSON'S SIGNATURE I authorize the release of any medical or other information necessary to process this claim. I also request payment of government benefits either to myself or to the party who accepts assignment below.

SIGNED ______ DATE ______

13. INSURED'S OR AUTHORIZED PERSON'S SIGNATURE I authorize payment of medical benefits to the undersigned physician or supplier for services described below.

SIGNED ______

PHYSICIAN OR SUPPLIER INFORMATION

14. DATE OF CURRENT: MM DD YY ILLNESS (First symptom) OR INJURY (Accident) OR PREGNANCY (LMP)

15. IF PATIENT HAS HAD SAME OR SIMILAR ILLNESS, GIVE FIRST DATE MM DD YY

16. DATES PATIENT UNABLE TO WORK IN CURRENT OCCUPATION FROM MM DD YY TO MM DD YY

17. NAME OF REFERRING PHYSICIAN OR OTHER SOURCE

17a. I.D. NUMBER OF REFERRING PHYSICIAN

18. HOSPITALIZATION DATES RELATED TO CURRENT SERVICES FROM MM DD YY TO MM DD YY

19. RESERVED FOR LOCAL USE

20. OUTSIDE LAB? YES NO $ CHARGES

21. DIAGNOSIS OR NATURE OF ILLNESS OR INJURY. (RELATE ITEMS 1,2,3 OR 4 TO ITEM 24E BY LINE)

1. ___ . __

2. ___ . __

3. ___ . __

4. ___ . __

22. MEDICAID RESUBMISSION CODE ORIGINAL REF. NO.

23. PRIOR AUTHORIZATION NUMBER

24. A DATE(S) OF SERVICE From MM DD YY	To MM DD YY	B Place of Service	C Type of Service	D PROCEDURES, SERVICES, OR SUPPLIES (Explain Unusual Circumstances) CPT/HCPCS MODIFIER	E DIAGNOSIS CODE	F $ CHARGES	G DAYS OR UNITS	H EPSDT Family Plan	I EMG	J COB	K RESERVED FOR LOCAL USE
1											
2											
3											
4											
5											
6											

25. FEDERAL TAX I.D. NUMBER SSN EIN

26. PATIENT'S ACCOUNT NUMBER

27. ACCEPT ASSIGNMENT? (For govt. claims, see back) YES NO

28. TOTAL CHARGE $

29. AMOUNT PAID $

30. BALANCE DUE $

31. SIGNATURE OF PHYSICIAN OR SUPPLIER INCLUDING DEGREES OR CREDENTIALS (I certify that the statements on the reverse apply to this bill and are made a part thereof.)

SIGNED DATE

32. NAME AND ADDRESS OF FACILITY WHERE SERVICES WERE RENDERED (If other than home or office)

33. PHYSICIAN'S, SUPPLIER'S BILLING NAME, ADDRESS, ZIP CODE & PHONE #

PIN # GRP#

(APPROVED BY AMA COUNCIL ON MEDICAL SERVICE 8/88) Form 1240LM

PLEASE PRINT OR TYPE

FORM HCFA-1500 (12-90) FORM OWCP-1500 FORM RRB-1500

Case Four, Form 15

Appointment Schedule

DAY: Mon. | Tue. | Wed. | Thu. | Fri. | Sat.

DATE	HUGHES, M.D.	LAWLER, M.D.	LOPEZ, M.D.
8 00			
8 10		NO ACUTE	NO NEW
8 20		OR	OB
8 30		NEW PATIENTS	
8 40			
8 50			
9 00	Sx-Blackburn	Johnson, Marvin	
9 10	Hosp.	555-921-3195	
9 20	Smith,	CPE	
9 30	Mariane		
9 40			
9 50		↓	
10 00		Seeburn, Kate	Richards, Mary
10 10		INFLUENZA 555-817-	↓ PAP 619-3191
10 20		↓ FLU 3615	Scheeler, Virginia
10 30		Butler, Carl	↓ PAP 721-9951
10 40		NEURO ✓ UP	
10 50	↓	↓ 555-331-9195	
11 00	Jefferson, Martha	Doyle, Mike 555-	Longfellow, Wilma
11 10	NEW OB 555-245-1790	↓ PROSTATE ✓ 277-	PAP, PE
11 20		Doyle, Hanah 1965	555-317-2198
11 30		↓ ✓ UP	
11 40			
11 50	↓		↓
12 00	Davis, Marvin 555-	HOSPITAL	
12 10	↓ ALLERGY 241-9200	ROUNDS	
12 20	Martin, Darlene 555-		LUNCH MTG
12 30	↓ SUT REM 917-1909		
12 40	Sorbin, John 555-		
12 50	↓ VACCINES 914-3190		
1 00	Shapiro, Ivan		Simpson, Lisa
1 10			3 MO PRENATAL
1 20			↓ 555-129-3190
1 30			Schmidt, Cindy
1 40			STD 555-377-
1 50	↓		↓ 2198
2 00	Docker, Millie 555-219-		
2 10	CHEST PAIN 7191		
2 20	↓		
2 30			
2 40			
2 50		↓	
3 00	Starvey, Jill 555-	AMA Mtg	Jessup, Carl 719-
3 10	↓ VACCINES 319-2191	Convention	↓ STRESS EKG 3307
3 20		Center	Lawson, Milton 331-
3 30		3:30 pm	↓ PROSTATE 9900
3 40			
3 50			
4 00	HOSPITAL		Geary, Leon 555-
4 10	ROUNDS		↓ VACCINE 498-3150
4 20			
4 30			
4 40			
4 50			
5 00			MED SOCIETY
5 10			MTG
5 20			5-7 pm
5 30			
5 40			
5 50	↓	↓	↓

Case Four, Form 16

ANDRUS/CLINI-REC® HEALTH HISTORY QUESTIONNAIRE

Chart No. ________

Identification Information

Today's Date 1/15/05

Name Lucille Ferguson Date of Birth 6/21/30

Occupation ________ Marital Status Widowed

PART A – PRESENT HEALTH HISTORY

I. CURRENT MEDICAL PROBLEMS

Please list the medical problems for which you came to see the doctor. About when did they begin?

Problems	Date Began
Pain when urinating	1 wk ago
Fever	Yesterday

What concerns you most about these problems?

____

If you are being treated for any other illness or medical problems by another physician, please describe the problems and write the name of the physician or medical facility treating you.

Illness or Medical Problem	Physician or Medical Facility	City
Osteoarthritis		

II. MEDICATIONS

Please list all medications you are now taking, including those you buy without a doctor's prescription (such as aspirin, cold tablets or vitamin supplements).

____

III. ALLERGIES AND SENSITIVITIES

List anything that you are allergic to such as certain foods, medications, dust, chemicals or soaps, household items, pollens, bee stings, etc., and indicate how each affects you.

Allergic To:	Effect	Allergic To:	Effect
None			

IV. GENERAL HEALTH, ATTITUDE AND HABITS

How is your overall health now?	Health now:	Poor ___ Fair ___ Good ✓ Excellent ___
How has it been most of your life?	Health has been:	Poor ___ Fair ___ Good ✓ Excellent ___
In the past year:		
Has your appetite changed?	Appetite:	Decreased ✓ Increased ___ Stayed same ___
Has your weight changed?	Weight:	Lost ___ lbs. Gained ___ lbs. No change ✓
Are you thirsty much of the time?	Thirsty:	No ✓ Yes ___
Has your overall 'pep' changed?	Pep:	Decreased ___ Increased ___ Stayed same ✓
Do you usually have trouble sleeping?	Trouble sleeping:	No ___ Yes ✓
How much do you exercise?	Exercise:	Little or none ___ Less than I need ✓ All I need ___
Do you smoke?	Smokes:	No ✓ Yes ___ If yes, how many years? ___
How many each day?		___ Cigarettes ___ Cigars ___ Pipesfull
Have you ever smoked?	Smoked:	No ___ Yes ✓ If yes, how many years? 15
How many each day?		30 Cigarettes ___ Cigars ___ Pipesfull
Do you drink alcoholic beverages?	Alcohol:	No ___ Yes ✓ I drink ___ Beers ✓ Glasses of wine 2 Drinks of hard liquor - per day
Have you ever had a problem with alcohol?	Prior problem:	No ✓ Yes ___
How much coffee or tea do you usually drink?	Coffee/Tea:	1 cups of coffee or tea a day
Do you regularly wear seatbelts?	Seatbelts:	No ___ Yes ✓

DO YOU:	Rarely/Never	Occasionally	Frequently
Feel nervous?	X		
Feel depressed?	X		
Find it hard to make decisions?	X		
Lose your temper?	X		
Worry a lot?	X		
Tire easily?		X	
Have trouble relaxing?	X		
Have any sexual problems?	X		

DO YOU:	Rarely/Never	Occasionally	Frequently
Ever feel like committing suicide?	X		
Feel bored with your life?	X		
Use marijuana?	X		
Use "hard drugs"?	X		

Do you want to talk to the doctor about a personal matter? No X Yes ___

C O N F I D E N T I A L

STOCK NO. 19-742-4 8/95 Page 1

Courtesy of Bibbero Systems, Inc., Petaluma, California.

PART A – PRESENT HEALTH HISTORY (continued)

IV. GENERAL HEALTH, ATTITUDE AND HABITS (continued)

Have you recently had any changes in your: / If yes, please explain:

	No	Yes	If yes, please explain
Marital status?	X		
Job or work?	X		
Residence?	X		
Financial status?	X		
Are you having any legal problems or trouble with the law?	X		

PART B – PAST HISTORY

I. FAMILY HEALTH

Please give the following information about your immediate family:

Relationship	Age, if Living	Age At Death	State of Health Or Cause of Death
Father		95	excellent
Mother		unknown	cancer
Brothers and Sisters			
	68		multiple sclerosis
Spouse			
Children			

Have any **blood relatives** had any of the following illnesses? If so, indicate relationship (mother, brother, etc.)

Illness	Family Members
Asthma	Brother
Diabetes	—
Cancer	Breast cancer-Mom
Blood Disease	—
Glaucoma	—
Epilepsy	—
Rheumatoid Arthritis	—
Tuberculosis	—
Gout	—
High Blood Pressure	—
Heart Disease	—
Mental Problems	—
Suicide	—
Stroke	—
Alcoholism	Uncle
Rheumatic Fever	—

II. HOSPITALIZATIONS, SURGERIES, INJURIES

Please list all times you have been hospitalized, operated on, or seriously injured.

Year	Operation, Illness, Injury	Hospital and City
1976	Appendix taken out	Mercy Hospital

III. ILLNESS AND MEDICAL PROBLEMS

Please mark with an (X) any of the following illnesses and medical problems you have or have had and indicate the year when each started. If you are not certain when an illness started, write down an approximate year.

Illness	(x)	(Year)
Eye or eye lid infection		
Glaucoma		
Other eye problems		
Ear trouble		
Deafness or decreased hearing		
Thyroid trouble		
Strep throat	X	as child
Bronchitis	X	several
Emphysema		
Pneumonia		
Allergies, asthma or hay fever		
Tuberculosis		
Other lung problems		
High blood pressure		
Heart attack		
High cholesterol	X	1991
Arteriosclerosis (Hardening of arteries)		
Heart murmur		
Other heart condition		
Stomach/duodenal ulcer		
Diverticulosis		
Colitis		
Other bowel problems		
Hepatitis		
Liver trouble		
Gallbladder trouble		

Illness	(x)	(Year)
Hernia		
Hemorrhoids	X	1955
Kidney or bladder disease		
Prostate problem (male only)		
Mental problems		
Headaches		
Head injury		
Stroke		
Convulsions, seizures		
Arthritis	X	now
Gout		
Cancer or tumor		
Bleeding tendency		
Diabetes		
Measles/Rubeola	X	child
German measles/Rubella		
Polio	X	child
Mumps	X	child
Scarlet fever		
Chicken pox	X	child
Mononucleosis		
Eczema		
Psoriasis		
Venereal disease		
Genital herpes		
HIV test		
AIDS		

CONFIDENTIAL

Case Four, Form 16

PART C – BODY SYSTEMS REVIEW

Please answer all of the following questions.

Circle any questions you find difficult to answer.

MEN: Please answer questions 1 through 12, then skip to question 18.

WOMEN: Please start on question 6.

MEN ONLY

1. Have you had or do you have prostate trouble?	No ____	Yes ____
2. Do you have any sexual problems or a problem with impotency?	No ____	Yes ____
3. Have you ever had sores or lesions on your penis?	No ____	Yes ____
4. Have you ever had any discharge from your penis?	No ____	Yes ____
5. Do you ever have pain, lumps or swelling in your testicles?	No ____	Yes ____

Check here if you wish to discuss any special problems with the doctor ☐

MEN & WOMEN

	Rarely/ Never	Occasionally	Frequently
6. Is it sometimes hard to start your urine flow?	X		
7. Is urination ever painful?			X
8. Do you have to urinate more than 5 times a day?	X		
9. Do you get up at night to urinate?	X		
10. Has your urine ever been bloody or dark colored?	X		
11. Do you ever lose urine when you strain, laugh, cough or sneeze?	X		
12. Do you ever lose urine during sleep?	X		

WOMEN ONLY

Do you:

	Rarely/ Never	Occasionally	Frequently
13. a. Have any menstrual problems?	X		
b. Feel rather tense just before your period?	X		
c. Have heavy menstrual bleeding?	X		
d. Have painful menstrual periods?	X		
e. Have any bleeding between periods?	X		
f. Have any unusual vaginal discharge or itching?	X		
g. Ever have tender breasts?	X		
h. Have any discharge from your nipples?	X		
i. Have any hot flashes?	X		

14. How many times, if any, have you been pregnant? 3
15. How many children born alive? 3
16. Are you taking birth control pills? No X Yes ____
17. Do you examine your breasts monthly for lumps? No ____ Yes Sometimes
17a. What was the date of your last menstrual period? Date 1980

Check here if you wish to discuss any special problem with the doctor ☐

MEN & WOMEN

	Rarely/ Never	Occasionally	Frequently
18. In the past year have you had any:			
a. Severe shoulder pain?	X		
b. Severe back pain?	X		
c. Muscle or joint stiffness or pain due to sports, exercise or injury?	X		
d. Pain or swelling in any joints not due to sports, exercise or injury?	X		

19. Do you have dry skin or brittle fingernails?	No X	Yes ____
20. Do you bruise easily?	No X	Yes ____
21. Do you have any moles that have changed in color or in size?	No X	Yes ____
22. Do you have any other skin problems?	No X	Yes ____
23. In the last 3 months have you had:		
a. A fever that lasted more than one day?	No ____	Yes X
b. Sores or cuts that were hard to heal?	No X	Yes ____
c. Any cold sores (fever blisters)?	No X	Yes ____
d. Any lumps in your neck, armpits or groin?	No X	Yes ____
e. Do you ever have chills or sweat at night?	No X	Yes ____
24. Have you traveled out of the country in the last 2 years?	No X	Yes, Traveled in: ____

25. Write in the dates for the shots you have had: Measles ____ Mumps ____ Polio ____ Smallpox ____ Tetanus ____ Typhoid ____

26. Have you had a tuberculin (TB) skin test?	No X	Yes ____	Date ____
If so, was it negative or positive?	Neg ____	Pos ____	
27. Have you had an HIV test for AIDS?	No X	Yes ____	Date ____
If so, was it negative or positive?	Neg ____	Pos ____	

 PLEASE TURN THIS PAGE STOCK NO. 19-742-4 8/95 Page 3

CONFIDENTIAL

BODY SYSTEMS REVIEW

REMOVE THIS PAGE AFTER COMPLETING QUESTIONNAIRE

					VISION / HEARING
28.	Do you wear eyeglasses?	No___	Yes X		Wears eyeglasses
29.	Do you wear contact lenses?	No X	Yes___		Wears contacts
30.	Has your vision changed in the last year?	No___	Yes X		Vision changes in last year
		Rarely/ Never	**Occasionally**	**Frequently**	
31.	How often do you have:				
	a. Double vision?		X		Double vision
	b. Blurry vision?		X		Blurred vision
	c. Watery or itchy eyes?			X	Watery/itchy eyes
32.	Do you ever see colored rings around lights?	X			Sees halos
33.	Do others tell you you have a hearing problem?		X		Hearing problem
34.	Do you have trouble keeping your balance?	X			Loses balance
35.	Do you have any discharge from your ears?	X			Discharge from ears
36.	Do you ever feel dizzy or have motion sickness?	X			Dizzy / motion sickness
37.	Do you have any problems with your hearing?	No X	Yes___	Hearing Problems	
38.	Do you ever have ringing in your ears?	No X	Yes___	Ringing in ears	

		Rarely/ Never	Occasionally	Frequently	NOSE / THROAT / RESPIRATORY
39.	How often do you have:				
	a. Head colds?		X		Head colds
	b. Chest colds?		X		Chest colds
	c. Runny nose?		X		Runny nose
	d. Stuffed up nose?		X		Head congestion
	e. Sore/hoarse throat?		X		Sore / hoarse throat
	f. Bad coughing spells?	X			Coughing spells
	g. Sneezing spells?	X			Sneezing spells
	h. Trouble breathing?	X			Trouble breathing
	i. Nose bleeds?	X			Nose bleeds
	j. Cough blood?	X			Cough blood
40.	Have you ever worked or spent time:				
	a. On a farm?	No___	Yes X	Worked on a farm	
	b. In a mine?	No X	Yes___	Worked in a mine	
	c. In a laundry or mill?	No X	Yes___	Worked in a laundry/mill	
	d. In very dusty places?	No X	Yes___	Worked in high dust concentrations	
	e. With or near toxic chemicals?	No X	Yes___	Exposed to toxic chemicals	
	f. With or near radioactive materials?	No X	Yes___	Exposed to radioactive materials	
	g. With or near asbestos?	No X	Yes___	Exposed to asbestos	

		Rarely/ Never	Occasionally	Frequently	CARDIOVASCULAR
41.	Do you get out of breath easily when you are active (like climbing stairs)?	X			Out of breath quickly when exercising
42.	Do you ever feel light-headed or dizzy?	X			Dizziness
43.	Have you ever fainted or passed out?	X			Fainted
44.	Do you sometimes feel your heart is racing or beating too fast?	X			Rapid heartbeat
45.	When you exercise do you ever get pains in your chest or shoulders?	X			Chest/shoulder pains in exercise
46.	Do you have any leg cramps or pain in your thighs or legs when walking?	X			Pain in thighs or legs when walking
47.	Do you ever have to sit up at night to breathe easier?	X			Sits up at night to breathe easier
48.	Do you use two pillows at night to help you breathe easier?	X			Breathing problems during sleep
49.	Would you say you are a restless sleeper?	X			Restless sleeper
50.	Are you bothered by leg cramps at night?	X			Leg cramps at night
51.	Do you sometimes have swollen ankles or feet?	X			Swollen ankles/feet

		Rarely/ Never	Occasionally	Frequently	DIGESTIVE
52.	How often, if ever:				
	a. Are you nauseated (sick to your stomach)?	X			Nauseated
	b. Do you have stomach pains?	X			Stomach pains
	c. Do you burp a lot after eating?	X			Burps after eating
	d. Do you have heartburn?	X			Heartburn
	e. Do you have trouble swallowing your food?	X			Trouble swallowing food
	f. Have you vomited blood?	X			Vomited blood
	g. Are you constipated?	X			Constipated
	h. Do you have diarrhea (watery stools)?	X			Diarrhea
	i. Are your bowel movements painful?	X			Painful bowel movements
	j. Are your bowel movements bloody?	X			Bloody bowel movements
	k. Are your bowel movements dark or black?	X			Dark bowel movements
53.	Have you ever had a sigmoidoscopy?	No X	Yes___	Date___	Date of last sigmoidoscopy?

PLEASE TURN TO BACK PAGE AND COMPLETE QUESTIONS ON NUTRITION.

Case Four, Form 16

Andrus/Clini-Rec®

BIBBERO SYSTEMS, INC.

COMPREHENSIVE
PHYSICAL EXAMINATION
MALE OR FEMALE
NEW OR ESTABLISHED PATIENT
CPT # 99201 - 99215

(For Office Use Only)

C O N F I D E N T I A L

NAME ______________________ AGE ________ YRS. OLD TODAY'S DATE ____________ DATE OF BIRTH ____________

Key: [O] Neg. Findings [+] Positive Findings [X] Omitted [✔] See Notes/CIRCLE WORDS OF IMPORTANCE & EXPLAIN

1 GEN. APPEARANCE	[ ]	Apparent Age/Nutrition/Development/Mental & Emotional Status/Gait/Posture/Distress/Speech –
2 HEAD / SCALP	[ ]	Size/Shape/Tender over Sinuses/Hair/Alopecia/Eruption/Masses/Bruit –
3 EYES	[ ]	Conjunct/Sclerae/Cornea/Pupils/EOM'S/Arcus/Ptosis/Fundi/Tension/Eyelids/Pallor/Light/Bruit –
4 EARS	[ ]	Ext. Canal/TM's/Perforation/Discharge/Tophi/Hearing Problem/Weber/Rinne –
5 NOSE / SINUSES	[ ]	Septum/Obstruction/Turbinates/Discharge –
6 MOUTH / THROAT	[ ]	Odor/Lips/Tongue/Tonsils/Teeth/Dentures/Gums/Pharynx –
7 NECK	[ ]	Adenopathy/Thyroid/Carotids/Trachea/Veins/Masses/Spine/Motion/Bruit –
8 BACK	[ ]	Kyphosis/Scoliosis/Lordosis/Mobility/CVA/Bone/Tenderness –
9 THORAX	[ ]	Symmetry/Movement/Contour/Tender –
10 BREASTS	[ ]	Size/Size-Consistency/Nipples/Areolar/Palpable Mass/Discharge/Tenderness/Nodes/Scars –
11 HEART	[ ]	Rate/Rhythm/Apical Impulse/Thrills/Quality of Sound/Intensity/Splitting/Extra Sounds/ Murmurs –
12 CHEST / LUNGS	[ ]	Excursion/Dullness or Hyperresonance to Percussion/Quality of Breath Sounds/Rales/Wheezing/ Rhonchi/Diaphragm/Rubs/Bruit –
13 ABDOMEN	[ ]	Bowel Sounds/Appearance/Liver/Spleen/Masses/Hernias/Murmurs/Contour/Tenderness/Bruit/ ING Nodes –
14 GROIN	[ ]	Hernia/Inguinal Nodes/Femoral Pulses –
15 MALE GENITALIA	[ ]	Penis/Testes/Scrotum Epididymis/Varicocele/Scars/Discharge –
16 FEMALE GENITALIA	[ ]	Vuvla/Vagina/Cervix/Uterus/Adnexae/Rectocele/Cystocele/Bartholin Gland/Urethra/ Discharge – Pap Smear (if done ✔) ☐
17 EXTREMITIES	[ ]	Deformity/Clubbing/Cyanosis/Edema/Nails/Peripheral Pulses/Calf Tenderness/Joints for Swelling/ ROM –
18 SKIN	[ ]	Color/Birthmarks/Scars/Texture/Rash/Eczema/Ulcers –
19 NEUROLOGICAL	[ ]	DTR's/Babinski/Cranial Nerves/Motor Abnormalities/Tremor/Paralysis/Sensory Exam – (touch, pin prick, vibration)/Coordination/Romberg –
20 MUSCULAR SYSTEM	[ ]	Strength/Wasting/Development –
21 RECTAL EXAM	[ ]	Sphincter Tone/Hemorrhoids/Fissures/Masses/Prostate/Stool Guaiac (if done ✔) ☐ Pos ☐ Neg –

Impression: ☐ Check If Normal Physical Examination

Summary: ____

____

____________________ Signature ____________________ Date ____________

Page 4

Case Four, Form 16

COMPREHENSIVE PHYSICAL EXAMINATION
(continued)

(For Office Use Only)

PHYSICIAN'S NOTES:

Body Area Number	REMARKS:

R L L R

R L

	VISION	AUDIOMETRIC TESTING	BLOOD PRESSURE
HEIGHT______	Without Glasses Far R 20/ L 20/ Near R 20/ L 20/	250 500 1000 R ___ ___ ___ L ___ ___ ___	Sitting R / L /
WEIGHT______			
BUILD ______	With Glasses R 20/ L 20/ R 20/ L 20/	2000 4000 8000 R ___ ___ ___ L ___ ___ ___	Standing R / L /
PULSE ______			
RESP. ______	Tonometry R______ L______ Colorvision__________	Gross Hearing __________	Lying R / L /
TEMP. ______	Peripheral Fields R____ L____		

Diagnostic Test:	Results:

The space below is provided for additional information when these data are being forwarded to a hospital, insurance company, a referral physician, etc.

Significant Comments / Recommendations:	
	Physician's Name __________
	Address __________
	__________
	Telephone (area code) __________

CONFIDENTIAL

NUTRITION AND DIET

1. How many meals do you eat each day? .... _______ Meals each day
2. Do you usually eat breakfast? .... ☐ No ☐ Yes Breakfast
3. Do you diet frequently and/or are you now dieting? .... ☐ No ☐ Yes Diets
4. Do you consider yourself .... ☐ Underweight ☐ Overweight ☐ Just right? Weight
5. Do you snack? .... ☐ More than once a day ☐ Usually daily ☐ Rarely? Snacks
6. Do you add salt to your food at the table? ..... ☐ Almost always ☐ Sometimes ☐ Rarely Salts food
7. Check the frequency you eat the following types of foods:

	More than once daily	Daily	3 times weekly	Once weekly	Twice monthly	Less or never
a. Whole grain or enriched bread or cereal						
b. Milk, cheese, or other dairy products						
c. Eggs						
d. Meat, Poultry, Fish						
e. Beans, Peas, or other legumes						
f. Citrus						
g. Dark green or deep yellow vegetables						

List any food supplements or vitamins you take regularly: ____________________

Additional Patient Comments: ____________________

CONFIDENTIAL

Thanks for completing this questionnaire. Please review for skipped questions, sign your name on the space to the right and return it to the physician or assistant. If you wish to add any information, please write it in the spaces provided above.

Patient's Signature ____________________

Physician's Notes: ____________________

To order, call or write:
Bibbero Systems, Inc.
1300 N. McDowell Blvd., Petaluma, CA 94954-1180
Toll Free: 800-BIBBERO (800 242-2376)
Or Fax: 800-242-9330
STOCK NO. 19-742-4 8/95

Case Four, Form 17

Patient Information Sheet

Blackburn Primary Care Associates
1990 Turquoise Drive
Blackburn, WI 54937
(555)555-1234

REGISTRATION
(PLEASE PRINT)

Home Phone: 555-819-7759

Today's Date: 1/15/00

PATIENT INFORMATION

Name FERGUSON (Last Name) LUCILLE (First Name) P (Initial) Soc. Sec.# 576-19-3130

Address 10 LONGVIEW CIRCLE

City BLACKBURN State WI Zip 54938

Single___ Married___ Widowed ✔ Separated___ Divorced___ Sex M___ F ✔ Age 75 Birthdate 6/21/24

Patient Employed by Retired Occupation ———

Business Address ___ Business Phone ___

By whom were you referred? ___

In case of emergency who should be notified? JAMES FERGUSON (Name) SON (Relation to Patient) Phone 555-811-2191

PRIMARY INSURANCE

Person Responsible for Account FERGUSON (Last Name) LUCILLE (First Name) P (Initial)

Relation to Patient self Birthdate ___ Soc. Sec.# ___

Address (if different from patient's) ___ Phone ___

City ___ State ___ Zip ___

Person Responsible Employed by ___ Occupation ___

Business Address ___ Business Phone ___

Insurance Company Medicare

Contract # ___ Group # ___ Subscriber # 576193130

Name of other dependents covered under this plan ___

ADDITIONAL INSURANCE

Is patient covered by additional insurance? ___Yes ✔ No

Subscriber Name ___ Relation to Patient ___ Birthdate ___

Address (if different from patient's) ___ Phone ___

City ___ State ___ Zip ___

Subscriber Employed by ___ Business Phone ___

Insurance Company ___ Soc. Sec.# ___

Contract # ___ Group # ___ Subscriber # ___

Name of other dependents covered under this plan ___

ASSIGNMENT AND RELEASE

I, the undersigned, certify that I (or my dependent) have insurance coverage with *Medicare* (Name of Insurance Company(ies)) and assign directly to Dr. *Blackburn Primary* insurance benefits, if any, otherwise payable to me for services rendered. I understand that I am financially responsible for all charges whether or not paid by insurance. I hereby authorize the doctor to release all information necessary to secure the payment of benefits. I authorize the use of this signature on all insurance submissions.

Lucille Ferguson (Responsible Party Signature) *Self* (Relationship) *1/15/00* (Date)

ORDER # 58-8426 • © 1996 BIBBERO SYSTEMS, INC. • PETALUMA, CALIFORNIA • TO REORDER CALL TOLL FREE: (800) 242-2376 OR FAX: (800) 242-9330
Courtesy of Bibbero Systems, Inc., Petaluma, California.

Case Four, Form 18

Patient Encounter Form

Blackburn Primary Care Associates

1990 Turquoise Drive
Blackburn, WI 54937
(555) 555-1234

FED. I.D. # 52-1963787

PAT. INFO.

ACCT. NO.	PATIENT'S LAST NAME	FIRST	M.I.	DATE OF BIRTH	SEX	TODAY'S DATE
	FERGUSON	LUCILLE	P	06/21/24	☐ M ☒ F	01/15/00

INSURANCE	COPAY	DISABILITY RELATED TO: ☐ ACCIDENT ☐ INDUSTRIAL ☐ ILLNESS ☐ OTHER
Medicare		DATES SYMPTOMS APPEARED, INCEPTION OF PREGNANCY, OR ACCIDENT OCCURRED: / /

✔	DESCRIPTION	CPT/MD	FEE
	OFFICE VISITS-NEW PATIENTS		
	Focused	99201	
	Expanded	99202	
	Detailed	99203	
X	Comprehensive	99204	
	Complex	99205	
	OFFICE VISITS - EST. PATIENTS		
	Minimal	99211	
	Focused	99212	
	Expanded	99213	
	Detailed	99214	
	Comprehensive	99215	
	PREVENTIVE HEALTH CARE NEW PT. EST. PT		
	Eval./Mgmt. > 1 Yr 99381	99391	
	Early Child 1 - 4 Yrs 99382	99392	
	Late Child 5 - 11 Yrs 99383	99393	
	Adolescent 12 - 17 Yrs 99384	99394	
	Eval./Mgmt. 18 - 39 Yrs 99385	99395	
	Eval./Mgmt. 40 - 64 Yrs 99386	99396	
	Eval./Mgmt. 65 - Over 99387	99397	
	HOSP./SNF/HOME VISITS		
	House Calls	99341	
	ER Visit	9928__	
	Init. Hosp. Care	99222	
	Sub. Hosp. Care	99232	
	SNF, Sub. Care	99312	
	INJECTIONS		
	Allergy	95125	
	B-12	J3420	
	Flu Shot	90724	
	Gamma Globulin	90741	
	Hormone		
	Depo Provera	J1055	
	Kenalog 40-60 mg	J3301	
	Morphine/Demerol	J2270	
	Phenergan	J2550	
	Celestone	J0700	
	Hep B, newborn to 11 years	90744	
	Hep B, 11 - 19 years	90745	
	Hep B, 20 years and above	90746	
	Rocephin/Claforan	J0696	
	Iron	J1760	
	Lidocaine NCL	J2000	
	Admin of INJ	J0110	
	Unlist INJ	90782	
	Drug		
	Dose		

✔	DESCRIPTION	CPT/MD	FEE
	SPECIAL SERVICES		
	Drivers Physical	99214	
X	Pelvic/Breast Exam	99214	30.00
	Industrial	99214	
	IMMUNIZATIONS		
	DtaP	90700	
	DPT	90701	
	DT	90702	
	Td (Tetanus Booster)	90703	
	MMR	90707	
	Mumps	90704	
	Pneumococcal	90732	
	Rubella	90706	
	Polio (TOPV)	90712	
	PPD	86580	
	TB Tine Test	86585	
	Hib	90737	
	OFFICE PROCEDURES		
	Audiometry	92551	
	Diathermy (Ultrasound)	97024	
	EKG Tracing & Interp.	93000	
	Intermed Joint Injection	20605	
	Major Joint Injection	20610	
	Nebulizer TX	94664	
	Rem. Impact. Cer.	69210	
	Spirometry	94010	
	Stress Test	93015	
	Trigger Pt. Inj.	20550	
	Eye Wash	65205*	
	LABORATORY		
	Throat Culture	87060	
	Glucose Blood	82947	
	Glucose Stick	82948	
	UA Pregnancy	81025	
	Occult Blood, Stool	82270	
	Rapid Strep	86588	
	Smear	88150	
X	UA Dip	81002	
	Urinalysis	81000	
X	Venipuncture	36415	
	Wet Mount, Smear	87210	
	Wet Mount KOH	87220	
	Collect/Handing	99000	
	MISCELLANEOUS		
	Pre-OP	993__	
	After Hours	99050	
	Sunday/Holidays	99054	
	Cast Removal	29705	
	Norplant Insertion	11975	
	Norplant Kit	99070	

✔	DESCRIPTION	CPT/MD	FEE
	SURGERY		
	Toenail Removal	11750	
	Cryosurgery	17200	
	I & D	10060	
	Drainage Paronychia	10060	
	Enucleation Ext. Hemorrhoid	46320	
	I & D Abscess/Cyst	10060	
	Podophyllom	17100	
	Removal Foreign Body	10120	
	Wart Removal	17110	
	Destr. Single Lesion Face	17000	
	2nd and 3rd Lesion Face	17001	
	Destr. Single Lesion Body	17106	
	2nd and 3rd Lesion Body	17003	
	Lesion Rem. Excision		
	Anoscopy	46600	
	Flex. Scope with Sig.	45330	
	Vasectomy	55250	
	Therapeutic Abor.	59840	
	Removal Foreign Body of Eye	65205	
	SUPPLIES		
	Ace Wrap	99070	
	Cast Material	99070	
	Cervical Collar	99070	
	Elastic Bandage	99070	
	Splint/Sling	99070	
	Sterile Dressing	99070	
	Surgical Tray	99070	

DIAGNOSIS: ICD-9

☐ Abscess Cellulitis 682.9
☐ Abdominal Pain 789.0
☐ Abrasions 919.0
☐ Acne 706.1
☐ ADD 314.00
☐ Alcoholism 303.90
☐ Allergic Rhinitis 477.9
☐ Allergy, Unsp 995.3
☐ Anemia 285.9
☐ Angina Pectoris 413.9
☐ Anxiety Depression 300.4
☐ Anxiety State 300.00
☐ ASCVD 429.2
☐ Asthma W/O Status Asthma 493.90
☐ Atten Surg. Dressing/Suture V58.3
☐ BCP Consult V25.9
☐ BPH 600
☐ Bronchitis, Acute 466.0
☐ Bronchitis, Chronic 491.9
☐ Burn _______ 949.0
☐ Bursitis 727.3
☐ C.T.S. 354.0
☐ CAD 746.85
☐ CA-Prostate 185
☐ Cardiac Arrhythmia 427.9
☐ Cataracts 366.9
☐ Chest Pain 786.50
☐ Congestive Heart Failure 428.0
☐ Conjunctivitis 372.30
☐ Constipation 564.0
☐ Consult Vasc. V65.8
☐ Convulsions 780.3
☐ COPD 496
☐ Coronary Atherosclerosis. 414.0
☐ CVA 436
☐ Cyst Sebaceous 706.2
☐ Dermatitis 692.9
☐ Diabetes, Uncomp. Adult 250.00
☐ Diabetes, Complicated .. 250.90
☐ Disc Degeneration 722.6
☐ Duodenal Ulcer 532.90
☐ Dysmenorrhea 625.3
☐ Fatigue 780.7
☐ Flu Shot Only V04.8
☐ Flu Vac V04.8
☐ Flu W/Resp. Manifest ... 487.1
☐ Folliculitis 704.8
☐ FX _______
☐ Gallbladder Disease 575.9
☐ Gastroenteritis 558.9
☐ Ganglion 727.43
☐ Gastroenteritis 558.9
☐ Gout 274.9
☐ Gyn Exam V72.3
☐ Headache Tension 307.81
☐ Hemorrhoids Ext. 455.3
☐ Hepatitis 573.3
☐ Hernia-Inguinal 550.90
☐ Herpes Zoster 053.9
☐ Hyperlipidemia 272.4
☐ Hypertension 401.9
☐ Hyperthyroidism 242.9
☐ Hypothyroidism 244.9
☐ Impacted Cerumen 380.4
☐ Impetigo 684
☐ Ingrown Toenail 703.0
☐ Internal Derangement Knee . 717.9
☐ Labyrinthitis 386.30
☐ Laceration Open Wound . 879.8__
☐ Levator Scapular Syndrome 726.90
☐ Menopausal Disorder ... 627.9
☐ Metabolic Diff. 277.8
☐ Migraine 346.90
☐ Mitral Valve Disorder ... 424.0
☐ Myalgia and Myositis ... 729.1
☐ Noninf. Gastroenterit. ... 558.9
☐ Obesity 278.0
☐ Osteoarthrosis 715.00
☒ Osteoporosis 733.00
☐ Otitis Externa 380.10
☐ Otitis Media 382.9
☐ P.I.D. 614.9
☐ Peptic Ulcer 533.90
☐ Pharyngitis, Acute 462
☐ Pneumonia, Viral 480.9
☐ Poison Oak 692.6
☐ Premarital B-Test V70.3
☐ Pregnancy Test, Unconf.. V72.4
☐ Prostatitis 601.9
☐ Psoriasis 696.1
☐ Rheumatoid Arthritis 714.0
☐ Sciatica 724.3
☐ Sacroiliac Sprain 846.1
☐ Sinusitis, Acute 461.9
☐ Smoking Cessation 305.10
☐ Sprain _______
☐ SQ. Cell CA-Face 173.3
☐ Sterilization V25.2
☐ Stye 373.11
☐ TB Exposure V01.1
☐ Tendonitis 726.90
☐ Tinea 110.9
☐ Tonsillitis, Acute 463
☐ URI, Acute 465.9
☐ Urine Tract Infection 599.0
☐ Vaginitis 616.10
☐ Well Adult Medical Exam V70.9
☐ Well Child Health Exam . V20.2

DIAGNOSIS (If not checked above) ICD-9	PHYSICIAN SIGNATURE	TODAY'S FEE	$
Kyphosis		PAYMENT	
PLEASE REMEMBER THAT PAYMENT IS YOUR OBLIGATION REGARDLESS OF INSURANCE OR OTHER THIRD PARTY INVOLVEMENT.	PAYMENT BY ☐ CASH ☐ CREDIT CARD ☐ CHECK # _______	BALANCE DUE	

Case Four, Form 19

FEE SCHEDULE

BLACKBURN PRIMARY CARE ASSOCIATES
1990 TURQUOISE DRIVE
BLACKBURN, WI 54937

Federal Tax ID Number: **52-1963787**

BCBS Group Number: **14982**
Medicare Group Number: **14982**

OFFICE VISIT, NEW PATIENT

Focused, 99201	$ 45.00
Expanded, 99202	$ 53.00
Detailed, 99203	$ 60.00
Comprehensive, 99204	$ 95.00
Complex, 99205	$195.00
Consultation, 99245	$250.00

OFFICE VISIT, ESTABLISHED PATIENT

Minimal, 99211	$ 40.00
Focused, 99212	$ 48.00
Expanded, 99213	$ 55.00
Detailed, 99214	$ 65.00
Comprehensive, 99215	$195.00

OFFICE PROCEDURES

EKG, 12 Lead, 93000	$ 55.00
Stress EKG, Treadmill, 93015	$295.00
Sigmoidoscopy, Flex., 45330	$145.00
Spirometry, 94010	$ 50.00
Cerumen Removal, 69210	$ 40.00
Collection & Handling	
Lab Specimen, 99000	$ 9.00
Venipuncture, 36415	$ 9.00
Urinalysis, 81000	$ 20.00
Urinalysis, 81002 (Dip Only)	$ 12.00
Influenza Injection, 90724	$ 20.00
Pneumococcal Injection, 90732	$ 20.00
Oral Polio, 90712	$ 15.00
DTaP, 90700	$ 20.00
Tetanus Toxoid, 90703	$ 15.00
MMR, 90707	$ 25.00
Hib, 90737	$ 20.00
Hepatitis B, newborn to age 11 years, 90744	$ 60.00
Hepatitis B, 11-19 years, 90745	$ 60.00
Hepatitis B, 20 years and above 90746	$ 60.00
Intramuscular Injection, 90788	
Penicillin	$ 30.00
Ceftriaxone	$ 25.00
Solu-Medrol	$ 23.00
Vitamin B-12	$ 13.00
Subcutaneous Injection, 90782	
Epinephrine	$ 18.00
Sus-Pherine	$ 25.00
Insulin, U-100	$ 15.00

COMMON DIAGNOSIS CODES

Ischemic Heart Disease	414.9
w/o myocardial infarction	411.89
w/ coronary occlusion	411.81
Hypertension, Malignant	401.0
Benign	401.1
Unspecified	401.9
w/ congest. heart failure	402.91
Asthma, Bronchial	493.9
w/ COPD	493.2
allergic, w/ S.A.	493.91
allergic, w/o S.A.	493.90
Kyphosis	737.10
w/ osteoporosis	733.0
Osteoporosis	733.00
Otitis Media, Acute	382.9
Chronic	382.9
Well Child Health Exam	V20.2
Well Adult Medical Exam	V70.9

Case Four, Form 20

PLEASE DO NOT STAPLE IN THIS AREA

APPROVED OMB-0938-0008

CARRIER

PICA

HEALTH INSURANCE CLAIM FORM

PICA

PATIENT AND INSURED INFORMATION

1. MEDICARE (Medicare #) MEDICAID (Medicaid #) CHAMPUS (Sponsor's SSN) CHAMPVA (VA File #) GROUP HEALTH PLAN (SSN or ID) FECA BLK LUNG (SSN) OTHER (ID)

1a. INSURED'S I.D. NUMBER (FOR PROGRAM IN ITEM 1)

2. PATIENT'S NAME (Last Name, First Name, Middle Initial)

3. PATIENT'S BIRTHDATE MM DD YY SEX M F

4. INSURED'S NAME (Last Name, First Name, Middle Initial)

5. PATIENT'S ADDRESS (No., Street)

6. PATIENT RELATIONSHIP TO INSURED Self Spouse Child Other

7. INSURED'S ADDRESS (No., Street)

CITY STATE

8. PATIENT STATUS Single Married Other

CITY STATE

ZIP CODE TELEPHONE (Include Area Code) ( )

Employed Full-Time Student Part-Time Student

ZIP CODE TELEPHONE (Include Area Code) ( )

9. OTHER INSURED'S NAME (Last Name, First Name, Middle Initial)

10. IS PATIENT'S CONDITION RELATED TO:

11. INSURED'S POLICY GROUP OR FECA NUMBER

a. OTHER INSURED'S POLICY OR GROUP NUMBER

a. EMPLOYMENT? (CURRENT OR PREVIOUS) YES NO

a. INSURED'S DATE OF BIRTH MM DD YY SEX M F

b. OTHER INSURED'S DATE OF BIRTH MM DD YY SEX M F

b. AUTO ACCIDENT? PLACE (State) YES NO

b. EMPLOYER'S NAME OR SCHOOL NAME

c. EMPLOYER'S NAME OR SCHOOL NAME

c. OTHER ACCIDENT? YES NO

c. INSURANCE PLAN NAME OR PROGRAM NAME

d. INSURANCE PLAN NAME OR PROGRAM NAME

10d. RESERVED FOR LOCAL USE

d. IS THERE ANOTHER HEALTH BENEFIT PLAN? YES NO *If yes, return to and complete item 9a-d.*

READ BACK OF FORM BEFORE COMPLETING & SIGNING THIS FORM.

12. PATIENT'S OR AUTHORIZED PERSON'S SIGNATURE I authorize the release of any medical or other information necessary to process this claim. I also request payment of government benefits either to myself or to the party who accepts assignment below.

SIGNED ____ DATE ____

13. INSURED'S OR AUTHORIZED PERSON'S SIGNATURE I authorize payment of medical benefits to the undersigned physician or supplier for services described below.

SIGNED ____

PHYSICIAN OR SUPPLIER INFORMATION

14. DATE OF CURRENT: MM DD YY ILLNESS (First symptom) OR INJURY (Accident) OR PREGNANCY (LMP)

15. IF PATIENT HAS HAD SAME OR SIMILAR ILLNESS, GIVE FIRST DATE MM DD YY

16. DATES PATIENT UNABLE TO WORK IN CURRENT OCCUPATION FROM MM DD YY TO MM DD YY

17. NAME OF REFERRING PHYSICIAN OR OTHER SOURCE

17a. I.D. NUMBER OF REFERRING PHYSICIAN

18. HOSPITALIZATION DATES RELATED TO CURRENT SERVICES FROM MM DD YY TO MM DD YY

19. RESERVED FOR LOCAL USE

20. OUTSIDE LAB? YES NO $ CHARGES

21. DIAGNOSIS OR NATURE OF ILLNESS OR INJURY. (RELATE ITEMS 1,2,3 OR 4 TO ITEM 24E BY LINE)

1. ____ . __

2. ____ . __

3. ____ . __

4. ____ . __

22. MEDICAID RESUBMISSION CODE ORIGINAL REF. NO.

23. PRIOR AUTHORIZATION NUMBER

24.	A DATE(S) OF SERVICE From MM DD YY	To MM DD YY	B Place of Service	C Type of Service	D PROCEDURES, SERVICES, OR SUPPLIES (Explain Unusual Circumstances) CPT/HCPCS MODIFIER	E DIAGNOSIS CODE	F $ CHARGES	G DAYS OR UNITS	H EPSDT Family Plan	I EMG	J COB	K RESERVED FOR LOCAL USE
1												
2												
3												
4												
5												
6												

25. FEDERAL TAX I.D. NUMBER SSN EIN

26. PATIENT'S ACCOUNT NUMBER

27. ACCEPT ASSIGNMENT? (For govt. claims, see back) YES NO

28. TOTAL CHARGE $

29. AMOUNT PAID $

30. BALANCE DUE $

31. SIGNATURE OF PHYSICIAN OR SUPPLIER INCLUDING DEGREES OR CREDENTIALS (I certify that the statements on the reverse apply to this bill and are made a part thereof.)

SIGNED DATE

32. NAME AND ADDRESS OF FACILITY WHERE SERVICES WERE RENDERED (If other than home or office)

33. PHYSICIAN'S, SUPPLIER'S BILLING NAME, ADDRESS, ZIP CODE & PHONE #

PIN # GRP#

(APPROVED BY AMA COUNCIL ON MEDICAL SERVICE 8/88) Form 1240LM

PLEASE PRINT OR TYPE

FORM HCFA-1500 (12-90) FORM OWCP-1500 FORM RRB-1500

Administrative Skills, Form 21

Patient Information Sheet

 **Blackburn Primary Care Associates** 

1990 Turquoise Drive
Blackburn, WI 54937
(555)555-1234

REGISTRATION
(PLEASE PRINT)

Home Phone: 555-997-1909 Today's Date: 1/15/00

PATIENT INFORMATION

Name LATHAM (Last Name) CHARLES (First Name) ___ (Initial) Soc. Sec.# 219 61 9002

Address 10971 Clarkbird Road

City Blackburn State WI Zip 54938

Single ___ Married ✓ Widowed ___ Separated ___ Divorced ___ Sex M ✓ F ___ Age 39 Birthdate 7/19/60

Patient Employed by self - LATHAM AUTO Occupation ___

Business Address 10971 Clarkbird Road Business Phone ___

By whom were you referred? ———

In case of emergency who should be notified? PEGGY LATHAM (Name) Wife (Relation to Patient) Phone 555-997-1920

PRIMARY INSURANCE

Person Responsible for Account Same (Last Name) ___ (First Name) ___ (Initial)

Relation to Patient ___ Birthdate ___ Soc. Sec.# ___

Address (if different from patient's) ___ Phone ___

City ___ State ___ Zip ___

Person Responsible Employed by Self Occupation ___

Business Address ___ Business Phone ___

Insurance Company U.S. Healthcare

Contract # ___ Group # LAT 3600 Subscriber # 1649701

Name of other dependents covered under this plan wife-as above

ADDITIONAL INSURANCE

Is patient covered by additional insurance? ___ Yes ✓ No

Subscriber Name ___ Relation to Patient ___ Birthdate ___

Address (if different from patient's) ___ Phone ___

City ___ State ___ Zip ___

Subscriber Employed by ___ Business Phone ___

Insurance Company ___ Soc. Sec.# ___

Contract # ___ Group # ___ Subscriber # ___

Name of other dependents covered under this plan ___

ASSIGNMENT AND RELEASE

I, the undersigned, certify that I (or my dependent) have insurance coverage with *US Healthcare* (Name of Insurance Company(ies)) and assign directly to Dr. *Blackburn Primary* insurance benefits, if any, otherwise payable to me for services rendered. I understand that I am financially responsible for all charges whether or not paid by insurance. I hereby authorize the doctor to release all information necessary to secure the payment of benefits. I authorize the use of this signature on all insurance submissions.

Charles Latham (Responsible Party Signature) *self* (Relationship) 1/15/00 (Date)

ORDER # 58-8426 • © 1996 BIBBERO SYSTEMS, INC. • PETALUMA, CALIFORNIA • TO REORDER CALL TOLL FREE: (800) 242-2376 OR FAX: (800) 242-9330
Courtesy of Bibbero Systems, Inc., Petaluma, California.

Administrative Skills, Form 22

Patient Encounter Form

Blackburn Primary Care Associates
1990 Turquoise Drive
Blackburn, WI 54937
(555) 555-1234

FED. I.D. # 52-1963787

PAT. INFO.	ACCT. NO.	PATIENT'S LAST NAME	FIRST	M.I.	DATE OF BIRTH	SEX	TODAY'S DATE
		LATHAM	CHARLES		07/19/60	☒ M ☐ F	01/15/00
	INSURANCE: US Healthcare		COPAY		DISABILITY RELATED TO: ☐ ACCIDENT ☐ INDUSTRIAL ☐ ILLNESS ☐ OTHER		
					DATES SYMPTOMS APPEARED, INCEPTION OF PREGNANCY, OR ACCIDENT OCCURRED: / /		

✓	DESCRIPTION	CPT/MD	FEE
	OFFICE VISITS-NEW PATIENTS		
	Focused	99201	
	Expanded	99202	
	Detailed	99203	
X	Comprehensive	99204	
	Complex	99205	
	OFFICE VISITS - EST. PATIENTS		
	Minimal	99211	
	Focused	99212	
	Expanded	99213	
	Detailed	99214	
	Comprehensive	99215	
	PREVENTIVE HEALTH CARE NEW PT. / EST. PT		
	Eval./Mgmt. > 1 Yr	99381 / 99391	
	Early Child 1 - 4 Yrs	99382 / 99392	
	Late Child 5 - 11 Yrs	99383 / 99393	
	Adolescent 12 - 17 Yrs	99384 / 99394	
	Eval./Mgmt. 18 - 39 Yrs	99385 / 99395	
	Eval./Mgmt. 40 - 64 Yrs	99386 / 99396	
	Eval./Mgmt. 65 - Over	99387 / 99397	
	HOSP./SNF/HOME VISITS		
	House Calls	99341	
	ER Visit	9928__	
	Init. Hosp. Care	99222	
	Sub. Hosp. Care	99232	
	SNF, Sub. Care	99312	
	INJECTIONS		
	Allergy	95125	
	B-12	J3420	
X	Flu Shot	90724	
	Gamma Globulin	90741	
	Hormone		
	Depo Provera	J1055	
	Kenalog 40-60 mg	J3301	
	Morphine/Demerol	J2270	
	Phenergan	J2550	
	Celestone	J0700	
	Hep B, newborn to 11 years	90744	
	Hep B, 11 - 19 years	90745	
	Hep B, 20 years and above	90746	
	Rocephin/Claforan	J0696	
	Iron	J1760	
	Lidocaine NCL	J2000	
	Admin of INJ	J0110	
	Unlist INJ	90782	
	Drug		
	Dose		

✓	DESCRIPTION	CPT/MD	FEE
	SPECIAL SERVICES		
	Drivers Physical	99214	
	Pelvic/Breast Exam	99214	
	Industrial	99214	
	IMMUNIZATIONS		
	DtaP	90700	
	DPT	90701	
	DT	90702	
	Td (Tetanus Booster)	90703	
	MMR	90707	
	Mumps	90704	
	Pneumococcal	90732	
	Rubella	90706	
	Polio (TOPV)	90712	
	PPD	86580	
	TB Tine Test	86585	
	Hib	90737	
	OFFICE PROCEDURES		
X	Audiometry	92551	35.00
	Diathermy (Ultrasound)	97024	
	EKG Tracing & Interp.	93000	
	Intermed Joint Injection	20605	
	Major Joint Injection	20610	
	Nebulizer TX	94664	
	Rem. Impact. Cer.	69210	
	Spirometry	94010	
	Stress Test	93015	
	Trigger Pt. Inj.	20550	
	Eye Wash	65205*	
	LABORATORY		
	Throat Culture	87060	
	Glucose Blood	82947	
	Glucose Stick	82948	
	UA Pregnancy	81025	
X	Occult Blood, Stool	82270	15.00
	Rapid Strep	86588	
	Smear	88150	
	UA Dip	81002	
X	Urinalysis	81000	
	Venipuncture	36415	
	Wet Mount, Smear	87210	
	Wet Mount KOH	87220	
	Collect/Handing	99000	
	MISCELLANEOUS		
	Pre-OP	993__	
	After Hours	99050	
	Sunday/Holidays	99054	
	Cast Removal	29705	
	Norplant Insertion	11975	
	Norplant Kit	99070	

✓	DESCRIPTION	CPT/MD	FEE
	SURGERY		
	Toenail Removal	11750	
	Cryosurgery	17200	
	I & D	10060	
	Drainage Paronychia	10060	
	Enucleation Ext. Hemorrhoid	46320	
	I & D Abscess/Cyst	10060	
	Podophyllom	17100	
	Removal Foreign Body	10120	
	Wart Removal	17110	
	Destr. Single Lesion Face	17000	
	2nd and 3rd Lesion Face	17001	
	Destr. Single Lesion Body	17106	
	2nd and 3rd Lesion Body	17003	
	Lesion Rem. Excision		
	Anoscopy	46600	
	Flex. Scope with Sig.	45330	
	Vasectomy	55250	
	Therapeutic Abor.	59840	
	Removal Foreign Body of Eye	65205	
	SUPPLIES		
	Ace Wrap	99070	
	Cast Material	99070	
	Cervical Collar	99070	
	Elastic Bandage	99070	
	Splint/Sling	99070	
	Sterile Dressing	99070	
	Surgical Tray	99070	

DIAGNOSIS: ICD-9

- ☐ Abscess Cellulitis 682.9
- ☐ Abdominal Pain 789.0
- ☐ Abrasions 919.0
- ☐ Acne 706.1
- ☐ ADD 314.00
- ☐ Alcoholism 303.90
- ☐ Allergic Rhinitis 477.9
- ☐ Allergy, Unsp 995.3
- ☐ Anemia 285.9
- ☐ Angina Pectoris 413.9
- ☐ Anxiety Depression 300.4
- ☐ Anxiety State 300.00
- ☐ ASCVD 429.2
- ☐ Asthma W/O Status Asthma 493.90
- ☐ Atten Surg. Dressing/Suture V58.3
- ☐ BCP Consult V25.9
- ☐ BPH 600
- ☐ Bronchitis, Acute 466.0
- ☐ Bronchitis, Chronic 491.9
- ☐ Burn __________ 949.0
- ☐ Bursitis 727.3
- ☐ C.T.S. 354.0
- ☐ CAD 746.85
- ☐ CA-Prostate 185
- ☐ Cardiac Arrhythmia 427.9
- ☐ Cataracts 366.9
- ☐ Chest Pain 786.50
- ☐ Congestive Heart Failure 428.0
- ☐ Conjunctivitis 372.30
- ☐ Constipation 564.0
- ☐ Consult Vasc V65.8
- ☐ Convulsions 780.3
- ☐ COPD 496
- ☐ Coronary Atherosclerosis. 414.0
- ☐ CVA 436
- ☐ Cyst Sebaceous 706.2
- ☐ Dermatitis 692.9
- ☐ Diabetes, Uncomp. Adult 250.00
- ☐ Diabetes, Complicated .. 250.90
- ☐ Disc Degeneration 722.6
- ☐ Duodenal Ulcer 532.90
- ☐ Dysmenorrhea 625.3
- ☐ Fatigue 780.7
- ☐ Flu Shot Only V04.8
- ☐ Flu Vac V04.8
- ☐ Flu W/Resp. Manifest ... 487.1
- ☐ Folliculitis 704.8
- ☐ FX __________
- ☐ Gallbladder Disease 575.9
- ☐ Ganglion 727.43
- ☐ Gastroenteritis 558.9
- ☐ Gout 274.9
- ☐ Gyn Exam V72.3
- ☐ Headache Tension 307.81
- ☐ Hemorrhoids Ext. 455.3
- ☐ Hepatitis 573.3
- ☐ Hernia-Inguinal 550.90
- ☐ Herpes Zoster 053.9
- ☐ Hyperlipidemia 272.4
- ☐ Hypertension 401.9
- ☐ Hyperthyroidism 242.9
- ☐ Hypothyroidism 244.9
- ☐ Impacted Cerumen 380.4
- ☐ Impetigo 684
- ☐ Ingrown Toenail 703.0
- ☐ Internal Derangement Knee . 717.9
- ☐ Labyrinthitis 386.30
- ☐ Laceration Open Wound. 879.8__
- ☐ Levator Scapular Syndrome 726.90
- ☐ Menopausal Disorder ... 627.9
- ☐ Metabolic Diff. 277.8
- ☐ Migraine 346.90
- ☐ Mitral Valve Disorder ... 424.0
- ☐ Myalgia and Myositis ... 729.1
- ☐ Noninf. Gastroenterit. ... 558.9
- ☐ Obesity 278.0
- ☐ Osteoarthrosis 715.00
- ☐ Osteoporosis 733.00
- ☐ Otitis Externa 380.10
- ☐ Otitis Media 382.9
- ☐ P.I.D. 614.9
- ☐ Peptic Ulcer 533.90
- ☐ Pharyngitis, Acute 462
- ☐ Pneumonia, Viral 480.9
- ☐ Poison Oak 692.6
- ☐ Premarital B-Test V70.3
- ☐ Pregnancy Test, Unconf.. V72.4
- ☐ Prostatitis 601.9
- ☐ Psoriasis 696.1
- ☐ Rheumatoid Arthritis 714.0
- ☐ Sciatica 724.3
- ☐ Sacroiliac Sprain 846.1
- ☐ Sinusitis, Acute 461.9
- ☐ Smoking Cessation 305.10
- ☐ Sprain __________
- ☐ SQ. Cell CA-Face 173.3
- ☐ Sterilization V25.2
- ☐ Stye 373.11
- ☐ TB Exposure V01.1
- ☐ Tendonitis 726.90
- ☐ Tinea 110.9
- ☐ Tonsillitis, Acute 463
- ☐ URI, Acute 465.9
- ☐ Urine Tract Infection 599.0
- ☐ Vaginitis 616.10
- ☒ Well Adult Medical Exam V70.9
- ☐ Well Child Health Exam . V20.2

DIAGNOSIS (If not checked above) ICD-9	PHYSICIAN SIGNATURE	TODAY'S FEE	$
	Ralph Lopez, MD	PAYMENT	
PLEASE REMEMBER THAT PAYMENT IS YOUR OBLIGATION REGARDLESS OF INSURANCE OR OTHER THIRD PARTY INVOLVEMENT.	PAYMENT BY ☐ CASH ☐ CREDIT CARD ☐ CHECK # __________	BALANCE DUE	

INSUR-A-BILL ® BIBBERO SYSTEMS, INC. • PETALUMA, CA • © 9/94 SB43006.01 (REV. 1/99)

Courtesy of Bibbero Systems, Inc., Petaluma, California.

FEE SCHEDULE

BLACKBURN PRIMARY CARE ASSOCIATES
1990 TURQUOISE DRIVE
BLACKBURN, WI 54937

Federal Tax ID Number: **52-1963787**

BCBS Group Number: **14982**
Medicare Group Number: **14982**

OFFICE VISIT, NEW PATIENT

Focused, 99201	$ 45.00
Expanded, 99202	$ 53.00
Detailed, 99203	$ 60.00
Comprehensive, 99204	$ 95.00
Complex, 99205	$195.00
Consultation, 99245	$250.00

OFFICE VISIT, ESTABLISHED PATIENT

Minimal, 99211	$ 40.00
Focused, 99212	$ 48.00
Expanded, 99213	$ 55.00
Detailed, 99214	$ 65.00
Comprehensive, 99215	$195.00

OFFICE PROCEDURES

EKG, 12 Lead, 93000	$ 55.00
Stress EKG, Treadmill, 93015	$295.00
Sigmoidoscopy, Flex., 45330	$145.00
Spirometry, 94010	$ 50.00
Cerumen Removal, 69210	$ 40.00
Collection & Handling	
Lab Specimen, 99000	$ 9.00
Venipuncture, 36415	$ 9.00
Urinalysis, 81000	$ 20.00
Urinalysis, 81002 (Dip Only)	$ 12.00
Influenza Injection, 90724	$ 20.00
Pneumococcal Injection, 90732	$ 20.00
Oral Polio, 90712	$ 15.00
DTaP, 90700	$ 20.00
Tetanus Toxoid, 90703	$ 15.00
MMR, 90707	$ 25.00
Hib, 90737	$ 20.00
Hepatitis B, newborn to age 11 years, 90744	$ 60.00
Hepatitis B, 11-19 years, 90745	$ 60.00
Hepatitis B, 20 years and above 90746	$ 60.00
Intramuscular Injection, 90788	
Penicillin	$ 30.00
Ceftriaxone	$ 25.00
Solu-Medrol	$ 23.00
Vitamin B-12	$ 13.00
Subcutaneous Injection, 90782	
Epinephrine	$ 18.00
Sus-Pherine	$ 25.00
Insulin, U-100	$ 15.00

COMMON DIAGNOSIS CODES

Ischemic Heart Disease	414.9
w/o myocardial infarction	411.89
w/ coronary occlusion	411.81
Hypertension, Malignant	401.0
Benign	401.1
Unspecified	401.9
w/ congest. heart failure	402.91
Asthma, Bronchial	493.9
w/ COPD	493.2
allergic, w/ S.A.	493.91
allergic, w/o S.A.	493.90
Kyphosis	737.10
w/ osteoporosis	733.0
Osteoporosis	733.00
Otitis Media, Acute	382.9
Chronic	382.9
Well Child Health Exam	V20.2
Well Adult Medical Exam	V70.9

PLEASE DO NOT STAPLE IN THIS AREA

APPROVED OMB-0938-0008

CARRIER

PICA

HEALTH INSURANCE CLAIM FORM

PICA

PATIENT AND INSURED INFORMATION

1. MEDICARE (Medicare #) MEDICAID (Medicaid #) CHAMPUS (Sponsor's SSN) CHAMPVA (VA File #) GROUP HEALTH PLAN (SSN or ID) FECA BLK LUNG (SSN) OTHER (ID)

1a. INSURED'S I.D. NUMBER (FOR PROGRAM IN ITEM 1)

2. PATIENT'S NAME (Last Name, First Name, Middle Initial)

3. PATIENT'S BIRTHDATE MM DD YY SEX M F

4. INSURED'S NAME (Last Name, First Name, Middle Initial)

5. PATIENT'S ADDRESS (No., Street)

6. PATIENT RELATIONSHIP TO INSURED Self Spouse Child Other

7. INSURED'S ADDRESS (No., Street)

CITY STATE

8. PATIENT STATUS Single Married Other

CITY STATE

ZIP CODE TELEPHONE (Include Area Code) ( )

Employed Full-Time Student Part-Time Student

ZIP CODE TELEPHONE (Include Area Code) ( )

9. OTHER INSURED'S NAME (Last Name, First Name, Middle Initial)

10. IS PATIENT'S CONDITION RELATED TO:

11. INSURED'S POLICY GROUP OR FECA NUMBER

a. OTHER INSURED'S POLICY OR GROUP NUMBER

a. EMPLOYMENT? (CURRENT OR PREVIOUS) YES NO

a. INSURED'S DATE OF BIRTH MM DD YY SEX M F

b. OTHER INSURED'S DATE OF BIRTH MM DD YY SEX M F

b. AUTO ACCIDENT? YES NO PLACE (State)

b. EMPLOYER'S NAME OR SCHOOL NAME

c. EMPLOYER'S NAME OR SCHOOL NAME

c. OTHER ACCIDENT? YES NO

c. INSURANCE PLAN NAME OR PROGRAM NAME

d. INSURANCE PLAN NAME OR PROGRAM NAME

10d. RESERVED FOR LOCAL USE

d. IS THERE ANOTHER HEALTH BENEFIT PLAN? YES NO *If yes, return to and complete item 9a-d.*

READ BACK OF FORM BEFORE COMPLETING & SIGNING THIS FORM.

12. PATIENT'S OR AUTHORIZED PERSON'S SIGNATURE I authorize the release of any medical or other information necessary to process this claim. I also request payment of government benefits either to myself or to the party who accepts assignment below.

SIGNED ______ DATE ______

13. INSURED'S OR AUTHORIZED PERSON'S SIGNATURE I authorize payment of medical benefits to the undersigned physician or supplier for services described below.

SIGNED ______

PHYSICIAN OR SUPPLIER INFORMATION

14. DATE OF CURRENT: MM DD YY ILLNESS (First symptom) OR INJURY (Accident) OR PREGNANCY (LMP)

15. IF PATIENT HAS HAD SAME OR SIMILAR ILLNESS, GIVE FIRST DATE MM DD YY

16. DATES PATIENT UNABLE TO WORK IN CURRENT OCCUPATION FROM MM DD YY TO MM DD YY

17. NAME OF REFERRING PHYSICIAN OR OTHER SOURCE

17a. I.D. NUMBER OF REFERRING PHYSICIAN

18. HOSPITALIZATION DATES RELATED TO CURRENT SERVICES FROM MM DD YY TO MM DD YY

19. RESERVED FOR LOCAL USE

20. OUTSIDE LAB? YES NO $ CHARGES

21. DIAGNOSIS OR NATURE OF ILLNESS OR INJURY. (RELATE ITEMS 1,2,3 OR 4 TO ITEM 24E BY LINE)

1. ___ . __

2. ___ . __

3. ___ . __

4. ___ . __

22. MEDICAID RESUBMISSION CODE ORIGINAL REF. NO.

23. PRIOR AUTHORIZATION NUMBER

24. A DATE(S) OF SERVICE From MM DD YY To MM DD YY	B Place of Service	C Type of Service	D PROCEDURES, SERVICES, OR SUPPLIES (Explain Unusual Circumstances) CPT/HCPCS MODIFIER	E DIAGNOSIS CODE	F $ CHARGES	G DAYS OR UNITS	H EPSDT Family Plan	I EMG	J COB	K RESERVED FOR LOCAL USE
1										
2										
3										
4										
5										
6										

25. FEDERAL TAX I.D. NUMBER SSN EIN

26. PATIENT'S ACCOUNT NUMBER

27. ACCEPT ASSIGNMENT? (For govt. claims, see back) YES NO

28. TOTAL CHARGE $

29. AMOUNT PAID $

30. BALANCE DUE $

31. SIGNATURE OF PHYSICIAN OR SUPPLIER INCLUDING DEGREES OR CREDENTIALS (I certify that the statements on the reverse apply to this bill and are made a part thereof.)

SIGNED DATE

32. NAME AND ADDRESS OF FACILITY WHERE SERVICES WERE RENDERED (If other than home or office)

33. PHYSICIAN'S, SUPPLIER'S BILLING NAME, ADDRESS, ZIP CODE & PHONE #

PIN # GRP#

(APPROVED BY AMA COUNCIL ON MEDICAL SERVICE 8/88)

Form 1240LM

PLEASE PRINT OR TYPE

FORM HCFA-1500 (12-90) FORM OWCP-1500 FORM RRB-1500

Administrative Skills, Form 25

Patient Information Sheet

 **Blackburn Primary Care Associates** 
1990 Turquoise Drive
Blackburn, WI 54937
(555)555-1234

REGISTRATION
(PLEASE PRINT)

Home Phone: 555-722-1975

Today's Date: 1/20/00

PATIENT INFORMATION

Name JORDAN (Last Name) MARRION (First Name) ___ (Initial) Soc. Sec.# 319-21-6115

Address 3242 BOSTON CIRCLE

City BLACKBURN State WI Zip 59767

Single ___ Married ___ Widowed ___ Separated ___ Divorced ✓ Sex M ___ F ✓ Age 29 Birthdate 3/16/70

Patient Employed by UNIVERSITY OF WISCONSIN Occupation TEACHER

Business Address ___ Business Phone 555-719-0011

By whom were you referred? RAYMOND JOHNSON

In case of emergency who should be notified? CAROL JORDAN (Name) mom (Relation to Patient) Phone 555-722-1919

PRIMARY INSURANCE

Person Responsible for Account JORDAN (Last Name) MARRION (First Name) ___ (Initial)

Relation to Patient self Birthdate 3/16/70 Soc. Sec.# 319216115

Address (if different from patient's) same Phone ___

City ___ State ___ Zip ___

Person Responsible Employed by as above Occupation ___

Business Address ___ Business Phone ___

Insurance Company BCBS

Contract # ___ Group # P2170 Subscriber # 319216115

Name of other dependents covered under this plan ___

ADDITIONAL INSURANCE

Is patient covered by additional insurance? ___ Yes ✓ No

Subscriber Name ___ Relation to Patient ___ Birthdate ___

Address (if different from patient's) ___ Phone ___

City ___ State ___ Zip ___

Subscriber Employed by ___ Business Phone ___

Insurance Company ___ Soc. Sec.# ___

Contract # ___ Group # ___ Subscriber # ___

Name of other dependents covered under this plan ___

ASSIGNMENT AND RELEASE

I, the undersigned, certify that I (or my dependent) have insurance coverage with BCBS (Name of Insurance Company(ies)) and assign directly to Dr. Blackburn Primary insurance benefits, if any, otherwise payable to me for services rendered. I understand that I am financially responsible for all charges whether or not paid by insurance. I hereby authorize the doctor to release all information necessary to secure the payment of benefits. I authorize the use of this signature on all insurance submissions.

Marrion Jordan (Responsible Party Signature) self (Relationship) 1/20/00 (Date)

Administrative Skills, Form 26

Patient Encounter Form

Blackburn Primary Care Associates
1990 Turquoise Drive
Blackburn, WI 54937
(555) 555-1234

FED. I.D. # 52-1963787

PAT. INFO.

ACCT. NO.	PATIENT'S LAST NAME	FIRST	M.I.	DATE OF BIRTH	SEX	TODAY'S DATE
	JORDAN	MARRION		03/16/70	☐ M ☒ F	01/20/00

INSURANCE	COPAY	DISABILITY RELATED TO: ☐ ACCIDENT ☐ INDUSTRIAL ☐ ILLNESS ☐ OTHER
BCBS		DATES SYMPTOMS APPEARED, INCEPTION OF PREGNANCY, OR ACCIDENT OCCURRED: / /

✓	DESCRIPTION	CPT/MD	FEE
	OFFICE VISITS-NEW PATIENTS		
	Focused	99201	
	Expanded	99202	
X	Detailed	99203	
	Comprehensive	99204	
	Complex	99205	
	OFFICE VISITS - EST. PATIENTS		
	Minimal	99211	
	Focused	99212	
	Expanded	99213	
	Detailed	99214	
	Comprehensive	99215	
	PREVENTIVE HEALTH CARE NEW PT.	EST. PT	
	Eval./Mgmt. > 1 Yr 99381	99391	
	Early Child 1 - 4 Yrs 99382	99392	
	Late Child 5 - 11 Yrs 99383	99393	
	Adolescent 12 - 17 Yrs 99384	99394	
	Eval./Mgmt. 18 - 39 Yrs 99385	99395	
	Eval./Mgmt. 40 - 64 Yrs 99386	99396	
	Eval./Mgmt. 65 - Over 99387	99397	
	HOSP./SNF/HOME VISITS		
	House Calls	99341	
	ER Visit	9928__	
	Init. Hosp. Care	99222	
	Sub. Hosp. Care	99232	
	SNF, Sub. Care	99312	
	INJECTIONS		
	Allergy	95125	
	B-12	J3420	
	Flu Shot	90724	
	Gamma Globulin	90741	
	Hormone		
X	Depo Provera	J1055	30.00
	Kenalog 40-60 mg	J3301	
	Morphine/Demerol	J2270	
	Phenergan	J2550	
	Celestone	J0700	
	Hep B, newborn to 11 years	90744	
	Hep B, 11 - 19 years	90745	
	Hep B, 20 years and above	90746	
	Rocephin/Claforan	J0696	
	Iron	J1760	
	Lidocaine NCL	J2000	
	Admin of INJ	J0110	
	Unlist INJ	90782	
	Drug		
	Dose		

✓	DESCRIPTION	CPT/MD	FEE
	SPECIAL SERVICES		
	Drivers Physical	99214	
	Pelvic/Breast Exam	99214	
	Industrial	99214	
	IMMUNIZATIONS		
	DtaP	90700	
	DPT	90701	
	DT	90702	
	Td (Tetanus Booster)	90703	
	MMR	90707	
	Mumps	90704	
	Pneumococcal	90732	
	Rubella	90706	
	Polio (TOPV)	90712	
	PPD	86580	
	TB Tine Test	86585	
	Hib	90737	
	OFFICE PROCEDURES		
	Audiometry	92551	
	Diathermy (Ultrasound)	97024	
	EKG Tracing & Interp.	93000	
	Intermed Joint Injection	20605	
	Major Joint Injection	20610	
	Nebulizer TX	94664	
	Rem. Impact. Cer.	69210	
	Spirometry	94010	
	Stress Test	93015	
	Trigger Pt. Inj.	20550	
	Eye Wash	65205*	
	LABORATORY		
	Throat Culture	87060	
	Glucose Blood	82947	
	Glucose Stick	82948	
X	UA Pregnancy	81025	22.00
	Occult Blood, Stool	82270	
	Rapid Strep	86588	
	Smear	88150	
	UA Dip	81002	
	Urinalysis	81000	
	Venipuncture	36415	
	Wet Mount, Smear	87210	
	Wet Mount KOH	87220	
	Collect/Handing	99000	
	MISCELLANEOUS		
	Pre-OP	993__	
	After Hours	99050	
	Sunday/Holidays	99054	
	Cast Removal	29705	
	Norplant Insertion	11975	
	Norplant Kit	99070	

✓	DESCRIPTION	CPT/MD	FEE
	SURGERY		
	Toenail Removal	11750	
	Cryosurgery	17200	
	I & D	10060	
	Drainage Paronychia	10060	
	Enucleation Ext. Hemorrhoid	46320	
	I & D Abscess/Cyst	10060	
	Podophyllom	17100	
	Removal Foreign Body	10120	
	Wart Removal	17110	
	Destr. Single Lesion Face	17000	
	2nd and 3rd Lesion Face	17001	
	Destr. Single Lesion Body	17106	
	2nd and 3rd Lesion Body	17003	
	Lesion Rem. Excision		
	Anoscopy	46600	
	Flex. Scope with Sig.	45330	
	Vasectomy	55250	
	Therapeutic Abor.	59840	
	Removal Foreign Body of Eye	65205	
	SUPPLIES		
	Ace Wrap	99070	
	Cast Material	99070	
	Cervical Collar	99070	
	Elastic Bandage	99070	
	Splint/Sling	99070	
	Sterile Dressing	99070	
	Surgical Tray	99070	

DIAGNOSIS: **ICD-9**

- ☐ Abscess Cellulitis 682.9
- ☐ Abdominal Pain 789.0
- ☐ Abrasions 919.0
- ☐ Acne 706.1
- ☐ ADD 314.00
- ☐ Alcoholism 303.90
- ☐ Allergic Rhinitis 477.9
- ☐ Allergy, Unsp 995.3
- ☐ Anemia 285.9
- ☐ Angina Pectoris 413.9
- ☐ Anxiety Depression 300.4
- ☐ Anxiety State 300.00
- ☐ ASCVD 429.2
- ☐ Asthma W/O Status Asthma 493.90
- ☐ Atten Surg. Dressing/Suture V58.3
- ☐ BCP Consult V25.9
- ☐ BPH 600
- ☐ Bronchitis, Acute 466.0
- ☐ Bronchitis, Chronic 491.9
- ☐ Burn ________ 949.0
- ☐ Bursitis 727.3
- ☐ C.T.S. 354.0
- ☐ CAD 746.85
- ☐ CA-Prostate 185
- ☐ Cardiac Arrhythmia 427.9
- ☐ Cataracts 366.9
- ☐ Chest Pain 786.50
- ☐ Congestive Heart Failure 428.0
- ☐ Conjunctivitis 372.30
- ☐ Constipation 564.0
- ☐ Consult Vasc. V65.8
- ☐ Convulsions 780.3
- ☐ COPD 496
- ☐ Coronary Atherosclerosis. 414.0
- ☐ CVA 436
- ☐ Cyst Sebaceous 706.2
- ☐ Dermatitis 692.9
- ☐ Diabetes, Uncomp. Adult 250.00
- ☐ Diabetes, Complicated .. 250.90
- ☐ Disc Degeneration 722.6
- ☐ Duodenal Ulcer 532.90
- ☒ Dysmenorrhea 625.3
- ☐ Fatigue 780.7
- ☐ Flu Shot Only V04.8
- ☐ Flu Vac V04.8
- ☐ Flu W/Resp. Manifest ... 487.1
- ☐ Folliculitis 704.8
- ☐ FX ________
- ☐ Gallbladder Disease 575.9
- ☐ Ganglion 727.43
- ☐ Gastroenteritis 558.9
- ☐ Gout 274.9
- ☐ Gyn Exam V72.3
- ☐ Headache Tension 307.81
- ☐ Hemorrhoids Ext. 455.3
- ☐ Hepatitis 573.3
- ☐ Hernia-Inguinal 550.90
- ☐ Herpes Zoster 053.9
- ☐ Hyperlipidemia 272.4
- ☐ Hypertension 401.9
- ☐ Hyperthyroidism 242.9
- ☐ Hypothyroidism 244.9
- ☐ Impacted Cerumen 380.4
- ☐ Impetigo 684
- ☐ Ingrown Toenail 703.0
- ☐ Internal Derangement Knee . 717.9
- ☐ Labyrinthitis 386.30
- ☐ Laceration Open Wound . 879.8__
- ☐ Levator Scapular Syndrome 726.90
- ☐ Menopausal Disorder ... 627.9
- ☐ Metabolic Diff. 277.8
- ☒ Migraine 346.90
- ☐ Mitral Valve Disorder ... 424.0
- ☐ Myalgia and Myositis ... 729.1
- ☐ Noninf. Gastroenterit. ... 558.9
- ☐ Obesity 278.0
- ☐ Osteoarthrosis 715.00
- ☐ Osteoporosis 733.00
- ☐ Otitis Externa 380.10
- ☐ Otitis Media 382.9
- ☐ P.I.D. 614.9
- ☐ Peptic Ulcer 533.90
- ☐ Pharyngitis, Acute 462
- ☐ Pneumonia, Viral 480.9
- ☐ Poison Oak 692.6
- ☐ Premarital B-Test V70.3
- ☐ Pregnancy Test, Unconf.. V72.4
- ☐ Prostatitis 601.9
- ☐ Psoriasis 696.1
- ☐ Rheumatoid Arthritis 714.0
- ☐ Sciatica 724.3
- ☐ Sacroiliac Sprain 846.1
- ☐ Sinusitis, Acute 461.9
- ☐ Smoking Cessation 305.10
- ☐ Sprain ________
- ☐ SQ. Cell CA-Face 173.3
- ☐ Sterilization V25.2
- ☐ Stye 373.11
- ☐ TB Exposure V01.1
- ☐ Tendonitis 726.90
- ☐ Tinea 110.9
- ☐ Tonsillitis, Acute 463
- ☐ URI, Acute 465.9
- ☐ Urine Tract Infection 599.0
- ☐ Vaginitis 616.10
- ☐ Well Adult Medical Exam V70.9
- ☐ Well Child Health Exam . V20.2

DIAGNOSIS (If not checked above) ICD-9	PHYSICIAN SIGNATURE	TODAY'S FEE	$
		PAYMENT	
PLEASE REMEMBER THAT PAYMENT IS YOUR OBLIGATION REGARDLESS OF INSURANCE OR OTHER THIRD PARTY INVOLVEMENT.	PAYMENT BY ☐ CASH ☐ CREDIT CARD ☐ CHECK # ________	**BALANCE DUE**	

INSUR-A-BILL ® BIBBERO SYSTEMS, INC. • PETALUMA, CA • © 9/94 SB43006.01 (REV. 1/99)

Courtesy of Bibbero Systems, Inc., Petaluma, California.

Administrative Skills, Form 27

FEE SCHEDULE

BLACKBURN PRIMARY CARE ASSOCIATES
1990 TURQUOISE DRIVE
BLACKBURN, WI 54937

Federal Tax ID Number: **52-1963787**

BCBS Group Number: **14982**
Medicare Group Number: **14982**

OFFICE VISIT, NEW PATIENT

Focused, 99201	$ 45.00
Expanded, 99202	$ 53.00
Detailed, 99203	$ 60.00
Comprehensive, 99204	$ 95.00
Complex, 99205	$195.00
Consultation, 99245	$250.00

OFFICE VISIT, ESTABLISHED PATIENT

Minimal, 99211	$ 40.00
Focused, 99212	$ 48.00
Expanded, 99213	$ 55.00
Detailed, 99214	$ 65.00
Comprehensive, 99215	$195.00

OFFICE PROCEDURES

EKG, 12 Lead, 93000	$ 55.00
Stress EKG, Treadmill, 93015	$295.00
Sigmoidoscopy, Flex., 45330	$145.00
Spirometry, 94010	$ 50.00
Cerumen Removal, 69210	$ 40.00
Collection & Handling	
Lab Specimen, 99000	$ 9.00
Venipuncture, 36415	$ 9.00
Urinalysis, 81000	$ 20.00
Urinalysis, 81002 (Dip Only)	$ 12.00
Influenza Injection, 90724	$ 20.00
Pneumococcal Injection, 90732	$ 20.00
Oral Polio, 90712	$ 15.00
DTaP, 90700	$ 20.00
Tetanus Toxoid, 90703	$ 15.00
MMR, 90707	$ 25.00
Hib, 90737	$ 20.00
Hepatitis B, newborn to age 11 years, 90744	$ 60.00
Hepatitis B, 11-19 years, 90745	$ 60.00
Hepatitis B, 20 years and above 90746	$ 60.00
Intramuscular Injection, 90788	
Penicillin	$ 30.00
Ceftriaxone	$ 25.00
Solu-Medrol	$ 23.00
Vitamin B-12	$ 13.00
Subcutaneous Injection, 90782	
Epinephrine	$ 18.00
Sus-Pherine	$ 25.00
Insulin, U-100	$ 15.00

COMMON DIAGNOSIS CODES

Ischemic Heart Disease	414.9
w/o myocardial infarction	411.89
w/ coronary occlusion	411.81
Hypertension, Malignant	401.0
Benign	401.1
Unspecified	401.9
w/ congest. heart failure	402.91
Asthma, Bronchial	493.9
w/ COPD	493.2
allergic, w/ S.A.	493.91
allergic, w/o S.A.	493.90
Kyphosis	737.10
w/ osteoporosis	733.0
Osteoporosis	733.00
Otitis Media, Acute	382.9
Chronic	382.9
Well Child Health Exam	V20.2
Well Adult Medical Exam	V70.9

PLEASE DO NOT STAPLE IN THIS AREA

APPROVED OMB-0938-0008

CARRIER

PICA

HEALTH INSURANCE CLAIM FORM

PICA

1. MEDICARE (Medicare #) MEDICAID (Medicaid #) CHAMPUS (Sponsor's SSN) CHAMPVA (VA File #) GROUP HEALTH PLAN (SSN or ID) FECA BLK LUNG (SSN) OTHER (ID)

1a. INSURED'S I.D. NUMBER (FOR PROGRAM IN ITEM 1)

2. PATIENT'S NAME (Last Name, First Name, Middle Initial)

3. PATIENT'S BIRTHDATE MM DD YY SEX M F

4. INSURED'S NAME (Last Name, First Name, Middle Initial)

5. PATIENT'S ADDRESS (No., Street)

6. PATIENT RELATIONSHIP TO INSURED Self Spouse Child Other

7. INSURED'S ADDRESS (No., Street)

CITY STATE

8. PATIENT STATUS Single Married Other

CITY STATE

ZIP CODE TELEPHONE (Include Area Code) ( )

Employed Full-Time Student Part-Time Student

ZIP CODE TELEPHONE (Include Area Code) ( )

9. OTHER INSURED'S NAME (Last Name, First Name, Middle Initial)

10. IS PATIENT'S CONDITION RELATED TO:

11. INSURED'S POLICY GROUP OR FECA NUMBER

a. OTHER INSURED'S POLICY OR GROUP NUMBER

a. EMPLOYMENT? (CURRENT OR PREVIOUS) YES NO

a. INSURED'S DATE OF BIRTH MM DD YY SEX M F

b. OTHER INSURED'S DATE OF BIRTH MM DD YY SEX M F

b. AUTO ACCIDENT? PLACE (State) YES NO

b. EMPLOYER'S NAME OR SCHOOL NAME

c. EMPLOYER'S NAME OR SCHOOL NAME

c. OTHER ACCIDENT? YES NO

c. INSURANCE PLAN NAME OR PROGRAM NAME

d. INSURANCE PLAN NAME OR PROGRAM NAME

10d. RESERVED FOR LOCAL USE

d. IS THERE ANOTHER HEALTH BENEFIT PLAN? YES NO *If yes, return to and complete item 9a-d.*

READ BACK OF FORM BEFORE COMPLETING & SIGNING THIS FORM.

12. PATIENT'S OR AUTHORIZED PERSON'S SIGNATURE I authorize the release of any medical or other information necessary to process this claim. I also request payment of government benefits either to myself or to the party who accepts assignment below.

SIGNED ______ DATE ______

13. INSURED'S OR AUTHORIZED PERSON'S SIGNATURE I authorize payment of medical benefits to the undersigned physician or supplier for services described below.

SIGNED ______

PATIENT AND INSURED INFORMATION

14. DATE OF CURRENT: MM DD YY ILLNESS (First symptom) OR INJURY (Accident) OR PREGNANCY (LMP)

15. IF PATIENT HAS HAD SAME OR SIMILAR ILLNESS, GIVE FIRST DATE MM DD YY

16. DATES PATIENT UNABLE TO WORK IN CURRENT OCCUPATION FROM MM DD YY TO MM DD YY

17. NAME OF REFERRING PHYSICIAN OR OTHER SOURCE

17a. I.D. NUMBER OF REFERRING PHYSICIAN

18. HOSPITALIZATION DATES RELATED TO CURRENT SERVICES FROM MM DD YY TO MM DD YY

19. RESERVED FOR LOCAL USE

20. OUTSIDE LAB? YES NO $ CHARGES

21. DIAGNOSIS OR NATURE OF ILLNESS OR INJURY. (RELATE ITEMS 1,2,3 OR 4 TO ITEM 24E BY LINE)

1. ___ . __
2. ___ . __
3. ___ . __
4. ___ . __

22. MEDICAID RESUBMISSION CODE ORIGINAL REF. NO.

23. PRIOR AUTHORIZATION NUMBER

24. A DATE(S) OF SERVICE From MM DD YY To MM DD YY	B Place of Service	C Type of Service	D PROCEDURES, SERVICES, OR SUPPLIES (Explain Unusual Circumstances) CPT/HCPCS MODIFIER	E DIAGNOSIS CODE	F $ CHARGES	G DAYS OR UNITS	H EPSDT Family Plan	I EMG	J COB	K RESERVED FOR LOCAL USE
1										
2										
3										
4										
5										
6										

25. FEDERAL TAX I.D. NUMBER SSN EIN

26. PATIENT'S ACCOUNT NUMBER

27. ACCEPT ASSIGNMENT? (For govt. claims, see back) YES NO

28. TOTAL CHARGE $

29. AMOUNT PAID $

30. BALANCE DUE $

31. SIGNATURE OF PHYSICIAN OR SUPPLIER INCLUDING DEGREES OR CREDENTIALS (I certify that the statements on the reverse apply to this bill and are made a part thereof.)

SIGNED DATE

32. NAME AND ADDRESS OF FACILITY WHERE SERVICES WERE RENDERED (If other than home or office)

33. PHYSICIAN'S, SUPPLIER'S BILLING NAME, ADDRESS, ZIP CODE & PHONE #

PIN # GRP#

PHYSICIAN OR SUPPLIER INFORMATION

(APPROVED BY AMA COUNCIL ON MEDICAL SERVICE 8/88)

PLEASE PRINT OR TYPE

FORM HCFA-1500 (12-90) FORM OWCP-1500 FORM RRB-1500

Form 1240LM

Administrative Skills, Form 29

Patient Information Sheet

 **Blackburn Primary Care Associates** 

1990 Turquoise Drive
Blackburn, WI 54937
(555)555-1234

REGISTRATION
(PLEASE PRINT)

Home Phone: 555-219-7676 Today's Date: 1/15/00

PATIENT INFORMATION

Name MINNOWITZ (Last Name) PRINNIE (First Name) ____ (Initial) Soc. Sec.# 197-24-6119

Address 16 A PARKTON ROAD

City BLACKBURN State WI Zip 54938

Single ___ Married ___ Widowed X Separated ___ Divorced ___ Sex M ___ F X Age 89 Birthdate 1/30/10

Patient Employed by ———— Occupation ____

Business Address ____ Business Phone ____

By whom were you referred? ____

In case of emergency who should be notified? Janice Selleman (Name) Daughter (Relation to Patient) Phone 555-219-7821

PRIMARY INSURANCE

Person Responsible for Account as above (Last Name) ____ (First Name) ____ (Initial)

Relation to Patient self Birthdate ____ Soc. Sec.# ____

Address (if different from patient's) ____ Phone ____

City ____ State ____ Zip ____

Person Responsible Employed by ____ Occupation ____

Business Address ____ Business Phone ____

Insurance Company Medicare

Contract # ____ Group # ____ Subscriber # 197246119 A

Name of other dependents covered under this plan ____

ADDITIONAL INSURANCE

Is patient covered by additional insurance? ___ Yes X No

Subscriber Name ____ Relation to Patient ____ Birthdate ____

Address (if different from patient's) ____ Phone ____

City ____ State ____ Zip ____

Subscriber Employed by ____ Business Phone ____

Insurance Company ____ Soc. Sec.# ____

Contract # ____ Group # ____ Subscriber # ____

Name of other dependents covered under this plan ____

ASSIGNMENT AND RELEASE

I, the undersigned, certify that I (or my dependent) have insurance coverage with Medicare (Name of Insurance Company(ies)) and assign directly to Dr. Blackburn Primary Care insurance benefits, if any, otherwise payable to me for services rendered. I understand that I am financially responsible for all charges whether or not paid by insurance. I hereby authorize the doctor to release all information necessary to secure the payment of benefits. I authorize the use of this signature on all insurance submissions.

Prinnie Minnowitz (Responsible Party Signature) self (Relationship) 1/15/00 (Date)

Patient Encounter Form

Blackburn Primary Care Associates
1990 Turquoise Drive
Blackburn, WI 54937
(555) 555-1234

FED. I.D. # 52-1963787

PAT. INFO.

ACCT. NO.	PATIENT'S LAST NAME	FIRST	M.I.	DATE OF BIRTH	SEX	TODAY'S DATE
	MINNOWITZ	PRINNIE		01/30/10	☐ M ☒ F	01/15/00

INSURANCE	COPAY	DISABILITY RELATED TO: ☐ ACCIDENT ☐ INDUSTRIAL ☐ ILLNESS ☐ OTHER
Medicare		DATES SYMPTOMS APPEARED, INCEPTION OF PREGNANCY, OR ACCIDENT OCCURRED: / /

✓	DESCRIPTION	CPT/MD	FEE
	OFFICE VISITS-NEW PATIENTS		
	Focused	99201	
	Expanded	99202	
X	Detailed	99203	
	Comprehensive	99204	
	Complex	99205	
	OFFICE VISITS - EST. PATIENTS		
	Minimal	99211	
	Focused	99212	
	Expanded	99213	
	Detailed	99214	
	Comprehensive	99215	
	PREVENTIVE HEALTH CARE NEW PT.	EST. PT	
	Eval./Mgmt. > 1 Yr 99381	99391	
	Early Child 1 - 4 Yrs 99382	99392	
	Late Child 5 - 11 Yrs 99383	99393	
	Adolescent 12 - 17 Yrs 99384	99394	
	Eval./Mgmt. 18 - 39 Yrs 99385	99395	
	Eval./Mgmt. 40 - 64 Yrs 99386	99396	
	Eval./Mgmt. 65 - Over 99387	99397	
	HOSP./SNF/HOME VISITS		
	House Calls	99341	
	ER Visit	9928__	
	Init. Hosp. Care	99222	
	Sub. Hosp. Care	99232	
	SNF, Sub. Care	99312	
	INJECTIONS		
	Allergy	95125	
	B-12	J3420	
	Flu Shot	90724	
	Gamma Globulin	90741	
	Hormone		
	Depo Provera	J1055	
	Kenalog 40-60 mg	J3301	
	Morphine/Demerol	J2270	
	Phenergan	J2550	
	Celestone	J0700	
	Hep B, newborn to 11 years	90744	
	Hep B, 11 - 19 years	90745	
	Hep B, 20 years and above	90746	
	Rocephin/Claforan	J0696	
	Iron	J1760	
	Lidocaine NCL	J2000	
	Admin of INJ	J0110	
	Unlist INJ	90782	
	Drug		
	Dose		

✓	DESCRIPTION	CPT/MD	FEE
	SPECIAL SERVICES		
	Drivers Physical	99214	
	Pelvic/Breast Exam	99214	
	Industrial	99214	
	IMMUNIZATIONS		
	DtaP	90700	
	DPT	90701	
	DT	90702	
	Td (Tetanus Booster)	90703	
	MMR	90707	
	Mumps	90704	
	Pneumococcal	90732	
	Rubella	90706	
	Polio (TOPV)	90712	
	PPD	86580	
	TB Tine Test	86585	
	Hib	90737	
	OFFICE PROCEDURES		
	Audiometry	92551	
	Diathermy (Ultrasound)	97024	
X	EKG Tracing & Interp.	93000	
	Intermed Joint Injection	20605	
	Major Joint Injection	20610	
	Nebulizer TX	94664	
	Rem. Impact. Cer.	69210	
	Spirometry	94010	
	Stress Test	93015	
	Trigger Pt. Inj.	20550	
	Eye Wash	65205*	
	LABORATORY		
	Throat Culture	87060	
X	Glucose Blood	82947	10.00
	Glucose Stick	82948	
	UA Pregnancy	81025	
	Occult Blood, Stool	82270	
	Rapid Strep	86588	
	Smear	88150	
X	UA Dip	81002	
	Urinalysis	81000	
	Venipuncture	36415	
	Wet Mount, Smear	87210	
	Wet Mount KOH	87220	
	Collect/Handing	99000	
	MISCELLANEOUS		
	Pre-OP	993__	
	After Hours	99050	
	Sunday/Holidays	99054	
	Cast Removal	29705	
	Norplant Insertion	11975	
	Norplant Kit	99070	

✓	DESCRIPTION	CPT/MD	FEE
	SURGERY		
	Toenail Removal	11750	
	Cryosurgery	17200	
	I & D	10060	
	Drainage Paronychia	10060	
	Enucleation Ext. Hemorrhoid	46320	
	I & D Abscess/Cyst	10060	
	Podophyllom	17100	
	Removal Foreign Body	10120	
	Wart Removal	17110	
	Destr. Single Lesion Face	17000	
	2nd and 3rd Lesion Face	17001	
	Destr. Single Lesion Body	17106	
	2nd and 3rd Lesion Body	17003	
	Lesion Rem. Excision		
	Anoscopy	46600	
	Flex. Scope with Sig.	45330	
	Vasectomy	55250	
	Therapeutic Abor.	59840	
	Removal Foreign Body of Eye	65205	
	SUPPLIES		
	Ace Wrap	99070	
	Cast Material	99070	
	Cervical Collar	99070	
	Elastic Bandage	99070	
	Splint/Sling	99070	
	Sterile Dressing	99070	
	Surgical Tray	99070	

DIAGNOSIS: ICD-9

- ☐ Abscess Cellulitis 682.9
- ☐ Abdominal Pain 789.0
- ☐ Abrasions 919.0
- ☐ Acne 706.1
- ☐ ADD 314.00
- ☐ Alcoholism 303.90
- ☐ Allergic Rhinitis 477.9
- ☐ Allergy, Unsp 995.3
- ☐ Anemia 285.9
- ☐ Angina Pectoris 413.9
- ☐ Anxiety Depression 300.4
- ☐ Anxiety State 300.00
- ☐ ASCVD 429.2
- ☐ Asthma W/O Status Asthma 493.90
- ☐ Atten Surg. Dressing/Suture V58.3
- ☐ BCP Consult V25.9
- ☐ BPH 600
- ☐ Bronchitis, Acute 466.0
- ☐ Bronchitis, Chronic 491.9
- ☐ Burn ______ 949.0
- ☐ Bursitis 727.3
- ☐ C.T.S. 354.0
- ☐ CAD 746.85
- ☐ CA-Prostate 185
- ☐ Cardiac Arrhythmia 427.9
- ☐ Cataracts 366.9
- ☐ Chest Pain 786.50
- ☐ Congestive Heart Failure 428.0
- ☐ Conjunctivitis 372.30
- ☐ Constipation 564.0
- ☐ Consult Vasc. V65.8
- ☐ Convulsions 780.3
- ☐ COPD 496
- ☐ Coronary Atherosclerosis 414.0
- ☐ CVA 436
- ☐ Cyst Sebaceous 706.2
- ☐ Dermatitis 692.9
- ☒ Diabetes, Uncomp. Adult 250.00
- ☐ Diabetes, Complicated 250.90
- ☐ Disc Degeneration 722.6
- ☐ Duodenal Ulcer 532.90
- ☐ Dysmenorrhea 625.3
- ☐ Fatigue 780.7
- ☐ Flu Shot Only V04.8
- ☐ Flu Vac V04.8
- ☐ Flu W/Resp. Manifest 487.1
- ☐ Folliculitis 704.8
- ☐ FX ______
- ☐ Gallbladder Disease 575.9
- ☐ Ganglion 727.43
- ☐ Gastroenteritis 558.9
- ☐ Gout 274.9
- ☐ Gyn Exam V72.3
- ☐ Headache Tension 307.81
- ☐ Hemorrhoids Ext. 455.3
- ☐ Hepatitis 573.3
- ☐ Hernia-Inguinal 550.90
- ☐ Herpes Zoster 053.9
- ☐ Hyperlipidemia 272.4
- ☐ Hypertension 401.9
- ☐ Hyperthyroidism 242.9
- ☐ Hypothyroidism 244.9
- ☐ Impacted Cerumen 380.4
- ☐ Impetigo 684
- ☐ Ingrown Toenail 703.0
- ☐ Internal Derangement Knee 717.9
- ☐ Labyrinthitis 386.30
- ☐ Laceration Open Wound 879.8__
- ☐ Levator Scapular Syndrome 726.90
- ☐ Menopausal Disorder 627.9
- ☐ Metabolic Diff. 277.8
- ☐ Migraine 346.90
- ☐ Mitral Valve Disorder 424.0
- ☐ Myalgia and Myositis 729.1
- ☐ Noninf. Gastroenterit. 558.9
- ☐ Obesity 278.0
- ☐ Osteoarthrosis 715.00
- ☐ Osteoporosis 733.00
- ☐ Otitis Externa 380.10
- ☐ Otitis Media 382.9
- ☐ P.I.D. 614.9
- ☐ Peptic Ulcer 533.90
- ☐ Pharyngitis, Acute 462
- ☐ Pneumonia, Viral 480.9
- ☐ Poison Oak 692.6
- ☐ Premarital B-Test V70.3
- ☐ Pregnancy Test, Unconf. V72.4
- ☐ Prostatitis 601.9
- ☐ Psoriasis 696.1
- ☐ Rheumatoid Arthritis 714.0
- ☐ Sciatica 724.3
- ☐ Sacroiliac Sprain 846.1
- ☐ Sinusitis, Acute 461.9
- ☐ Smoking Cessation 305.10
- ☐ Sprain ______
- ☐ SQ. Cell CA-Face 173.3
- ☐ Sterilization V25.2
- ☐ Stye 373.11
- ☐ TB Exposure V01.1
- ☐ Tendonitis 726.90
- ☐ Tinea 110.9
- ☐ Tonsillitis, Acute 463
- ☐ URI, Acute 465.9
- ☒ Urine Tract Infection 599.0
- ☐ Vaginitis 616.10
- ☐ Well Adult Medical Exam V70.9
- ☐ Well Child Health Exam V20.2

DIAGNOSIS (If not checked above) ICD-9	PHYSICIAN SIGNATURE	TODAY'S FEE	$
		PAYMENT	
PLEASE REMEMBER THAT PAYMENT IS YOUR OBLIGATION REGARDLESS OF INSURANCE OR OTHER THIRD PARTY INVOLVEMENT.	PAYMENT BY ☐ CASH ☐ CREDIT CARD ☐ CHECK # ______	BALANCE DUE	

Administrative Skills, Form 31

FEE SCHEDULE

BLACKBURN PRIMARY CARE ASSOCIATES
1990 TURQUOISE DRIVE
BLACKBURN, WI 54937

Federal Tax ID Number: **52-1963787**

BCBS Group Number: **14982**
Medicare Group Number: **14982**

OFFICE VISIT, NEW PATIENT

Focused, 99201	$ 45.00
Expanded, 99202	$ 53.00
Detailed, 99203	$ 60.00
Comprehensive, 99204	$ 95.00
Complex, 99205	$195.00
Consultation, 99245	$250.00

OFFICE VISIT, ESTABLISHED PATIENT

Minimal, 99211	$ 40.00
Focused, 99212	$ 48.00
Expanded, 99213	$ 55.00
Detailed, 99214	$ 65.00
Comprehensive, 99215	$195.00

OFFICE PROCEDURES

EKG, 12 Lead, 93000	$ 55.00
Stress EKG, Treadmill, 93015	$295.00
Sigmoidoscopy, Flex., 45330	$145.00
Spirometry, 94010	$ 50.00
Cerumen Removal, 69210	$ 40.00
Collection & Handling	
Lab Specimen, 99000	$ 9.00
Venipuncture, 36415	$ 9.00
Urinalysis, 81000	$ 20.00
Urinalysis, 81002 (Dip Only)	$ 12.00
Influenza Injection, 90724	$ 20.00
Pneumococcal Injection, 90732	$ 20.00
Oral Polio, 90712	$ 15.00
DTaP, 90700	$ 20.00
Tetanus Toxoid, 90703	$ 15.00
MMR, 90707	$ 25.00
Hib, 90737	$ 20.00
Hepatitis B, newborn to age 11 years, 90744	$ 60.00
Hepatitis B, 11-19 years, 90745	$ 60.00
Hepatitis B, 20 years and above 90746	$ 60.00
Intramuscular Injection, 90788	
Penicillin	$ 30.00
Ceftriaxone	$ 25.00
Solu-Medrol	$ 23.00
Vitamin B-12	$ 13.00
Subcutaneous Injection, 90782	
Epinephrine	$ 18.00
Sus-Pherine	$ 25.00
Insulin, U-100	$ 15.00

COMMON DIAGNOSIS CODES

Ischemic Heart Disease	414.9
w/o myocardial infarction	411.89
w/ coronary occlusion	411.81
Hypertension, Malignant	401.0
Benign	401.1
Unspecified	401.9
w/ congest. heart failure	402.91
Asthma, Bronchial	493.9
w/ COPD	493.2
allergic, w/ S.A.	493.91
allergic, w/o S.A.	493.90
Kyphosis	737.10
w/ osteoporosis	733.0
Osteoporosis	733.00
Otitis Media, Acute	382.9
Chronic	382.9
Well Child Health Exam	V20.2
Well Adult Medical Exam	V70.9

PLEASE DO NOT STAPLE IN THIS AREA

APPROVED OMB-0938-0008

CARRIER

PICA

HEALTH INSURANCE CLAIM FORM

PICA

1. MEDICARE (Medicare #) | MEDICAID (Medicaid #) | CHAMPUS (Sponsor's SSN) | CHAMPVA (VA File #) | GROUP HEALTH PLAN (SSN or ID) | FECA BLK LUNG (SSN) | OTHER (ID)

1a. INSURED'S I.D. NUMBER (FOR PROGRAM IN ITEM 1)

2. PATIENT'S NAME (Last Name, First Name, Middle Initial)

3. PATIENT'S BIRTHDATE MM DD YY — SEX M F

4. INSURED'S NAME (Last Name, First Name, Middle Initial)

5. PATIENT'S ADDRESS (No., Street)

6. PATIENT RELATIONSHIP TO INSURED — Self Spouse Child Other

7. INSURED'S ADDRESS (No., Street)

CITY — STATE

8. PATIENT STATUS — Single Married Other

CITY — STATE

ZIP CODE — TELEPHONE (Include Area Code) ( )

Employed — Full-Time Student — Part-Time Student

ZIP CODE — TELEPHONE (Include Area Code) ( )

9. OTHER INSURED'S NAME (Last Name, First Name, Middle Initial)

10. IS PATIENT'S CONDITION RELATED TO:

11. INSURED'S POLICY GROUP OR FECA NUMBER

a. OTHER INSURED'S POLICY OR GROUP NUMBER

a. EMPLOYMENT? (CURRENT OR PREVIOUS) — YES NO

a. INSURED'S DATE OF BIRTH MM DD YY — SEX M F

b. OTHER INSURED'S DATE OF BIRTH MM DD YY — SEX M F

b. AUTO ACCIDENT? — YES NO — PLACE (State)

b. EMPLOYER'S NAME OR SCHOOL NAME

c. EMPLOYER'S NAME OR SCHOOL NAME

c. OTHER ACCIDENT? — YES NO

c. INSURANCE PLAN NAME OR PROGRAM NAME

d. INSURANCE PLAN NAME OR PROGRAM NAME

10d. RESERVED FOR LOCAL USE

d. IS THERE ANOTHER HEALTH BENEFIT PLAN? — YES NO *If yes, return to and complete item 9a-d.*

READ BACK OF FORM BEFORE COMPLETING & SIGNING THIS FORM.

12. PATIENT'S OR AUTHORIZED PERSON'S SIGNATURE I authorize the release of any medical or other information necessary to process this claim. I also request payment of government benefits either to myself or to the party who accepts assignment below.

SIGNED ______ DATE ______

13. INSURED'S OR AUTHORIZED PERSON'S SIGNATURE I authorize payment of medical benefits to the undersigned physician or supplier for services described below.

SIGNED ______

PATIENT AND INSURED INFORMATION

14. DATE OF CURRENT: MM DD YY — ILLNESS (First symptom) OR INJURY (Accident) OR PREGNANCY (LMP)

15. IF PATIENT HAS HAD SAME OR SIMILAR ILLNESS, GIVE FIRST DATE MM DD YY

16. DATES PATIENT UNABLE TO WORK IN CURRENT OCCUPATION — FROM MM DD YY TO MM DD YY

17. NAME OF REFERRING PHYSICIAN OR OTHER SOURCE

17a. I.D. NUMBER OF REFERRING PHYSICIAN

18. HOSPITALIZATION DATES RELATED TO CURRENT SERVICES — FROM MM DD YY TO MM DD YY

19. RESERVED FOR LOCAL USE

20. OUTSIDE LAB? — YES NO — $ CHARGES

21. DIAGNOSIS OR NATURE OF ILLNESS OR INJURY. (RELATE ITEMS 1,2,3 OR 4 TO ITEM 24E BY LINE)

1. ___ . __
2. ___ . __
3. ___ . __
4. ___ . __

22. MEDICAID RESUBMISSION CODE — ORIGINAL REF. NO.

23. PRIOR AUTHORIZATION NUMBER

24. A DATE(S) OF SERVICE From MM DD YY To MM DD YY	B Place of Service	C Type of Service	D PROCEDURES, SERVICES, OR SUPPLIES (Explain Unusual Circumstances) CPT/HCPCS MODIFIER	E DIAGNOSIS CODE	F $ CHARGES	G DAYS OR UNITS	H EPSDT Family Plan	I EMG	J COB	K RESERVED FOR LOCAL USE
1										
2										
3										
4										
5										
6										

25. FEDERAL TAX I.D. NUMBER — SSN EIN

26. PATIENT'S ACCOUNT NUMBER

27. ACCEPT ASSIGNMENT? (For govt. claims, see back) — YES NO

28. TOTAL CHARGE $

29. AMOUNT PAID $

30. BALANCE DUE $

31. SIGNATURE OF PHYSICIAN OR SUPPLIER INCLUDING DEGREES OR CREDENTIALS (I certify that the statements on the reverse apply to this bill and are made a part thereof.)

SIGNED — DATE

32. NAME AND ADDRESS OF FACILITY WHERE SERVICES WERE RENDERED (If other than home or office)

33. PHYSICIAN'S, SUPPLIER'S BILLING NAME, ADDRESS, ZIP CODE & PHONE #

PIN # — GRP#

PHYSICIAN OR SUPPLIER INFORMATION

(APPROVED BY AMA COUNCIL ON MEDICAL SERVICE 8/88)

Form 1240LM

PLEASE PRINT OR TYPE

FORM HCFA-1500 (12-90)
FORM OWCP-1500 FORM RRB-1500

Appendix B

Record of Procedures Completed

Directions: Keep an ongoing record of all procedures you have performed successfully. When you have achieved a satisfactory score for the procedure in your educational program, your instructor should write his or her initials and the date in the box labeled *Classroom.* When you are considered independent in performing the procedure at your externship, your externship supervisor should write his or her initials and the date in the box marked *Externship.* If you are placed at more than one externship site, have the supervisor use the additional boxes on the form.

EXAMPLE:

7–1 Answering Incoming Calls	*SH* *7/8/01*	*PF* *4/26/01*	*JT* *5/23/01*	

NAME OF STUDENT				
UNIT III: PREPARING FOR THE PATIENT	**Classroom**	**Externship**	**Externship**	**Externship**
TELEPHONE TECHNIQUES				
7–1 Answering Incoming Calls				
7–2 Taking a Telephone Message				
7–3 Taking Requests for Medication or Prescription Refills				
7–4 Procedure for Emergency Calls				
7–5 Activating the Emergency Medical Services (EMS) System				
7–6 Placing Outgoing Telephone Calls				

UNIT III: PREPARING FOR THE PATIENT (*Continued*)	Classroom	Externship	Externship	Externship
SCHEDULING APPOINTMENTS				
9–1 Setting Up the Appointment Matrix				
9–2 Making an Appointment				
MEDICAL RECORDS AND FILING SYSTEMS				
10–1 Preparing a Medical Record for a New Patient				
10–2 Setting Up a Tickler File				
10–3 Filing Reports or Other Material in Patient Record				
10–4 Filing Patient Records				
MAINTAINING THE MEDICAL OFFICE				
11–1 Taking a Supply Inventory				
11–2 Stocking the Supply Cabinet				
11–3 Preparing a Purchase Order				
OPENING THE OFFICE AND CHECKING PATIENTS IN				
12–1 Taking Messages from an Answering Machine				
12–2 Taking Messages from an Answering Service				
12–3 Checking Patients In				

UNIT IV: THE PATIENT VISIT	Classroom	Externship	Externship	Externship
MEDICAL ASEPSIS AND INFECTION CONTROL				
13–1 Medical Aseptic Handwashing				
13–2 Removing Soiled Gloves				
13–3 Sanitizing Soiled Instruments				
13–4 Wrapping an Instrument for Sterilization				
13–5 Operating the Autoclave				

UNIT IV: THE PATIENT VISIT (*Continued*)	Classroom	Externship	Externship	Externship
PREPARING THE PATIENT FOR EXAMINATION				
14–1 Assisting a Patient to Transfer to and from a Wheelchair				
14–2 Obtaining and Recording a Patient History				
TAKING MEASUREMENTS AND VITAL SIGNS				
15–1 Measuring Height				
15–2 Measuring Weight Using a Balance-Beam Scale				
15–3 Measuring Oral Temperature Using a Glass-Mercury Thermometer				
15–4 Measuring Oral Temperature Using an Electronic Thermometer				
15–5 Measuring Oral Temperature Using a Disposable Thermometer				
15–6 Measuring Aural Temperature Using a Tympanic Thermometer				
15–7 Measuring Rectal Temperature				
15–8 Measuring Axillary Temperature				
15–9 Measuring the Radial Pulse				
15–10 Measuring the Apical Pulse				
15–11 Measuring Respirations				
15–12 Measuring Blood Pressure				
ASSISTING WITH THE PATIENT EXAMINATION				
16–1 Assisting with the Physical Examination				
16–2 Assisting with the Pap Test and Pelvic Examination				
16–3 Measuring Distance Visual Acuity Using a Snellen Chart				

UNIT IV: THE PATIENT VISIT *(Continued)*	Classroom	Externship	Externship	Externship
ASSISTING WITH THE PATIENT EXAMINATION *(Continued)*				
16–4 Ishihara Test of Color Vision				
16–5 Measuring Hearing Using a Manual Audiometer				
16–6 Testing Stool for Occult Blood				
16–7 Assisting with Flexible Sigmoidoscopy				
ASSISTING WITH SURGICAL PROCEDURES				
17–1 Surgical Aseptic Handwash				
17–2 Sterile Gloving				
17–3 Opening a Sterile Barrier Field				
17–4 Opening a Sterile Surgical Pack				
17–5 Adding Sterile Solution to the Sterile Field				
17–6 Preparing the Skin for Minor Surgery				
17–7 Assisting with Minor Surgery				
17–8 Applying a Tubular Gauze Bandage				
17–9 Changing a Sterile Dressing				
17–10 Suture Removal				
TAKING ELECTROCARDIOGRAMS				
18–1 Taking Electrocardiograms				
18–2 Applying a Holter Monitor				
ASSISTING WITH DIAGNOSTIC PROCEDURES				
19–1 Performing Spirometry to Measure Lung Volume				
19–2 Obtaining a Sputum Specimen				
19–3 Performing Urinary Catheterization on a Female				
19–4 Performing Sperm Washing				

UNIT IV: THE PATIENT VISIT (*Continued*)	Classroom	Externship	Externship	Externship
ASSISTING WITH DIAGNOSTIC PROCEDURES (*Continued*)				
19–5 Assisting with the Neurologic Exam				
19–6 Assisting with Lumbar Puncture				
ASSISTING WITH TREATMENTS				
21–1 Performing an Eye Irrigation				
21–2 Instilling Eye Medication				
21–3 Performing an Ear Irrigation				
21–4 Instilling Ear Medication				
21–5 Instructing a Patient to Use a Metered-Dose Inhaler				
21–6 Applying Warm Moist Compresses				
21–7 Applying an Ice Pack				
21–8 Assisting with Cast Application				
21–9 Applying a Sling Using a Triangular Bandage				
PREPARING AND ADMINISTERING MEDICATION				
22–1 Administering Oral Medications				
22–2 Drawing Up Medication from an Ampule				
22–3 Drawing Up Medication from a Vial				
22–4 Reconstituting a Powdered Medication				
22–5 Administering a Subcutaneous Injection				
22–6 Selecting a Site for an Intramuscular Injection				
22–7 Administering an Intramuscular Injection				
22–8 Administering a Z-Track Injection				
22–9 Administering an Intradermal Injection				
22–10 Administering a Tine or Mantoux Test				

UNIT V: THE LABORATORY AND LABORATORY TESTS	Classroom	Externship	Externship	Externship
THE PHYSICIAN'S OFFICE LABORATORY				
23–1 Using a Microscope				
URINALYSIS				
24–1 Collecting a Clean-Catch Midstream Urine Specimen				
24–2 Collecting a 24-Hour Urine Specimen				
24–3 Measuring Urine Specific Gravity Using a Refractometer				
24–4 Chemical Testing of Urine Using Reagent Strip Method				
24–5 Urine Testing Using the Clinitest 5-Drop Method				
24–6 Urine Testing Using Acetest Method				
24–7 Urine Testing Using Icotest Method				
24–8 Preparing Urine for Microscopic Examination				
PHLEBOTOMY, HEMATOLOGY, AND COAGULATION STUDIES				
25–1 Drawing Blood Using the Evacuated-Tube Method				
25–2 Drawing Blood Using the Syringe Method				
25–3 Drawing Blood Using the Butterfly Method				
25–4 Obtaining a Capillary Blood Specimen Using a Finger Stick				
25–5 Obtaining a Capillary Blood Specimen Using a Heel Stick				
25–6 Obtaining a Capillary Blood Specimen for PKU Testing				
25–7 Preparing a Peripheral Blood Smear				

UNIT V: THE LABORATORY AND LABORATORY TESTS (*Continued*)	Classroom	Externship	Externship	Externship
PHLEBOTOMY, HEMATOLOGY, AND COAGULATION STUDIES (*Continued*)				
25–8 Testing Hemoglobin Using a Hemoglobinometer				
25–9 Performing a Microhematocrit				
MICROBIOLOGY, IMMUNOLOGY, CHEMISTRY				
26–1 Obtaining a Wound Specimen for Microbiological Testing				
26–2 Obtaining a Throat Specimen for Microbiological Testing				
26–3 Preparing a Wet Mount and Hanging Drop Slide				
26–4 Preparing a Dry Smear for Staining				
26–5 Inoculating a Culture Plate				
26–6 Performing a Urine Culture Using a Dip Slide Kit				
26–7 Urine Pregnancy Testing				
26–8 Performing a Rapid Strep Test				
26–9 Testing for Glucose Using a Glucometer Elite Analyzer				

UNIT VI: SPECIAL POPULATIONS	Classroom	Externship	Externship	Externship
PEDIATRICS				
27–1 Measuring an Infant's Length				
27–2 Measuring an Infant's Weight				
27–3 Measuring Head Circumference of an Infant				
27–4 Measuring Chest Circumference of an Infant				
27–5 Measuring the Apical Pulse of an Infant				

UNIT VI: SPECIAL POPULATIONS (*Continued*)	Classroom	Externship	Externship	Externship
PEDIATRICS (*Continued*)				
27–6 Measuring the Respirations of an Infant				
27–7 Obtaining a Urine Specimen from an Infant				
OBSTETRICS				
29–1 Assisting with the First Prenatal Visit				
29–2 Assisting with Follow-Up Prenatal Visits				
29–3 Assisting with Postpartum Visits				
EMERGENCY CARE				
31–1 Checking Contents of Emergency Box/ Crash Cart				
31–2 Assisting the Choking Victim				
31–3 Administering Oxygen by Nasal Cannula/Face Mask				
31–4 Caring for Burns				
31–5 Controlling Bleeding				
31–6 Applying a Splint				
31–7 Cleaning Minor Wounds				

UNIT VII: PATIENT TEACHING AND FOLLOW-UP	Classroom	Externship	Externship	Externship
TEACHING PATIENTS IN THE MEDICAL OFFICE				
32–1 Teaching a Patient to Use a Cane				
32–2 Teaching a Patient to Use Crutches				
32–3 Teaching a Patient to Use a Walker				
MAINTAINING HEALTH: NUTRITION, EXERCISE, AND SELF-EXAMINATION				
33–1 Teaching Range-of-Motion Exercises				
33–2 Teaching Breast Self-Examination				
33–3 Teaching Testicular Self-Examination				

UNIT VII: PATIENT TEACHING AND FOLLOW-UP (*Continued*)	Classroom	Externship	Externship	Externship
ORAL FOLLOW-UP				
34–1 Scheduling Diagnostic Tests				
34–2 Scheduling a Surgical Procedure				
34–3 Completing a Referral Form for Managed Care				
WRITTEN FOLLOW-UP				
35–1 Composing a Business Letter				
35–2 Addressing an Envelope				
35–3 Transcribing a Dictated Letter or Report				
35–4 Preparing Outgoing Mail				
35–5 Sending a Fax				
35–6 Preparing Copies of Multiple-Page Documents				

UNIT VIII: FINANCIAL MANAGEMENT AND HEALTH INSURANCE	Classroom	Externship	Externship	Externship
MANAGING PRACTICE FINANCES				
36–1 Preparing Charge Slips for the Day's Patients				
36–2 Completing an Encounter Form (Superbill) for a Patient				
36–3 Posting Charges to the Patient Ledger				
36–4 Posting Payments and/or Adjustments				
36–5 Recording a Patient's Visit on the Day Sheet				
36–6 Balancing the Day Sheet				
36–7 Preparing a Bank Deposit				
36–8 Reconciling a Bank Statement				
36–9 Writing Checks to Pay Bills				

UNIT VIII: FINANCIAL MANAGEMENT AND HEALTH INSURANCE *(Continued)*	**Classroom**	**Externship**	**Externship**	**Externship**
CODING				
37–1 Looking Up a CPT-4 Code				
37–2 Looking Up a HCPCS Code				
37–3 Looking Up an ICD-9-CM Code				
HEALTH INSURANCE				
38–1 Completing the HCFA-1500 Form for Insurance Reimbursement				
BILLING AND COLLECTIONS				
39–1 Creating and Examining an Accounts Aging Record				
39–2 Writing a Collection Letter				

Appendix C

Using Lytec Medical 2001

The Lytec Medical 2001 computer program is contained on the CD-ROM included with the textbook *Saunders Fundamentals of Medical Assisting.* Lytec Medical 2001 is a Windows-based medical practice management program. In addition to workbook activities and activities on the CD-ROM, students have the opportunity to install and use this program to perform many administrative tasks of the medical office, such as:

- Recording demographic and insurance information for patients
- Entering patient charges
- Entering payments
- Creating receipts, bills, and insurance billing
- Performing electronic claims submission
- Creating reports such as day sheets and account aging reports
- Scheduling appointments.

INSTALLATION AND SETUP

To install Lytec Medical 2001, refer to the User Guide or the "readme" file on the CD-ROM.

INSTRUCTIONS TO ACCOMPANY CHAPTER 36—MANAGING PRACTICE FINANCES

Create Your Own Practice

First you will want to create your own practice file. Under the **File** menu go to the **Open Practice** window, right click your mouse on Blackburn Primary Care Associates, and select **Copy.** Next, click in the space beneath and select **Paste.** This will copy the original Blackburn Primary Care Associates file. Next, rename the copy file. This creates your personal "lpf" file so that you can save your work. Note: Do NOT make or save changes to the original Blackburn Primary Care Associates file.

Open Practice

Click on the **File** menu to see the options. Move your mouse to highlight and click **Open Practice.** When the **Open Practice** window appears, select and open your personal "lpf" file.

Finding a Patient

To determine what patients already have records in your practice, click the **Lists** menu. These records are equivalent to the ledger cards you have been asked to create manually. Move your mouse to highlight and click **Patients.** One of the patient records will be displayed. Click the magnifying glass at the right of the number in the top field (Patient Chart) to see a list of patients. Click on the patient whose record you wish to display and click **OK.** The patients in this chapter identified as established patients will have records.

Entering Data for a New Patient

You must create a record for each new patient. Click the button labeled **New** at the top right of the **Patients** window. Enter the patient number in the top field labeled **Patient Chart.** Below the chart number you will notice several tabs: **Patient Information** (the screen to which the dialog box opens automatically), **Primary Insurance, Secondary Insurance, Tertiary Insurance, Associations, Claim Information, and Diagnosis/Hold Codes.**

Patient Information Tab

Fill in the following fields with information from your workbook: **Last Name, First Name, Middle Initial** (if any), **Street Address, City, State, Zip Code, Home Phone, Work Phone, Birth Date, Social Security Number, Sex,** and **Marital Status.** You will notice an arrow to the right of some fields (such as **Sex** or **Marital Status**). If you click on the arrow, a drop down box will appear with the choices for that field. You can highlight and click on your choice.

Leave the field labeled **Recall Date** blank.

If the patient has Standard Health HMO insurance, enter $10.00 in the **Copay** field. Otherwise leave it blank.

In the **Fee Schedule** field, select 1 if the patient has Standard Health HMO insurance. Select 2 if the patient has Standard Health Care Indemnity Insurance. Select 3 if the patient has Medicare insurance.

Leave the **Patient Code** and **Patient Type** fields blank.

Select the **Primary Insurance** tab located beside the **Patient Information** tab. Click the magnifying glass beside the Insurance Code field to identify the code for the patient's insurance company.

In the **Type** field, click on the arrow and choose Employer (meaning that the patient has insurance from employment) for most patients in this exercise. If the patient has Medicare insurance, choose Medicare. Enter the patient's policy number in the **Policy Number** field.

For this exercise, leave the **ID Number** box blank.

Click the small white box beside **Bill insurance automatically** and **Accept assignment** for each patient in this exercise.

In the **Relation to Insured** field, **Self** is selected automatically. When you enter data for Marie Richards, a new patient of Dr. Lopez, note that her husband is the insured person. Click the arrow to the right of the field and select Spouse. Then click the **Set Insured** button to the right of the **Relation to Insured** field. When the **Insured** window opens, click the circle to the left of the **Guarantor** field. Then click the magnifying glass to the right of the field. When the **Find Guarantor** window opens, click the **Add** button on the right. This allows you to set up a billing account for the insured person, who is currently not a patient of Blackburn Primary Care Associates. Leave the **Guarantor Code** box blank and the program will assign a code. Enter the information you have about John

Richards assuming that he has the same address and telephone number as Marie Richards. Click the **OK** button on the **Quick Add Guarantor** window, the **Find Guarantor** window, and the **Insured** window.

Select the **Associations** tab located in the row above the **Patient Information** tab to link the patient to his or her primary care physician. In the **Provider** field, click the magnifying glass to the right. Highlight the number of the patient's physician and click **OK.**

NOTE: When you have entered all information or new information about a patient, click the Save button.

Entering Charges and Payments

Find the **Charges and Payments** icon on the toolbar. It is a rectangular box with a grid of nine squares. As you run your mouse over the toolbar, the name of the feature that each icon will open appears. Click the icon to open the box.

Click the magnifying glass to the right of the **Patient Chart** field, then highlight the patient for whom you wish to enter charges, and click **OK.** Tab to the **Billing** field. A number appears automatically. If you want to edit a previous entry, you can click the magnifying glass to search through all the billings entered for a patient.

The code for the patient's physician should automatically be entered in the **Provider** column of the **Detail Icons** section. If the patient was seen by another doctor in the practice, you need to change the code manually.

Tab to the **Created** field. Enter the date 10/12/2000, which is the date used for the exercises in the workbook.

Tab to the **Copay** field. If the patient has Standard Health HMO insurance, enter $10.00. If the patient has Standard Health Indemnity insurance, enter $15.00.

Enter check marks in the **Bill To** box beside patient and the primary insurance company.

Under **Detail Items** change the date to 10/12/2000. Enter each charge and payment on a separate line. Press **Enter** until you get to the **Code** column. Use the magnifying glass to find the list of codes. Select the correct code for a charge (by CPT-4 procedure code number) or payment (check). Press **Enter** twice and enter 11 in the **POS** (place of service) box for each charge. The program should provide the charge and units (always 1 for this exercise). You can change the charge or enter a charge manually from the fee schedule in your workbook if the program fails to provide it. If you keep pressing **Enter** to accept information, the program will provide a new line for another charge or payment. When you have entered all charges and payments for the patient, click the **Save** button at the bottom of the window.

Entering Insurance Payments

To enter the insurance payment for June St. Cyr, click the **Patient Ledger** icon on the toolbar. Find the ledger card for June St. Cyr by clicking the magnifying glass to the right of the **Patient** field. Note that June St. Cyr has a balance of $53.00 for charges on 7/22/00. She has additional charges that you entered for services on 10/12/00. Close the window.

Click the **Charges and Payments** icon on the toolbar. Find June St. Cyr by using the magnifying glass to the right of the **Patient Chart** field. Find the charge for procedure 99212 using the magnifying glass to the right of the **Billing** dialog box and then select it. Create a new line to enter the payment by clicking in one of the boxes of the current billing (such as the Units colunn) and pressing **Enter** until a new line appears. Click the **Date From** column and change the date to 10/12/00. Press **Enter** until the cursor is in the **Code** column. Use the magnifying glass to locate and select the code for an insurance payment. Press **Enter** until the cursor is in the **Amount** column. Enter $43.00. Press **Enter** until a new line appears. If the practice wants to keep track of insurance payments for specific procedures, click the **Detail** button and select **Pay Item.** Enter the CPT code to which the payment should be applied; the Lytec program can keep track of the amount of reimbursement by code.

Press **Enter** until the cursor is in the **Code** column of the new line. You need to adjust the account so that all charges for 7/22/00 are considered paid. Although the Lytec program can be set up to do this automatically, for the purposes of this tutorial, you will make the adjustment in order to understand the process. Using the magnifying glass to the right of the **Code** column, locate and select the code for an **Insurance Write Off.** This is a type of adjustment where the balance of the bill is adjusted to zero after applying the copayment and insurance payment according to the terms of the contract with the insurance company. Press **Enter** until the cursor is in the **Amount** column. Enter $10.00, which is the difference between June St. Cyr's balance (including billing for procedure 90703) and the insurance payment for services on 7/22/00. Click the **Save** button to post the payment and adjustment. Click the **Patient Ledger** icon and select June St. Cyr to review your work. Her balance should now be $39.00, to reflect the charges that you entered for 10/12/00.

Enter the insurance payments for Mary Ann St. Cyr and James Winston as instructed in your workbook.

Printing a Day Sheet

Open the **Reports** menu. Highlight and click **Print a Day Sheet.** Click the **Close after Printing** (checkbox) on the **Options** tab to remove the check mark; otherwise, you will not be able to reprint a day sheet for the selected date. In a real medical practice, this box normally stays checked so that the data for a given day cannot be changed. Click the circle next to **Service Date.** Click the **Ranges** tab. Highlight the first **Dates of Service** field and enter 10/12/2000 in both boxes. Click the **Preview** button to see the report on your screen. Click the **Print** button to print a copy. Compare the computer version to the manual day sheet you created in Chapter 36.

INSTRUCTIONS TO ACCOMPANY CHAPTER 38—HEALTH INSURANCE

Adding Permanent Diagnosis Codes to Patient Records

Open the **Lists** menu, highlight, and click **Patients** (or click the **Patients** icon on the toolbar). Locate the patient for whom you want to enter permanent diagnosis codes, select him or her, and click the **Diagnosis/Hold Codes** tab. Using the magnifying glass, locate and select the codes for the following permanent diagnosis codes:

June St. Cyr	Arteriosclerosis
Robert Ricigliano	Hypertension, benign
	Hyperplasia of the prostate
Mary Ann St. Cyr	Asthma
James Winston	Atrioventricular heart block, first degree

Adding Temporary Diagnosis Codes to Patient Billing

Locate and click the **Charges and Payments** icon on the toolbar. Locate the patient for whom you want to add a diagnosis using the magnifying glass. Select the billing number for 10/12/2000. Highlight the **Diagnosis** box on the first line of the billing. Click the **Detail** button at the bottom of the screen and select **More Detail.** To identify the diagnosis code that corresponds to each procedure code, look at the encounter form. Then enter all diagnoses for the patient in the boxes, putting the diagnosis that justifies the procedure being billed first. Putting this diagnosis first is important to ensure that the program fills out the insurance form correctly. For example, Robert Ricigliano has four diagnoses: angina pectoris on exertion; hypertension, benign; hyperplasia of the prostate; and post void dribbling. He needs to have diagnoses in at least two organ systems to justify the comprehensive office visit, so it is important for them to be printed on the insurance form. The diagnosis that justifies the EKG is angina pectoris on exertion, so that code must be listed first for that procedure.

Enter the diagnosis codes for all patients listed in Question 4 under Practical Applications. Be sure to enter the details for each patient for each charge dated 10/12/2000. It is not necessary to enter diagnosis codes for payments or adjustments.

Note that this computer program is capable of linking diagnosis codes so that you do not have to enter them for each charge each time.

Printing Insurance Forms

Locate and click the **Charges and Payments** icon on the toolbar. Using the magnifying glass, locate the patient whose insurance form you want to create. Select the billing number for 10/12/2000. Click the box under **Print** to put a check mark next to every item that you want to include on the insurance form. Be sure that there are also check marks in the **Bill To** checkboxes for the patient and the primary insurance company. Then click the **Print** button at the bottom of the window. Highlight and click **Primary Insurance.** A window will open to locate the insurance form you want to use. You may need to click the **Up One Level** icon to enter the general Lytec folder where the forms are located. Find and highlight the document labeled **HCFA-Standard (With Form).LCI.** Click **Open.** You can now preview the form and/or print it.

Preview and print forms for 10/12/2000 for June St. Cyr, Robert Ricigliano, Marie Richards, Mary Ann St. Cyr, and James Winston. Compare them to the forms you created manually and discuss any discrepancies.

INSTRUCTIONS TO ACCOMPANY CHAPTER 39—BILLING AND COLLECTIONS

Printing a Patient Statement

You can print an individual statement using the same method as printing insurance forms, but click on **Statement** after clicking the large rectangular **Print** box. A dialog box will open to locate the statement form you want to use. You may need to scroll over or click the **Up One Level** icon to enter the general Lytec folder where the statement forms are located. Find, highlight, and open the document labeled **STATEMENT-STANDARD.LCS.** In the **Print Statement** field, enter the date for which you want to print the statement. The statement date will print at the top of the statement.

To print statements for all patients with charges outstanding, click the **Billing** menu and select **Print Statements.** Find, highlight, and open the document labeled **STATEMENT-STANDARD.LCS.** Enter the date for which you wish to print the statements. You can view the statements on screen by clicking **Preview,** or you can print them by clicking **Print.**

Creating an Accounts Aging Report

Click on the **Reports** menu, highlight **Aging,** and select **Patient Aging** from the drop down menu to the right. Enter the date 11/24/2001 in the **Age From** field. You can view the report on screen by clicking **Preview,** or you can print it by clicking **Print.** Compare the total amounts at the end of the report to the report you generated manually.

OTHER FUNCTIONS

Lytec 2001 is capable of performing many other functions to facilitate scheduling and record keeping in the medical office. Be sure to check the CD-ROM for additional documents related to the program. You can also obtain more information from the website http://www.lytec.com.